Moshe Zarhy
Health Facilities in Israel

Moshe Zarhy
Health Facilities in Israel

Edited by Peter R. Pawlik

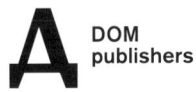
DOM
publishers

Contents

7
Papers

8
Appendix

1

"The planning of large hospital and university centres called for a more thorough study and survey of the programmatic aspects: functional, professional and psychological .... I was convinced we had to strive to design in a straight, modest and simple way, which is paradoxically the most intricate and difficult method".
Arieh Sharon in his book "Kibbutz+Bauhaus", 1972

Preface

For a long time it has been suggested to honour Moshe Zarhy, born in 1923, by a monograph. He counts among the second generation of architects, who have contributed decisively to shaping the face of today's modern state of Israel. By his functional, aesthetical and unadorned style he can be seen in direct succession to the founding fathers of Israeli architecture, who – in the twenties and thirties of the twentieth century – laid the foundation for the settlement of Palestine, largely undeveloped until then. The necessary new beginning for immigrants mostly from Europe was to make them forget all their previous experiences; virtually everything was to be made different and better than in their native countries. That created a good basis for realizing recent insights, in social but, of course, particularly in architectural respects. Born in 1923, Moshe Zarhy was, strictly speaking, not among the founding generation of what was to become Israel, but he grew up in the environment moulded by "the Big Three", the architects Dov Karmi, Zeev Rechter and Arieh Sharon, popularly known as "The Three Animals". Moshe Zarhy has known all of them personally. A particular relationship developed with Zeev Rechter leading to a partnership with this influential and successful Israeli architect.

The strong European influence on Israeli architecture is probably due to the origins as well as the education of many immigrants. This can be briefly exemplified by the backgrounds of the three above-mentioned architects. Karmi (1905–1962), born in Odessa/Ukraine, took up studies in Art and Design in Jerusalem before deciding to study architecture in Ghent/Belgium. Rechter (1899–1960), equally of Ukrainian origin, came to Palestine in 1919 and first worked in different offices before establishing himself as a self-employed architect. In 1926 he went to Rome for a year and came into touch with Russian constructivism. He gained further "European" experience from 1929 to 1933 in Paris. Arieh Sharon (1900–1984), of Polish origin, emigrated to Palestine in 1920 and first worked as an apiculturist in a kibbutz, but also contributed to planning the main building. The kibbutz community sent him to Germany for a year, where he met Walter Gropius in Weimar and was imparted the new, ground-breaking education of architects.

In 1919 the Bauhaus had taken up its reformist academic education in Weimar in Germany and formulated the basic principle: "The ultimate aim of all creative activity is the construction". Students were given a comprehensive education, not only intended to sharpen their senses of colour and form, but also to teach them the adequate use of materials. It is particularly these qualities that were of great importance with the first generation of immigrants. The difficult economic conditions forced them to think and act rationally and functionally. So it is not by chance that the first structures of buildings and towns in Palestine – at that time still under British mandate – were determined by the ideas of the Bauhaus.

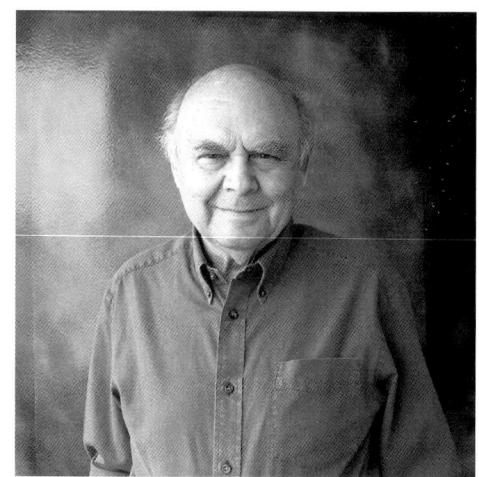

Photo of Moshe Zarhy in 2009

"The founding fathers, members of the first generation engaging in Israeli architecture, devoted considerable efforts to education and to the creation of a new Hebrew tradition – a society and a culture unique to this country. The melting pot of the Zionist revolution was intended to purify the values of the past in order to extract a new Jew from them, the absolute antithesis of a diaspora Jew – more handsome, muscular and a warrior." Ram Karmi (son of Dov Karmi).

It is in this modern architectural environment that Moshe Zarhy, himself a son of immigrants, grew up in Palestine. In his life as an architect he has achieved supreme international recognition. Numerous national as well as international distinctions were conferred upon him, his architectural work comprises practically every task that can ever be asked from an architect. It spans from single-family houses to Hi-Tech buildings and science based industries of the highest complexity; he has built schools and convention centres, museums, sports centres and synagogues. One field of work, however, has been of particular interest to Moshe Zarhy since the beginning of his activities: Health Facilities! It is in this field that he has achieved mastery by a multitude of outstanding and groundbreaking hospitals.

Meanwhile, at the age of ninety, Moshe Zarhy can look back on a life's achievement that is virtually unparalleled. He has authored many publications about his projects. In key functions, among others as Vice-President of the UIA, he has given numerous lectures in many countries. In these context he has often pointed out the specific requirements for Israeli architecture and its particular challenges, challenges that have their roots – inter alia – in the multicultural composition

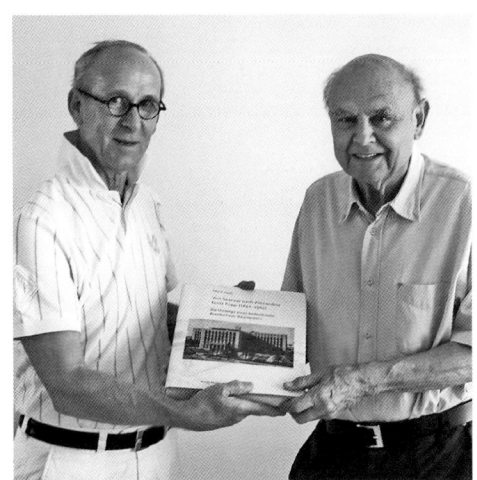

Tel Aviv, July 2013: Moshe Zarhy (right) receives a book about the German Hospital Architect Ernst Kopp from Peter R. Pawlik (left) in 2013

of the country's population. Different languages (Hebrew, Arab, English, Russian), different religions, and myriad conceptions of community require a mindset that leads to new planning processes from one project to the next. For years Moshe Zarhy has dedicated himself to the task of working out this "Israeli way" in the field of Health Facilities. In previous years he published a work entitled "Health Facilities in Israel". Zarhy himself has revised and expanded this work with the accumulated knowledge of over sixty years of professional activity. This version will form the core of the present book (chapter 4).

But this book will also recount the life story of Mosche Zarhy. The son of European immigrants, this life is so exemplary of the extremely difficult conditions and the exciting early days of the state of Israel, whose history was influenced by visionary characters, among whom architects can undoubtedly be counted. In addition to the projects of his speciality, the construction of hospitals, I will also give insight into the other fields of his substantial work.

How did this book project arise? In May 1992 the XIIIth International Public Health Seminar took place in Buenos Aires / Argentina, organized by the UIA (International Union of Architects) – Public Health Group, then under the direction of the German architect Richard Joachim Sahl. Moshe Zarhy, who had been a committed member of this group for a long time, gave a lecture entitled "The Health Facilities in the Continuous Quality Improvement in Israel". It was my first meeting with this successful architect, which was to be followed by so many more in various places all over the world in the following years. During his regular visits to Berlin, together with his wife Vera Ronnen-Zarhy, there arose not only a professional exchange of ideas, the couples Zarhy and Pawlik also found common ground in their enthusiasm for classical music.

Moshe Zarhy initially only sought support for finding a publisher for his book. After several conversations in Berlin and Tel Aviv, the common idea of producing more than just the new edition of the Health Facilities in Israel was born. Moshe Zarhy's confidence in me as a co-author was apparently due to the fact that I had already written two monographs about the German (hospital) architects Hermann Distel and Ernst Kopp. It is an honour and a pleasure for me to be allowed to participate in this book, written in large parts by Moshe Zarhy himself.

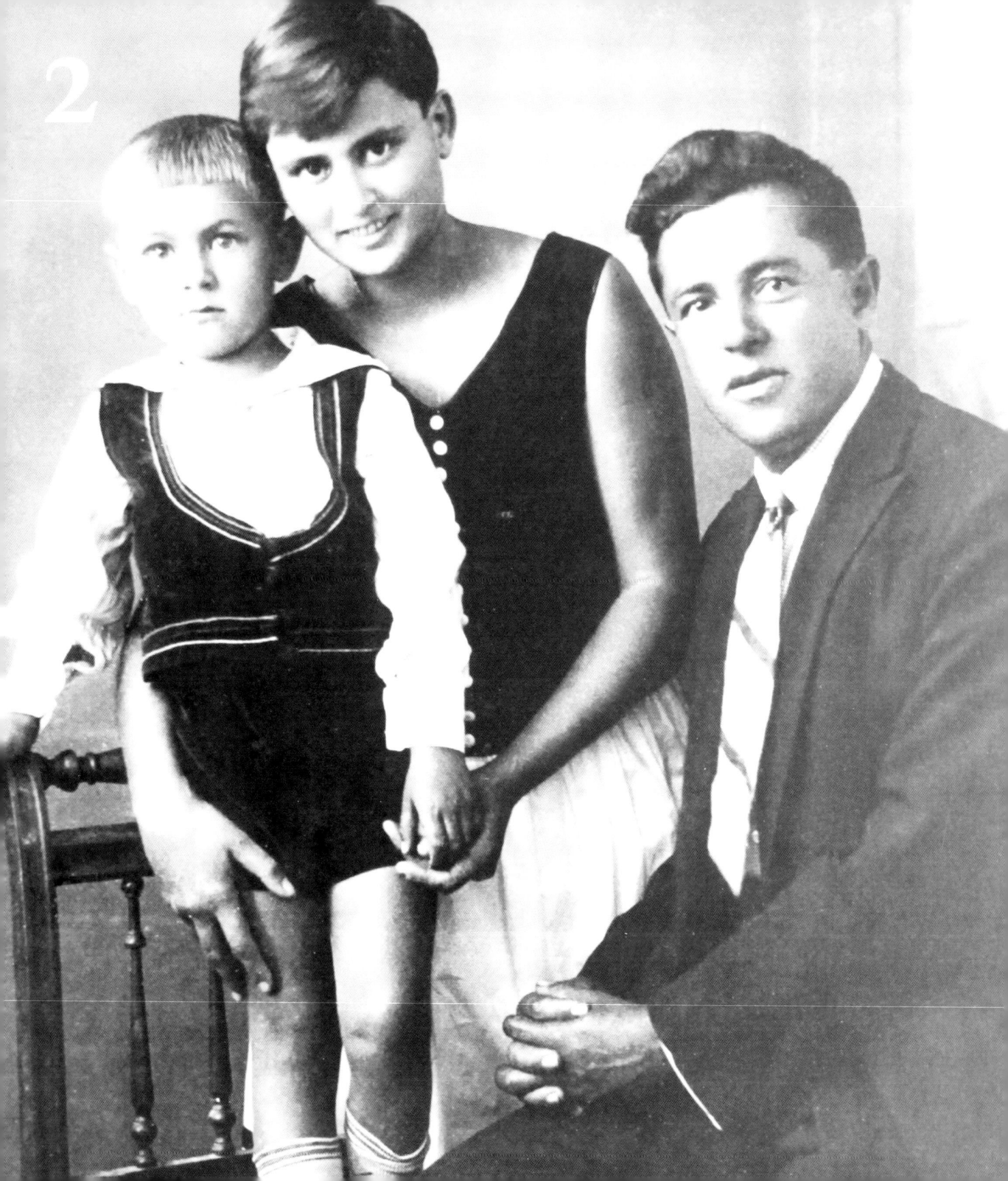

The Early Years

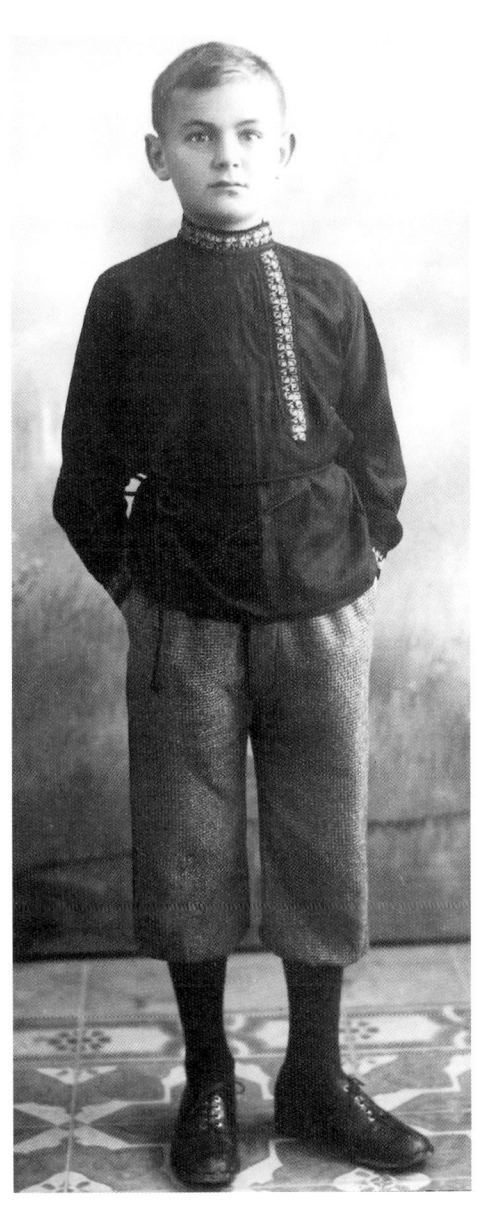

Moshe 1930

Left page: Moshe with his parents Rebecca and David 1926

At the age of only 20 years David Zarhy saw no more future prospects in his home town, Vitecs in Russia. It was not only since the Russian October Revolution in 1917, but principally so in the ensuing civil war, which lasted until 1921, that the Jewish population was no longer safe in various regions of Russia. In the Balfour Declaration of November 2nd, 1917 Great Britain had agreed to support Zionist efforts to establish a national home for the Jewish people in Palestine. This gave many persecuted Jews, who had lost their prospects in Russia, the opportunity of a new beginning in a "new homeland". When David Zarhy came to Jaffa / Tel Aviv in 1919, he had completed his training as a mechanical engineer. He married Rebecca Flexer, who came from Kamjanez-Podilsky in Western Ukraine.

On November 24th 1923 Rebecca gave birth to their first child, Moshe. At that time the family lived in Jerusalem. For the first 9 years of his life Moshe remained the only child of the Zarhy family until his brother Zvi was born in 1932. Father David earned his money as driver of an excavator. During the week, he worked at different construction sites, but every weekend he returned to the family. Mother Rebecca ran the household and raised the children. Moshe tells of a harmonious childhood. He attended High School Palestine in Jerusalem, walking distance from his home, from which he graduated in 1939.

Two events tragically overshadowed the otherwise happy childhood. In 1932, on their way back to Tel Aviv from a trip, the taxi transporting the whole Zarhy family collided with a train at a level crossing. Moshes' mother was killed instantly, father David, Moshe and the baby Zvi survived. From now on the two were raised by their grandmother, Haia Flexer, Rebecca's mother. In 1941, Moshes' father David was also killed in a car accident, near to the place where the brothers had lost their mother, nine years earlier. The two boys, aged 18 and 9 years, were orphans.

When asked about his hobbies, Moshe recalls that as a child he loved drawing and painting, the talent for which had been placed in his cradle. Consequently, he enrolled for architecture studies at the only Israeli university where this subject was taught, studying from 1939 to 1945 at the Technion – The Israel Institute of Technology in Haifa.

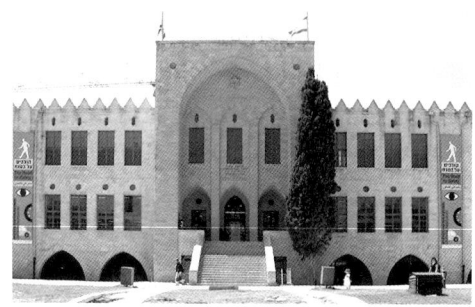

Technion Haifa, Architect Hans Baerwald, built from 1912–1924. Today: The Israeli National Museum of Science, Technology and Space

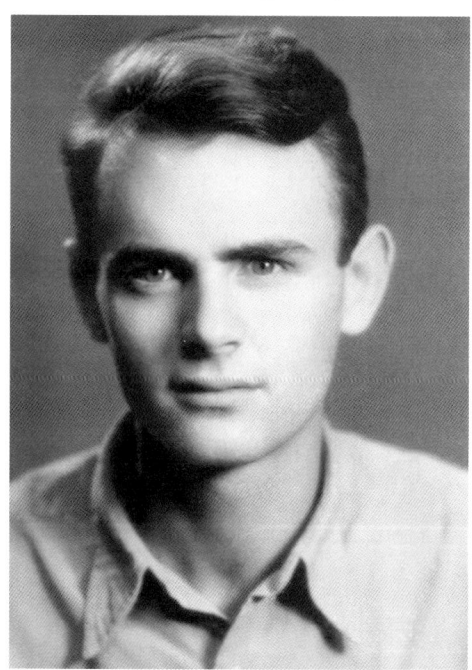

Moshe Zarhy as student 1943

From 1940 to 1943 he performed his military service in the British Army in the Haifa region, a duty which nevertheless enabled him to continue his studies at the Technion.

One of his fellow students at that time was Yaakov Rechter, the son of the famous architect Zeev Rechter. Zeev Rechter also had two daughters: Aviva and Tuti. Though Yaakov Moshe got to know the Rechter family and fell in love with Aviva. The website of Rechter Architects modestly mentions the founding father: "Rechter Architects was founded in 1930 by Zeev Rechter after his return to Israel from studies in Paris. Zeev designed various buildings and Master Plans that were to become icons of Israeli modernism. His scope of work ranged across the architectural discipline, from planning housing complexes in Tel Aviv to kibbutzim and major public buildings such as the Kalia Hotel in the dead sea and the Jerusalem international convention center and concert hall." Rechter's social milieu included poets, artists and actors, the Tel Aviv bohemians. He built private homes for the poet and writer Esther Raab in 1927 and Chana Orloff in Paris. He was involved in house building and in the Kibbutz movement. Some of his Bauhaus projects in Tel Aviv, such as Engel House and Soskin House, are equally outstanding. His hospital projects will be dealt with later, as they fall into a time when Moshe Zarhy was already a colleague and partner of Rechter. Mosche was married to Aviva Rechter, daughter of Zeev Rechter in 1944.

After completing his studies Moshe and his fellow student Yaakov Rechter accepted the honourable offer of Zeev Rechter to take their first steps as young architects in his renowned architect's office at Rabin Square in Tel Aviv. With his very first project in this office Moshe got into contact with hospital building, which was to become his special field. He was involved in planning a hospital complex in

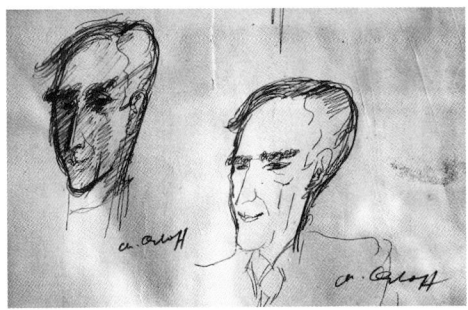

Sketch of Zeev Rechter by Chana Orloff

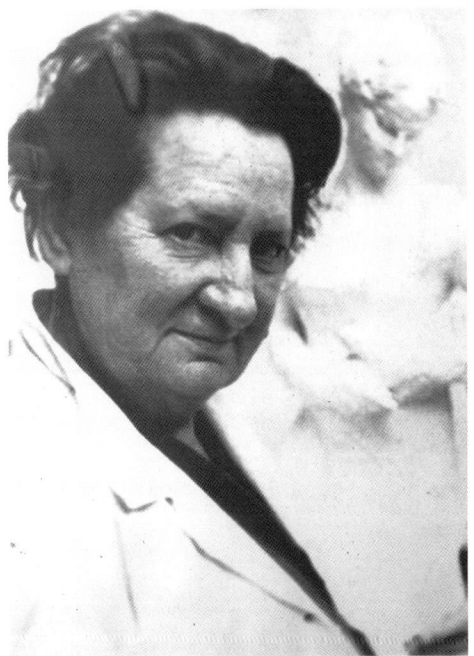

Photo of Chana Orloff, 1960s, hanging in Moshe Zarhy's office

Kfar-Saba, where initially a school of nurses and a tuberculosis hospital were planned. During the construction process the plans were changed and a General Hospital was built (later known as Meir Hospital).

In 1949, after a few years of office work, Moshe felt the need for further training in the area of Town Planning. At that time, one of the most prestigious universities in that area was the Ecole d'Urbanisme at the Sorbonne in Paris. There he studied from 1949 to 1950, enlarging not only his knowledge of architecture and urban development, but also quenching his thirst for knowledge in the field of fine arts.

Zarhy's "teacher" in the arts was the internationally renowned Chana Orloff, whom Moshe had already met in Israel. "When I went to Paris in 1949 with Aviva, Chana Orloff adopted me and she told me a lot about Paris. She also informed me about arts in Paris. I painted at that time and she told me, how to do it. In her sculptures she worked with wood, stone and bronze." This is what Moshe said in an interview in July 2013. Chana Orloff was born in Kostjantyniwka in Ukraine in 1888 and, in 1904, immigrated to British Mandate Palestine following pogroms in Ukraine. From 1910 she studied arts and sculpture in Paris. There she was in contact with the artistic avantgarde, among others Amedeo Modigliani, Jean Cocteau, Alexandre Archipenko and Ida Chagall. From 1928 she exhibited her sculptures in New York, Zurich, Tel Aviv and Paris. After the Second World War, she made a great breakthrough and achieved international recognition.

The proximity to this great sculptor influenced Moshe Zarhy's artistic development decisively. In 1950 he returned to Tel Aviv full of new ideas and, as a 28-year-old architect, received an offer to become a partner in Zeev Rechter's office. His apprenticeship was over. The remarkable career story of an inspired architect was now underway.

3

The Architect and high ranking official

The Architect and high ranking official

Even as a young graduate Moshe had worked for four years in Zeev Rechter's office after completing his studies at the Technion, interrupted by the military service in the British Army. He had enriched his knowledge in the areas of urban planning and art in Paris and now, at the age of 28, was offered a partnership as an architect in one of the most renowned offices in Israel. Beside the experienced master Zeev Rechter, his son Yaakov and Moshe Zarhy became members of the partnership **Rechter-Zarhy-Rechter**. Moshe's main occupation was planning the big Medical Centre in Kfar-Saba, which he had already worked on during the years before his stay in Paris. We will see later that this was to become a life's task, for until today, the office "Zarhy Architects" has been involved in building projects there. Rechter had already created exemplary architectural icons in all fields, in urban planning, the construction of Kibbutz settlements, public works and medical institutions. The young partners benefited from the good reputation of the office and had the opportunity of developing independently under the eyes of the master.

In 1960 Zeev Rechter died at the age of 61. The remaining junior partners now took the engineer Michael Peri into their office community and as a member of the family, for Michael Peri had married Zeev Rechter's second daughter, Tuti. The son and two sons-in-law now continued the successful work of the eminent architect Zeev Rechter, who had significantly contributed to shaping the foundations of architecture in Palestine and the young State of Israel.

The successful work of this three-partner office continued for 13 years. The number of staff had risen to approximately 80 people and had already necessitated dividing the projects among the different partners. This fact prompted Moshe to separate from his partners and found his own office, **Zarhy Architects,** in 1973. They continued working in the same building.

After his father-in-law, Zeev Rechter, Moshe Zarhy now represented the second generation of architects. Continuity was already provided, for at the time when Zarhy Architects Ltd. was founded, David, son of Moshe and Aviva, was studying architecture at the Technion in Tel Aviv, just like his father before him. From 1974 to 1978 he worked as

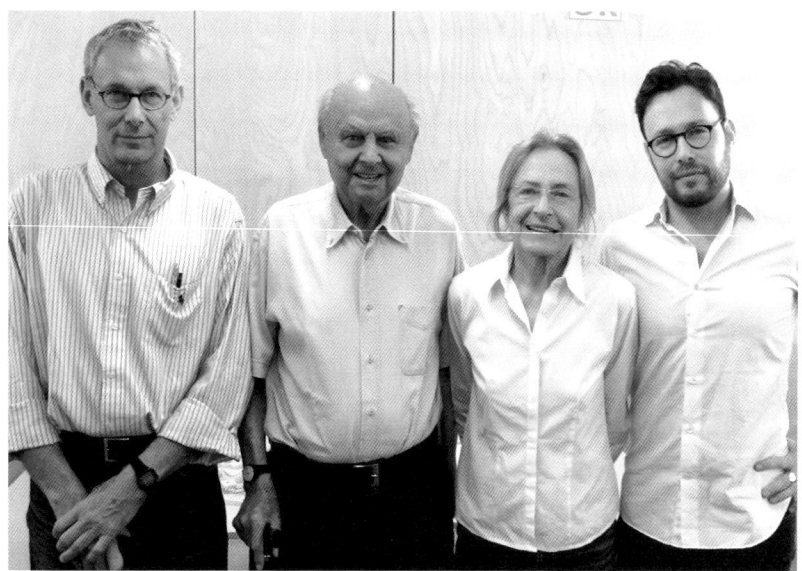

Three generations of architects with Zarhy Architects, from the left: David, Moshe, Anat-Patrycha and Daniel. Photo: Peter R. Pawlik 2013

an architect in the IDF (Israel Defense Forces). In 1978 he and his wife Anat-Patrycha Zarhy were included as partners in the office Zarhy Architects Ltd., constituting the third generation in the architectural office. Patrycha and David also have a son, who studied architecture at the Technion and has since gained international experience in the prestigious offices of Rem Koolhaas in Rotterdam / Netherlands and Herzog & de Meuron in Basel.

He now works as a freelance architect as well as for Zarhy Architects, and continues the family's architectural tradition in the fourth generation.

Moshe Zarhy is the Founder of Zarhy Architects. He was joined at the firm by his son, the architect David Zarhy and architect Anat Patrycha Zarhy in 1978. They currently run the firm. Zarhy Architects number about 30 employees including architects, architectural draft persons and support personnel. The firm is active in all areas of architectural planning: public institutions, housing projects, urban planning, private homes, education buildings, hotels and commercial buildings, sports facilities and IDF (Israel Defense Forces) projects. Special emphasis has been put on planning and developing Medical Centers, Health Facilities, Science and High-Tech facilities. These include:

3. The Architect and high ranking official

- Tchad – Etude D'Urbanisation des centres urbains et régionaux de la République du Tchad (Urbanization survey of the urban and regional centers of the Republic of Tchad), at the request of the government of Tchad in 1962.
- Sierra Leone – Proposal for the construction of a new national Medical Center for Sierra Leone at the request of the government of Sierra Leone in 1962.
- Central African Republic – Etudes des structures existantes des concentrations urbaines de la République Centre Africaine (Survey of the existing structures of the urban centers of the Central African Republic) at the request of the government of the Central African Republic in 1963.
- Venezuela – Medical Centers – Consulting at the request of the Venezuelan Ministry of Health in 1971.
- South Africa – Design of a five star hotel (not built) in 1975.
- Ireland – Appointed as assessor in the competition for the design of a major new hospital at Tallaght, Ireland; nominated by the International Union of Architects (UIA) in 1984–1985.
- The Annual Seminar of the International Union of Architects – Public Health Group (Paris and Düsseldorf) – Organizing the seminar in Israel on the subject of: "Computer assisted planning and operation of health and hospital care facilities" in 1986.

Sheba Medical Center (S.M.C) Ramat Gan – Greater Tel Aviv Area
- The General Hospital
- The Women Hospital
- Rehabilitation Hospital
- The Psychiatric Hospital
- Medical Training and Teaching Institute
- Public Health Research Institute

The Safed General Hospital – Upper Galilee.
- Nurses Training School – Safed Upper Galilee

School of Dental Medicine – Tel Aviv University

Meir Medical Center – Kfar Saba, Sharon Area
- Meir School for Nurses – Kfar Saba, Sharon Area

The Weizman Medical Multi Use Center – Tel Aviv.

During 60 years of professional experience Moshe Zarhy has provided comprehensive architectural services for numerous major building projects. He is the author of many professional papers. His projects have been widely documented and published in international professional press. He has been involved in the International Union of Architects' (UIA) activities since the mid-sixties. As a voting member of the Public Health Working Group, Zarhy has represented the Israeli National Section in all UIA Congresses since 1969. He was UIA Council Member during the years 1990–1993, was elected UIA vice President Region II for the terms of 1993–1996–1999, and has served as Director of the UIA Work Programme "Architecture for Science and Hi-Tech Facilities" since 1999. Moshe Zarhy has been elected as FAIA-Fellow of American Institute of Architects. He is a planner of large Medical Centers in Israel and largely responsible for several new architectural concepts in Israel Medical Centers."

Zarhy Architects work for numerous clients in Israel. Representative are: Israel Ministries of Health, Industry and Commerce (Mischarve'asia) and Housing and Construction, Histadrut Labor Federation "Kupat Holim" Sick Fund, Jewish Agency Jerusalem, Municipalities of Jerusalem and Tel Aviv, Rafael – Israel Armaments Development Authority, Israel Military Industries, Tel Aviv University, Technion – Israel Institute of Technology, Hebrew University of Jerusalem, Weizman Institute of Science, Africa-Israel Investment Corp. Ltd., Pecker Industries Lt., Clal Corporation Ltd. and National Semi-Conductor (Israel) Ltd.

Considering the abundance of his long-term professional commitments as well as his international presence it is not surprising that Moshe Zarhy has received a number of honours and awards. These include:

2012: Award given at the 1st international conference on medicine and Architecture in the 21st Century. Technion / Tel Aviv

2009: Senior Member of Israeli Top Executive Business Leadership of 2009

2000: Letter of evaluation from the Isreali Architects' Association.

2000: Vice President of the UIA Region 2

2004: Honorary Fellowship in the American Institute of Architects (AIA)

2004: Honorable Member of the "KAZGOR" Design Academy, Republic of Kazakhstan

1998: Honorary member of the Moscow Branch of the International Academy of Architecture.

1998: Letter of evaluation. Academy of the Architects of Russia

1996: Honoring with the Insignia of the higher council of the Spanish Architects

1996: Letter of evaluation. Architects of Russia

1996: Silver badge of Catalonian Architects

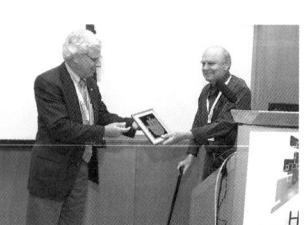

Moshe Zarhy (on the right) receives a "Hamsa" from Prof. Kalay.
Photo: Technion Spokesman

As director of the UIA Work Programme "Architecture for Science and HI-Tech Facilities" Moshe Zarhy has participated significantly in the following events:

- **First Annual Seminar and Founding Meeting**
  Theme: "Architecture for Science and High-Tech Facilities – A Comprehensive Outlook" Under the auspices patronage of the Israeli Association of United Architects and ISCAR Industries, at Tefen, one of the largest industrial parks in Israel. The meeting also included 2 tours to visit Israeli high-tech facilities in the greater Tel Aviv area and in Jerusalem.

- **Participation in the UIA congress.**
  Theme: "Architectural issue of planning for science and Hi-Tech facilities in our era. Seminar and 90-minute slide presentation, with a display of panels at the Architectural Exhibition depicting realizations of the high-tech facilities projects in various member countries.

- **Second International Seminar and Annual Members' Meeting under the auspices of the BDA / Germany and organized by Arch. Daniel Goessler (+)**
  Theme: "Science and the High-Tech Campus in the Urban Context Today"
  The focal point of the meeting was the Berlin-Adlershof "City of Science and Economy". The schedule of the meeting included a guided tour of the new architecture of Berlin, a tour of the Adlershof, and a symposium attended by architects, developers and city officials who were involved with its development.

- **Third International Seminar and Annual Members' Meeting**
  Theme: "Technopolis – the Town of Science" Under the auspices of and organized by the Union of Architects of Russia (UAR) and our Work Russia Program, Russian member Prof. Vsevolod Koulich, the Seminar included architectural tours of Moscow, Science Institutes and the Russian Science City of Chernogolovka. Co-organizers of this event were: The Russian Academy of Architecture and Construction Sciences (RAACS), the Russian Academy of Sciences (RAS) and the Moscow Architectural Institute / State Academy (MARCHI).

- **Participation in the UIA Congress**
  Theme: "Architectural issue of planning for Science and High-Tech facilities in our Era" Seminar and Exhibition emphasizing the increasing importance and relevance of the architectural issue of planning for science

3. The Architect and high ranking official

and high-tech facilities in our era. The Seminar attracted many architects and took place in front of a full auditorium. The events were organized by the colleague Daniel Goessler (+), under the auspices of the BDA / Germany.

- **Fourth International Seminar and Annual Members' Meeting**
Theme: "The Principles of Architecture for Science and High-Tech Facilities"
The organizer was our member Brian A. Spencer, AAI / IAA, Architect, and the co-organizers were: AIA-USA American Institute of Architects, the Frank Lloyd Wright Foundation, and the School of Architecture at the Arizona State University (ASU).
- **Fifth International Seminar and Annual Members' Meeting**
Theme: "Science and Hi-Tech Facilities – Contribution of Regional environment"
The meeting included visits to recently built Science and High-Tech Facilities in China. The event was organized by our Work Program member from Macau, Francisco Vizeu Pinheiro.
- **Sixth International Seminar and Annual Members' Meeting held within the context of the XXII World Congress.**
Theme: "Location of the High-Tech Facility Campus Within the City"
A study tour to visit the Gebze Institute of Technology was organized by our Work Program member Dr. Ahmet Vefik Alp.
- **Seventh International Seminar and Annual Members' Meeting**
Theme: "The Hi-Tech Campus in the city – The Eco-Technological dilemma".
A study tour was made to visit The Graphisoft Technology Park. The Meeting took place at the Budapest University of Technology and Economics and was co- hosted by the Association of the Hungarian Architects.
The organizer of the 2006 meeting WP member in Hungary, Gabor Becker.
- **Eighth International Seminar and Annual Members' Meeting Theme: "Life Sciences Facilities I Animal Breeding Laboratories".**
The meeting took place at the Central Office of the Max Planck-Society. The organizer of the 2007 meeting was WP member in Germany, Dieter Groemling.
- **Ninth International Seminar and Annual Members' Meeting**
This meeting is scheduled to take place in Turin, Italy, in the frame work of the "23rd Congress of the International Union of Architects (UIA) ".

Moshe lost his first wife Aviva in 1993, who died at the age of 72. Moshe married Vera Ronnen-Zarhy in 1994. She is an artist, working in vitreous enamel on steel, on site-specific installations in architecture all over the world. They lived together at Moshe's residence in Ramat Hasharon untill 2013, and recently they moved to their new home at Arlozorov 150 in Tel Aviv, the same address as Zarhy Architects office.

In the next chapter Moshe Zarhy shares his long experience in his specialty, the planning and construction of health facilities, with his readers.

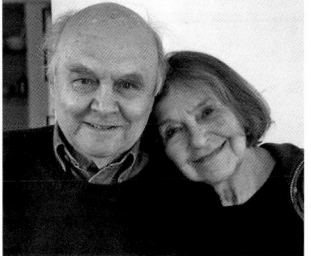

Portrait of Moshe Zarhy with his wife Vera Ronnen-Zarhy in 2009

4

Health Facilities
in Israel

Introduction

Prior to the establishment of the State of Israel health services and hospitalization were covered by various institutions controlled by the Mandatory Government, the Workers' Federation (Histadrut) Sick Fund, the Hadassah Organization and missionary and private bodies. Final responsibility for health matters rested with the British Mandatory Government. Maintenance of hospitals was the responsibility of the various sponsors.

When the State of Israel was founded, many immediate problems had to be solved by improvisation. One such problem was to provide health services for the country's expanding population. The makeshift solution in the case was to locate them in whatever buildings were available. These were often old and unsuited for their intended new purpose; in some cases abandoned World War II army camps were used. Very few new buildings were erected- insufficient to cover actual need. There was no comprehensive planning: no master plan. Serious planning of health services and hospitals only really commenced towards the end of the first decade of the State's existence. The construction work presently being carried out is the fruit of that initial development programme. It covers the erection of hospitals, 5,000 beds for general hospitals, 5.000 beds for psychiatric hospitals and 1,750 beds for rehabilitation centre and hospitals for chronic diseases.

Construction of these health centres is based on a hospitalization programme covering the whole country. As in other countries, there is the well-known tendency towards quantity and quality increases in large medical institutions, generally urban, with the simultaneous problem of insufficient rural density not supporting health and other services of an adequate standard. Since health centres which are too small cannot maintain modern health services of a reasonable level, they are unsatisfactory. The tendency to concentrate hospitalization services gives rise to the attendant problem of large distances separating them from the people for whom they are intended. Medical staff prefers to work in large institutions, contributing to an increase in professional standards in these places. A serious difficulty exists in attracting staff to small hospitals.

Another group of problems which manifest themselves in hospital design in Israel is specific to the country. These include actual dispersal of population and the anticipation of population increase (since planning and building of hospitals is a lengthy process, the time factor is also an important element to be taken into consideration). Limited budgets, coordination with local authorities, political pressures such as may be exerted by local inhabitants, problems of national security, particularly with regard to border settlements, national characteristics customs and population attitudes, all play their part in colouring the overall picture.

The above-mentioned factors are only a few of those influencing the acceptable hospital plan in Israel. It is impossible to enumerate here all the factors that have influenced and are still influencing the general concept of the hospital. I have asked myself more than once whether there exists a unique, Israeli "hospital concept." Years of planning medical institutions, constant contact with medical, administrative, technical staff and builders, following-up life in medical institutions and comparing facts that have materialized against preliminary planning of these institutions, visiting hospitals abroad and comparing them with those in Israel- all these have let me what can indeed be termed "the Israeli hospital concept." This collective effort began at the turn of the century, when doctors and others dealing with medical administration were few, but performed their jobs in a pioneering spirit, as did others at that time.

They worked in those days under very stringent conditions and only their inner strength enabled them to carry on. Several personalities who have become legendary figures, like Mr. Soroka and Dr. Sheba, dedicated themselves until their last days to advancing medical services in Israel. They faced many hardships, but achieved impressive results.

Over the years the tools have improved and the few become many. Organizations have been established. Many medical institutions have been built. Some of them have developed, but usually their development was not anticipated by their founders. Reality was the strongest factor. The initiators, planners and operators have learned their lessons from reality. Each "generation" of medical institutions has learned from previous experience and has added to our overall knowledge. Thus the thought of those dealing with the erection of medical institutions has crystallized until it has reached a point which can be termed "general perception." It is difficult to define anything connected with life which is based on actual multilateral reality; therefore, it is difficult to define the concept being discussed.

However, there is no doubt that any designer planning a medical institution in Israel today relies on previous experience. He has a common language with the visionaries and the founders of the policy of the institution which is going to be erected, and he begins his planning on the basis of perceptions and data which are available to all – the collective creation.

In this spirit, I have compiled projects that were planned in our office and are connected in one way or another with medical institutions: hospitals, convalescent homes, research institutions, polyclinics, etc. and I hope that their presentation will express the background upon which they were created. In addition, I thought that from all the medical facilities I should choose and describe an average Israeli hospital, let us say, a hospital of about 400–500 beds. With regards to optimal size, it is impossible to draw hard-and-fast conclusions, but present-day experience in Israel has shown that 400–500 beds with balanced medical and health services provides a sound basis for an effective, efficiently administered regional hospital. Hospitals of this size can support medical and health services of a generally acceptable standard.

I have chosen to describe not a particular medical institution but rather thoughts about the general structure of such an institution, thoughts about the various departments comprising the hospital as they were expressed in many hours of debate with many persons involved in one way or another in the planning of medical institutions on Israel. It is impossible, of course, to describe all the opinions and streams of thought. The description is subjective. It often expresses requests regarding planning as I have understood them. I have chosen to describe only from personal experience, or experience acquired in our office. I have sometimes gone into minute detail, hoping that a multilateral description of the problem and of its solutions will give the reader a general picture and will express the spirit and state of mind that have brought about these solutions, for as Le Corbusier put it, "Architecture is not a profession, it is a state of mind."

The Main Functional Divisions
of the Hospital

As with any complex problem it is difficult to determine whether the problem should be described first generally or in great detail.

I have chosen to describe first the main categories of functions to be considered in the planning of hospitals in Israel:

1. Hospitalization services
2. Medical services
3. Administrative services and miscellaneous
4. Supply services
5. Outpatient department

1. Hospitalization services

The main element in this function is the ward, which repeats itself with minor variation. Israel's experience shows that a ward of 35–40 beds is an optimum nursing unit. After experimenting with different-sized rooms, optimum size is thought to be a 2–3 bedded patients' room, which is also economical. However, a number of private rooms (1-bedded) must be provided in each ward for serious cases and other special purposes.

Generally, patients' toilet facilities adjoin rooms and are arranged so that they can be shared by pairs of rooms. Centrally located in the ward are the nurses' station, their workrooms, treatment and ancillary rooms. Ambulatory patients may use a day room. Attached to each ward there are the usually four doctors' rooms. Minor variations of the standard ward pattern enable it to meet special requirements such as for surgery, internal medicine, ear, nose and throat, eye diseases, etc. The fact that wards are standard provides flexibility for changes which may become necessary in the course of time. Slightly different in function are pediatrics, obstetrics and gynaecology wards. In a 400–500 bed hospital there will be 12–14 wards.

The building housing the wards usually takes the form of a superstructure served by one, two or three circulation cores. The ward block is often the dominating architectural element in the building. Although this is the least changing of the functional element, it is still important to allow for additional units.

4. Health Facilities in Israel

2. Medical services

These are usually concentrated in one or two floors, at, or directly accessible from ground level. The main medical department are: casualty department, diagnostic radiology, operating theatres, clinical and research laboratories, physiotherapy, occupational therapy, cardiology, etc. The medical services are under constant pressure, both from the great demands being made upon them and due to changes arising out of advances and technological developments in medicine. Flexibility, growth and change are integral requirements for this part of the building; new demands are not an unusual occurrence. It is, therefore, an advantage if each department can be expanded independently and at will without disturbing the functioning of the hospital as a whole. The element of change creates a planning system which is the essence of the character of this section of the hospital.

3. Administrative services and miscellaneous

According to the Israeli concept the administrative services include the administration and reception office for incoming patients. The administration section is responsible for the general management as well as the medical administration of the hospital. Because of its relationship to the general public it should be located in such a way, that people from outside have easy access to it, but cannot enter either the hospital proper or the special "closed" sections from this area without permission. The administration office serves the patients or the people that accompany them, and it processes the files of incoming patients and those being released. Therefore it must be located close to the casualty and admission section. Certain aspects of the process of admitting patients are Israeli in character and differ in many ways from those in European or American hospitals.

Functional areas and rooms, like the entrance hall, synagogue, circumcision hall, etc., which are not an integral part of the medical and supply services, can be classified as miscellaneous.

4. Supply services

To a certain degree the supply services are influenced by local Israeli conditions, such as the types of food, its manner of preparation and conditions of supply; the need for larger cold storage facilities than in countries having more temperate climates; and the lack, to this day, of centralized cooking on a large scale. The design of the central sterile supply depends to a large extent on the methods and systems used,

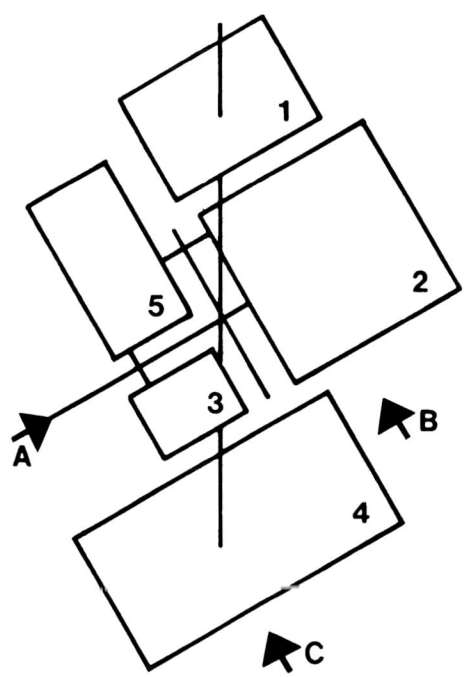

The interrelationship of the main functional divisions of the hospital.
1. Hospitalization services
2. Medical services
3. Administrative services and miscellaneous
4. Supply services
5. Outpatient department
A. Main entrance
B. Entrance to casualty department
C. Service entrance

on the way in which work is organized and upon whether it serves the operating theatres. Design is further affected by the fact that no conclusions have as yet been arrived at, concerning the advantages and disadvantages of using disposable materials. Different types of supply services, based on the various prevalent theories, can be found in Israel Supply storerooms and workshops are a subject which should receive separate consideration.

The main supply services are: food supply, general stores, maintenance workshops, bed centre, engine room (heat and refrigeration production), medical gases centre etc. It should be pointed out that experience has shown that all the supply services should be designed in the most flexible way, with possibility for expansion. A certain difficulty arises from the fact that these services, like others, are connected to the traffic cores of the hospital. In some hospitals, the supply services are located in the basement floor, close to the vertical traffic cores. In these hospitals it is difficult to expand this section. In other hospitals, the supply services form a block. The only difficulty in this case is to solve problems of traffic circulation.

5. Outpatient department

The outpatient department serves the patients coming for examination and short-term treatment. In many cases these patients are being followed up after hospitalization. The entrance to the outpatient department should be, therefore, from the outside or through the main entrance hall of the hospital.

The outpatient department makes use of the various medical services of the hospital. These are referred to in Israel as "Institutes" and include radiology (in Israel, the Radiology Institute), cardiology, physiotherapy, etc.

The above considerations dictate the location of the outpatient department within the hospital. Usually this wing is located on the ground floor or the medical services floor, so that there is a direct entrance from the outside but no passage through the clinics to the hospital itself. The outpatient department includes examination rooms, waiting rooms and treatment rooms.

The Master Plan

Master plan of Chaim Sheba Medical Centre

The Master Plan is comprised of the existing hospital which was housed, about twenty-five years ago, in a deserted army camp, and the new hospital which is under construction. The plan takes into account the fact that the existing hospital's function cannot cease, and that after completion of the new hospital, the building process will continue in the remaining areas and in the areas now occupied by the existing hospital.

1. Main building – wards
2. Radiology
3. Outpatient department
4. Entrance hall and public services
5. Entrance level – casualty and admission
   Ground level – administration
6. Entrance level – nephrology
   Ground level – night duty staff
7. Entrance level – operating theatres
   Ground level – central cloakrooms,
   central sterile supply dept.,
   underground casualty unit
8. Entrance level – lecture hall, library
   Ground level – pharmacy
9. Service maintenance and
   central power supply
   Entrance level – dining room
   Ground level – kitchen, central storerooms,
   workshops, boiler room, central gas supply
10. Research laboratories
11. Mortuary
A. Main entrance
B. Entrance to casualty department
C. Entrance to underground casualty unit
D. Service entrance
E. New road
F. Main parking
G. Helicopter landing pad
H. Future development
I. Children's hospital
J. Future expansion area
K. Existing hospital

The Importance of the Master Plan

The master plan of the hospital defines the main traffic routes, the location of the various buildings or wings, the connections between them and the direction of the institution's expansion in its various stages. We have divided the area into five categories, according to their designation, so as to simplify the problem. It is understandable that in reality there are many exceptions to this division and it is presented here only to aid discussions of the desirable connections between these categories or the various wings. We must emphasize here the importance

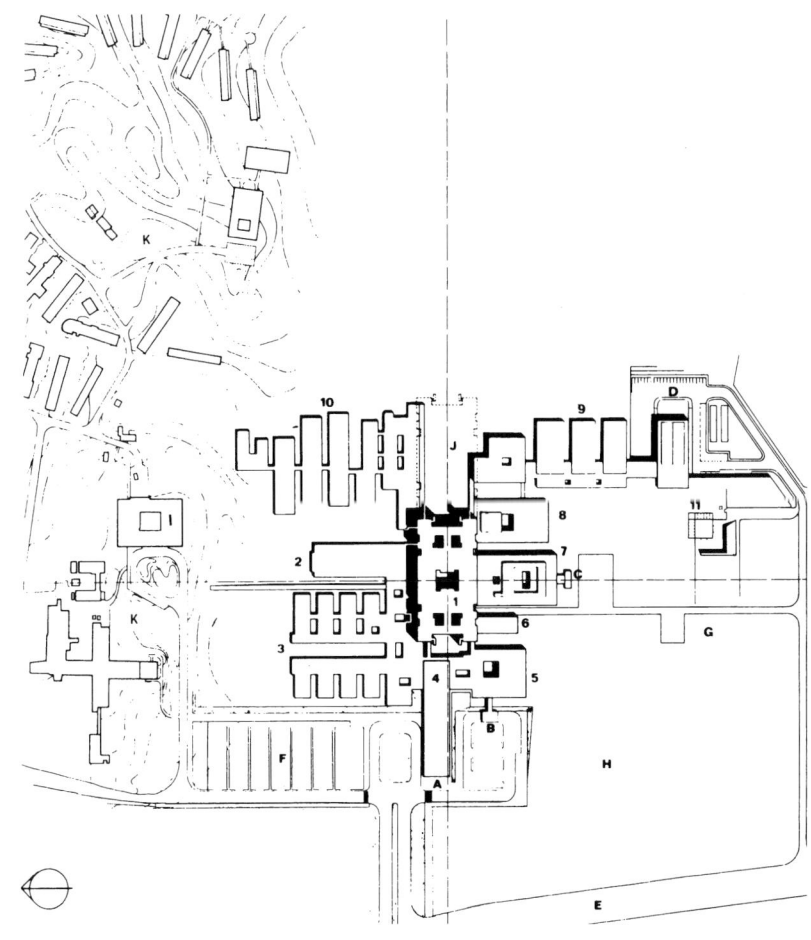

of the master plan. This plan forms the outline, upon which the hospital plan is built. With the passing of time the interior divisions or even the designations of the wards and wings may change, while the main traffic axes exist, usually, for the lifetime of the institutions. Although this traffic system grows and branches during the years, it is very difficult to change the location of the vertical and horizontal traffic axes. In other words, it is difficult to change the concept or the principles of planning after they have been set. Hence the master plan is of decisive importance.

The Pavilion Hospital Concept
During the last decades, several Israeli hospitals and health institutions were located in pavilions while others, of necessity, functioned out of the huts of deserted army camps.
In health institutions housed in pavilions of one or two storeys, there is a pleasant contact between the sick and the immediate landscape. This is a noticeable advantage which is hard to achieve in another building concept. On the other hand, in these "pavilion institutions" there are problems of transporting patients, personnel traffic, parking and accessibility to the different pavilions, distribution of food and medical supplies, scattering of visitors over the whole area, maintenancy problems, electromechanical problems, waste of land reserves and inability to control traffic within the institution's limits. These problems and others brought the pavilion concept to a dead end.
In reality, except for the problems listed above, there is no possibility of controlling the "building framework" of the health institution. Every day "additions" are being built and the general image of the health institution is being spoiled to the point that it can be termed an Institutional "slum". It is possible to visualize a hospital of up to 200 beds, but above this size it becomes too complex, distances are too great, etc. As an architect I can judge this occurrence with mixed feelings. There exists, of course, the physical possibility of sporadic additions as the need arises, but it seems to have been proven that this advantage turns into a stumbling block because minor, ununified additions are made, usually in an unprofessional manner.
We said that the pavilion concept has come to a dead end. This statement can be further strengthened because of the fact that most of the areas in which institutions are being built are becoming built-up urban areas, and the land reserve is dwindling until this concept becomes impossible to execute. It is very doubtful if any institution

4. Health Facilities in Israel

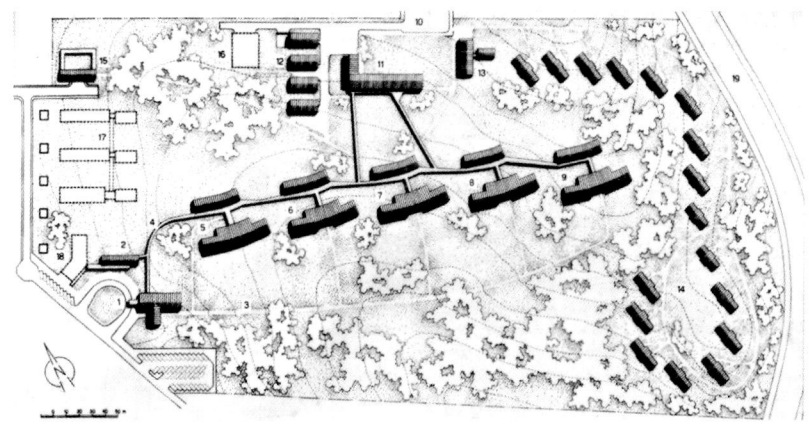

Site plan of Kaplan Pavilion Hospital 1954

would choose to go this way today. On the other hand, observation of life, problems and improvisations in these institutions has enabled us to examine, in an experimental manner, functions which could not have been examined otherwise.

We have learned the advantage of having medical and administrative services on the ground floor, the advantages of planning wards and complex services without limitations that are dictated by the other floors, the advantageous possible additions to services, etc.

The phenomena which do not cease to surprise me are the dynamism and vitality which are expressed freely in these institutions, and which ease, perhaps, the absorption of professionals and the development of new departments.

The thought which arises at the sight of the developments in these institutions, some of which have been built without planning or planners, is as follows: If we could give a planned institution the advantages of preplanning and add this to what we have learned in the experimentation field, i.e. give it the "dynamism" quality, then this quality will become a value and will dictate the building's composition. Its master plan would then be harmonious and lead to peaceful coexistence between the needs of the wings and their shape.

The Compact Hospital Concept
Other health institutions were built during these years in centralized buildings. This is an opposing approach to the pavilion concept. Here, all the wards and services are centralized in one building. In cases of severe land limitations there is often no choice but to centralize all the

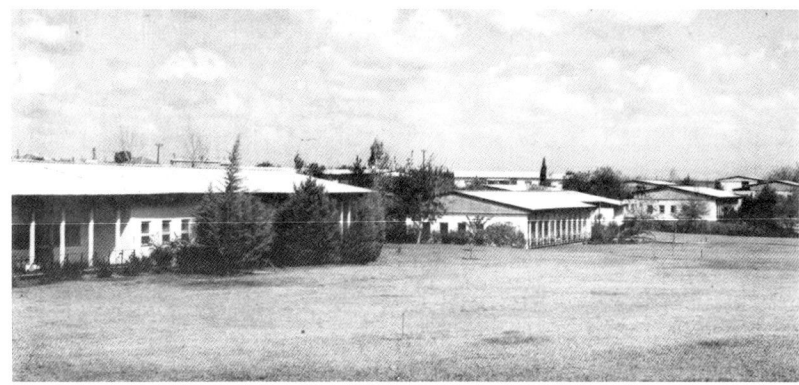

Photo of Kaplan Pavilion Hospital 1954

departments in one block, However, certain limitations are inherent in this compact hospital concept, for example those resulting from placement of one floor directly on top of another. There are services that do not fit into the floor area, whereas for some services the floor area is too large. It happens sometimes that a department or service unit is arranged on two floors and there is no possibility of efficiently performing the service. The differences in the needs of each floor make it impossible to plan identical electromechanical systems. In order to solve problems of electromechanical systems in a centralized building, an "empty floor" may be planned between each floor, to be used as a technical space for passage of systems. This is an extremely expensive solution which may be justified in certain science buildings where the systems are undergoing changes, repairs and constant control, but it seems too extreme and too expensive in our case.

Usually, in the compact hospital, the traffic route system is based on vertical traffic circulation. This is a rapid and technically reliable system, which enables direct communication between different departments without complications. It should be noted, however, that personal contact among the staff is "weaker" in a building with a vertical communication system.

I have presented two opposing concepts – that of the pavilion hospital – and that of the compact hospital. There are some who seek a golden path between these two concepts – a compromise which combines the advantages of the two systems. The intention here, however, is not to create a magic formula, but a principle or set of principles upon which one can plan in various ways according to the particular needs and circumstances of the site and the programme.

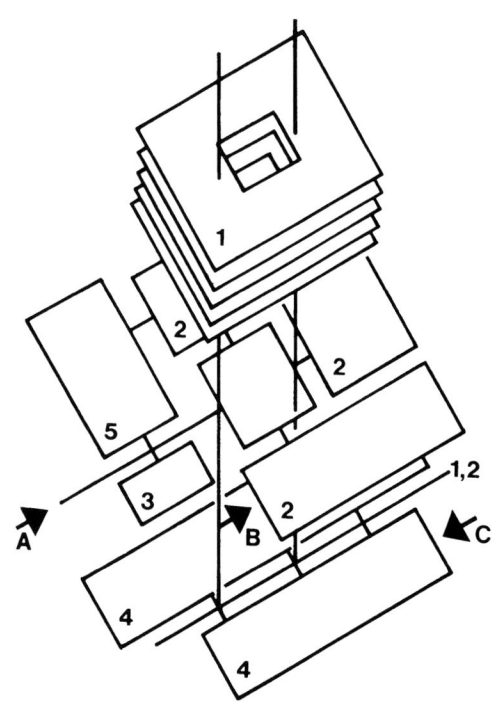

The "compact" hospital concept
1. Hospitalization services
2. Medical services
3. Administrative services and miscellaneous
4. Supply services
5. Outpatient department
A. Main entrance
B. Entrance to casualty department
C. Service entrance

4. Health Facilities in Israel

The Balanced Integrated Hospital Concept

As already stated, the least changing of the hospital wings is the inpatient department. The demands for alterations in this wing are small in comparison with that of medical and supply services where the changes and expansions are more frequent. However, in hospitalization services, the inpatient department repeats itself several times. This fact enables the planner to locate the inpatient departments on top of each other without special complications. The result is a building block of several storeys. Vertical traffic cores connect the floors. There is an advantage in having horizontal connections between medical services because of the attachment of various services to one another, as well as the attachment of certain medical services to the casualty department (in emergency cases). As previously mentioned, changes and additions in the medical and supply services are frequent and therefore the advantage of having them close to the ground floor is great.

It is necessary that the visitors' passage from the main entrance to the hospitalization services will not cross the traffic route system of the medical services. It is also desirable that food and medical supplies reach the various department without having to cross too many of the traffic axes of the medical services. It is therefore necessary to create a scheme, an infrastructure – flexible and universal as well as practical – which will withstand the changes occurring in the working systems of the various services.

The relationship between the vertical and horizontal traffic route systems can take several forms. As in Meir Hospital, Kfar Saba, it can take the form of one vertical transportation core, serving two wards on each floor, and a horizontal traffic route system comprised of one "main road" and branching "side roads" perpendicular to it.

The horizontal system pattern chosen for main traffic axes on the medical services floor depends upon the specific conditions of the site for which the hospital is planned, the specific programme of this institution, the dimensions and topography of the site, etc. In any case, simplicity and clarity of the scheme must be achieved.

We can compare this problem to a town planning problem on a small scale. The main traffic flows along the main traffic routes, while traffic to the various departments branches into the "cul-de-sacs." It seems that there are two systems of traffic axes – the vertical one of the inpatient services, and the horizontal one of the medical and supply services.

The balanced integrated hospital concept
1. Hospitalization services
2. Medical services
3. Administrative services and miscellaneous
4. Supply services
5. Outpatient department
A. Main entrance
B. Entrance to casualty department
C. Service entrance

The relationship of these systems to one another creates the -"skeleton" of the master plan

The horizontal system can comprise a "main road" and "side-roads" perpendicular to it, or it can be a system of two parallel main roads and perpendicular "side-roads." These are examples of "linear" options that enable us to start construction in the first phase on a small scale, and then expand and enlarge the complex according to a pre-set principle.

Still another possibility is to plan a "main road" in the shape of a closed rectangle, from which branch the "side-roads."

The building, based on the chosen "road" system, can be a continuous or a wing building. In a wing building, there is a certain planning freedom, analogous perhaps to the "freedom" which exists in a pavilion hospital.

The solution we have to strive for depends on the size of the institution. In a small building there is no possibility of creating wings – comprised, sometimes, of a small number of rooms. On the other hand, in a large building the orientation feeling is damaged if there is no division into wings.

While it cannot be stated decisively that only the general layout of the hospital is important or that the main thing is the planning and function of the various departments as independent units, it is impossible to conclude without repeating and emphasizing that in the end the hospital is planned as one unified entity and that the various departments are only different limbs of one body.

In Carmel Hospital there are two vertical transportation cores: one serves mainly visitors, and the other serves the internal traffic of the hospital, i.e. patient and staff traffic. The horizontal traffic route system has the form of a closed rectangle from which branch the side-roads. In the new hospital – Chaim Sheba Medical Centre – the horizontal traffic route system consists of two parallel main roads and branching perpendicular side-roads. Each side-road leads to a building designed to house a medical service. Each wing is independent and can be expanded.

There are actually three levels of horizontal traffic route systems: the upper one serves visitors (access to vertical transportation cores), the intermediate one interconnects all medical services, and the lower one connects the supply wings with the hospital.

The vertical transportation cores connect all levels of horizontal systems with the wards.

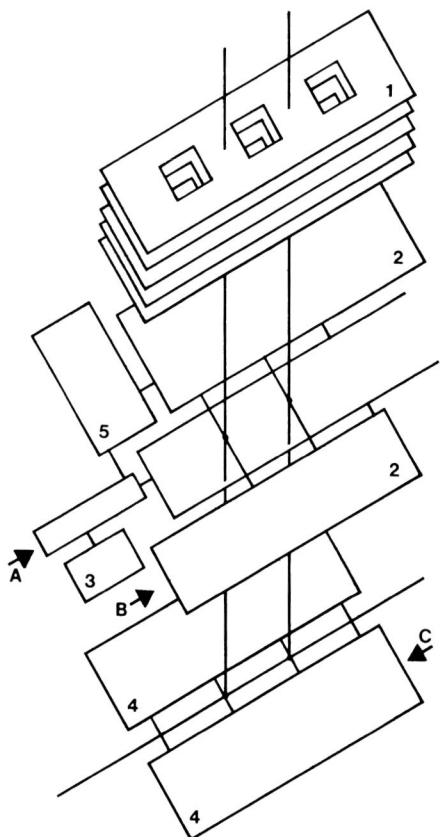

The balanced integrated hospital concept scheme (Carmel Hospital)
1. Hospitalization services
2. Medical services
3. Administrative services and miscellaneous
4. Supply services
5. Outpatient department
A. Main entrance
B. Entrance to casualty department
C. Service entrance

Main Entrance Hall and Facilities

Past attempts to fence in the hospital grounds and channel all access through a gatekeeper's lodge have not proved successful. Certain wings must be open to the public, and some of them, like the admission ward, must be open day and night. Visitors' access to inpatient wards is limited to visiting hours. Other sections are out of bounds for visitors. In planning a hospital, these facts must be taken into account and the plans must be drawn up in such a fashion, that visitors cannot pass through the "open" sections to the wards or other parts of the hospital that are accessible only at certain hours. There is therefore no point in setting up a double barrier, one at the outer gate and then again inside the hospital. Moreover, fencing-in the hospital has a repellent effect incompatible with the trend toward integrating the hospital into the surrounding community.

The general appearance, approaches and entrances of the hospital should reflect the tenet that "the hospital belongs to the Community". Most hospitals have therefore adopted the philosophy of one single main entrance for staff, ambulatory patients and visitors. This hall is freely accessible to the general public. From the hall, there should be easy access to the administrative wing, the patients' reception office, the admission ward, and free access to outpatient clinics.

In the entrance hall, a control and information desk is provided. Everyone who wishes to enter the system of main passages to the medical or maintenance services, the wards, or other parts of the hospital that are not open to the public, must pass this control paint. The entrance hall is an intersection for pedestrian traffic and serves a variety of purposes: it is an entrance, control point, waiting room, a place for obtaining information and directions, a meeting point, and so forth, The number of persons passing through it can be calculated as a function of the size of the hospital: it will always be in the order of thousands per day. For all these – patients, staff and visitors – the necessary facilities must be provided.

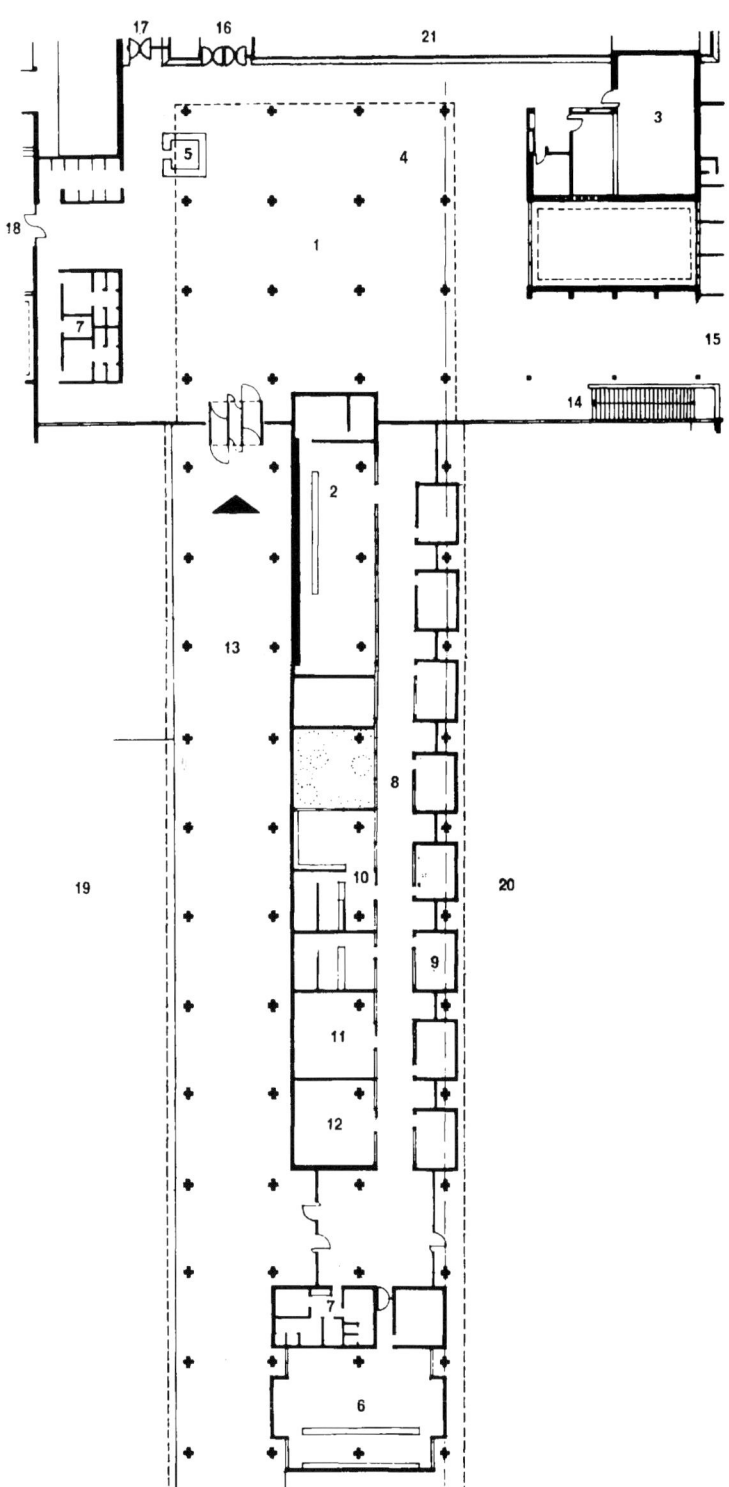

Main entrance wing to the Sheba Medical Centre.
North of this wing is the main entrance place and main parking (19) including a bus station for loading and unloading passengers. A covered entrance (13) leads to the hospital's main entrance. South of the wing is the entrance square to the casualty department. The main entrance hall (1) is designated for personnel, ambulatory patients and visitors. The public has free access to this hall which includes waiting areas. From the hall there is a direct link down to administration (14), reception and casualty departments (15). A control and information station (5) overlooks a ramp for visitors to wards and allows personnel access to the main hospital corridors (17). From the main entrance hall there is free access to the outpatient departments (18). The synagogue (3) and various services, which are arranged along a shopping arcade (8) and include a buffet (2), canteen (6), gift shops (9) (books, flowers, beauty parlour, etc.), post office (12) and library (10). The above services bear the character of a small community centre serving the hospital visitors, personnel and of course ambulatory patients.

1. Entrance hall
2. Cafeteria
3. Synagogue
4. Waiting
5. Information
6. Soldiers' cafeteria
7. Rest rooms
8. Shopping arcade
9. Shops
10. Library and reading room
11. Record-playing room
12. Post office
13. Main entrance to the hospital
14. Down to administration
15. To reception and casualty department
16. Ramp for visitors to wards
17. Main hospital corridors
18. To outpatient department
19. Main entrance and main parking
20. Entrance to casualty department
21. Patio

4. Health Facilities in Israel

Safed Hospital
Main entrance hall
1. Waiting patio
2. Main entrance hall
3. Information
4. Lifts
5. Buffet
6. Administration
7. Ambulance entrance
8. Casualty department
9. Admittance and connection
   to casualty department
10. Outpatient department

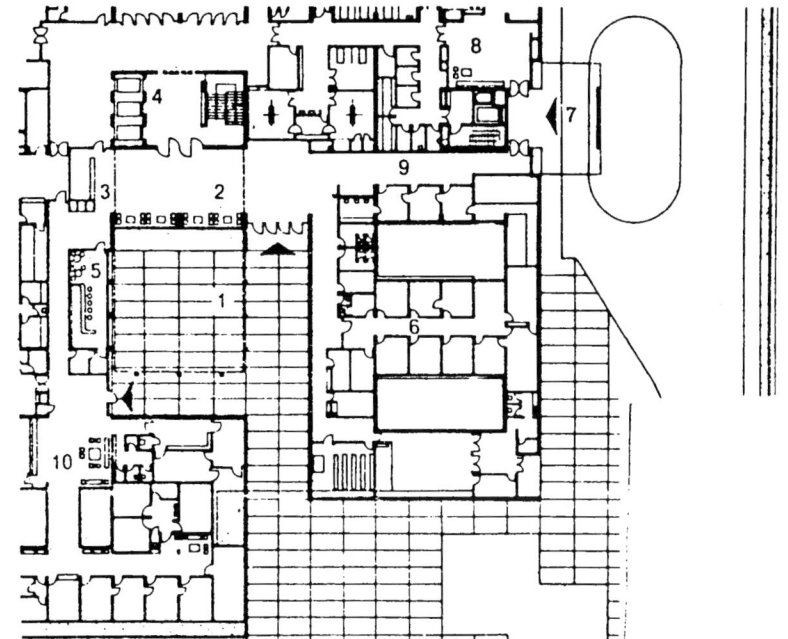

These facilities include an information desk, telephones, gift, flower and book shops, a post office, a taxi rank, an adequate number of toilets, etc. In addition ambulatory patients tend to look for a place where the atmosphere is not that of the hospital, and we must therefore try to give the entrance area a "civilian" look.

In addition to all of these functions, the entrance hall is, according to regulations, required to serve as an emergency admission station.

For a number of reasons, including emergency conditions, vehicles must be able to drive up to the main entrance. The entrance section is integrated with a system of approach roads, entrances and parking lots. From the parking lots for staff and visitors, a pedestrian passage leads to the main entrance. Particularly important is access by bus. The bulk of the visitors arrive by bus, and a suitable alighting and departure point must be planned.

Before visiting hours, there is usually quite a varied population waiting in the main entrance hall: Israeli old-timers, newcomers, multilanguage speakers, Arabs and other minority groups. Some arrive much before the appointed time and a waiting area must be provided for them – like the waiting patio in the Safed Hospital. The visitor ratio, according to experience, is about 1–2 visitors per patient.

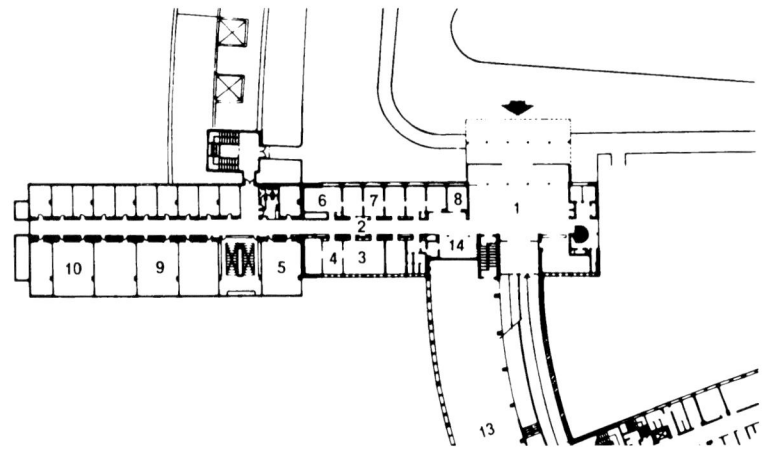

Meir Hospital
Main entrance hall
1. Main entrance hall
2. Administration
3. Director's office
4. Director's secretary
5. Conference room
6. Administrator
7. Chief assistant administrator's office
8. Chief social worker
9. Library
10. Records office
11. Main kitchen
12. Service lifts
13. Dining room
14. Waiting

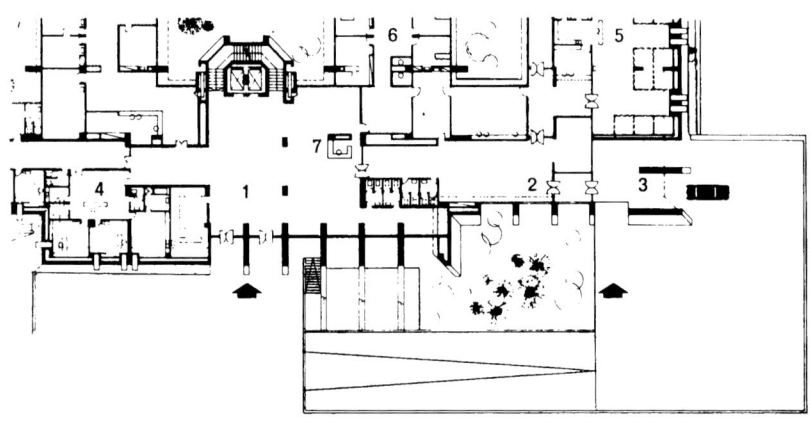

Carmel Hospital
Main entrance hall
1. Main entrance hall
2. Patients' entrance
3. Ambulance entrance
4. Children's admittance
5. Casualty department
6. Administration
7. Information

Meir Hospital – covered entrance
In the main entrance hall, before visiting hours, there is quite a varied population waiting: Israeli old-timers, new-comers, multi-language speakers, Arabs and other minority groups. Some arrive much before the appointed time and a waiting area must be provided for them – like the Waiting Patio in the Safed Hospital. Likewise, visitors have to be directed to the Inpatient departments. The visitors ratio, according to experience, is about 1–2 visitors per patient.

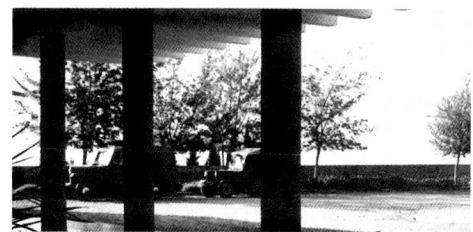

4. Health Facilities in Israel

Hospitalization Services

Standard ward

The standard ward contains, according to accepted customs and routine in Israel, between thirty and forty beds. The number of beds per standard unit has been determined empirically, based on the number of patients who can be handled from one nursing station. In most hospitals, hospitalization units are planned as standard units, each including patients' rooms, conveniences for patients, a day and dining room for ambulatory patients, doctors' and treatment rooms, a nurses' station and service rooms. Specialization of hospitalization units such as wards for internal medicine, surgical wards, urology, ENT, etc., is generally undertaken during the finishing stage of the building. The changes required for such specialization are not substantial, and the uniform structure of the hospitalization unit has great advantages.

The ward is the place where the patient spends most of his time in hospital. This is where the relation of the patient to the hospital building and the hospital environment is, in effect, established. The planner's purpose must be to make the patient feel as comfortable as possible. A feeling of comfort is of great importance for the patients' recovery. Making the hospital room face in the right direction (which differs from place to place), landscaping the immediate surroundings which can be seen from the patients' rooms, planning the patients' room, its dimensions and its openings correctly – these are only a few of the factors that will determine not only the patients' impression of the ward, but the shape of the ward as well.

The patients' room

The arrangement of the patients' room has gone through many stages. Generally, the standard three-bedded room is now thought to be the best compromise under local conditions. In recently-built Israeli hospitals, most wards have therefore been planned so that rooms have a depth which allows space for three beds, with a few one-bedded rooms for serious or special cases. Obviously, the depth of the rooms determines the length of the ward's passage, and there is a connection between this question and that of the cumulative distance walked by the nurse. But the search for balance between different factors such as

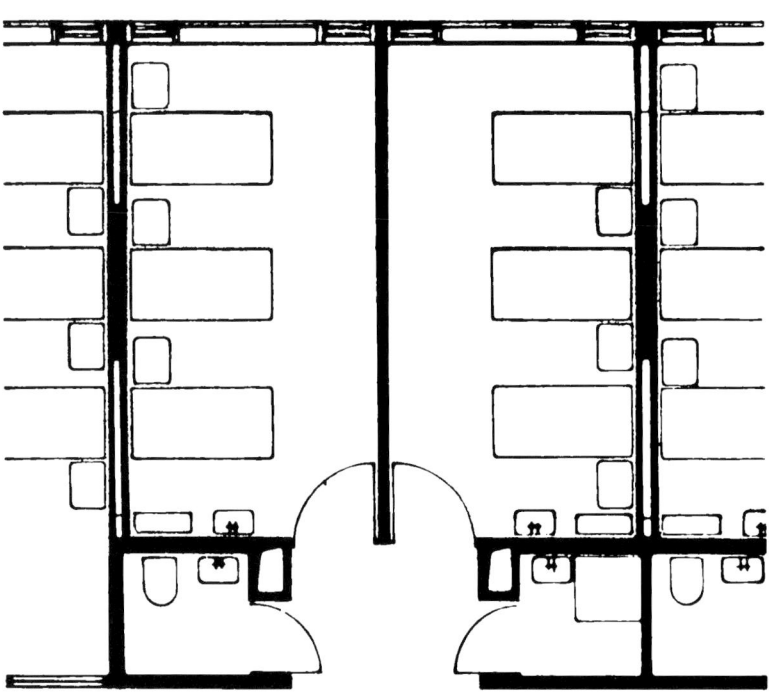

Sheba Medical Centre
Typical 3-bedded room

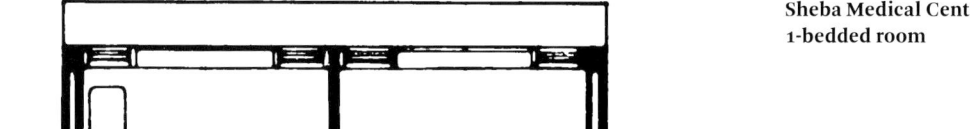

Sheba Medical Centre
1-bedded room

4. Health Facilities in Israel

climate, light, the impression made by the room, patients' psychological problems connected with the number of patients in the room, the choice of the room's measurements so as to give the staff easy access to the patient for examination and treatment, and so forth, have led most planners to the conclusion that a depth of three beds strikes the optimum balance between the different factors. Since the measurements of the hospital bed and the necessary distances between the beds are fixed, and the possibilities of arranging the beds within the room are closely limited, the dimensions of the room are obtained by an analysis of measurements and operations. The accepted axial measurements are 3.60 × 7.20 m. It is not easy to add a fourth bed in a room with such measurements, since they are the minimum necessary.

Location of nurses' station in the ward

In the course of time it was realized that the nurses' station should be an open room as opposed to the closed one that was used years ago. The possibility of effective supervision is in practice determined by the location of the nurses' station in relation to the patients' rooms. The nurse is, of course, in continuous motion while answering patients' calls or carrying out her other duties on the ward. A simple calculation shows that the total length of the distance walked by the nurse depends on the location of the station in relation to the patients. Locating the station at the end of the ward will make the total distance walked almost twice as long as if the station was located in the middle of the ward. To shorten this walking distance, every possible measure must be taken: location of the station, arrangement the rooms according to their number of beds and their function in ward (serious cases, special cases, etc.), so that the rooms there is most work are closest to the nurses' station. In several hospitals, oral communication between the ward nurse and patients is planned, so as to avoid unnecessary trips.

Control of entrance to the ward by the nurse

The nurse must be able to check who enters or leaves the ward. The station must therefore be located near the entrance to the ward, or at least the entrance to the ward must be visible from the station.

Easy access from station to service rooms

The nurse must frequently enter the ward service rooms, such as the linen room, instruments and bedpan room, the nurses' workroom (which is usually connected with the station), storerooms, etc. These rooms should therefore, by preference, be located near the station and be easily accessible from it. This is particularly important in the case of the nurses' workroom.

Continuity of patients' rooms and auxiliary rooms in the ward
In planning the arrangement of rooms within the ward, the manner of combining the wards on a typical floor must be taken into account. Continuity of rooms with the identical function permits greater elasticity in dividing wards into sections and sub-sections. There is therefore an advantage in a plan which allows for continuity between patients' rooms, service rooms and doctors' rooms of one ward, with the corresponding rooms of the adjacent ward.

Separation of traffic routes
In the ward passage, patients, staff, visitors, supply personnel and maintenance personnel intermingle; separating these categories of traffic in the ward passage is impossible. The question is where and for which categories of traffic, separate routes should be planned. Opinions on this subject are divided. It is generally agreed that food transport, removal of beds or corpses and service traffic should be separated from patients' and medical staff traffic and that separate lifts should be provided for these categories. But according to some opinions, maximum efficiency can be obtained by having one single group of lifts to serve patients, medical staff and visitor traffic, while others believe that visitor traffic at peak hours may interfere with other essential traffic. From the technical viewpoint, there is an advantage in concentrating the lifts within one single core.

Area of ward
If we divide the total area of the hospital by the number of beds, we obtain the area per bed in sqm. This key figure will be found to increase from year to year. In hospitals planned lately in Israel it amounts to more than 100 sqm. per bed. The additional area is mainly accounted for by medical and ancillary services. In the existing hospitals, medical and other services are added from time to time which increase the number of sqm. per bed. The ward area has also increased in comparison with wards planned several years ago; the additional area is accounted for, mainly by additional service rooms. Since it is very difficult to add rooms to a ward once the planning is completed, the programme for the unit must therefore be considered with great care.

4. Health Facilities in Israel

Sheba Medical Centre
Vertical transportation core
In the Sheba Medical Centre there is a concentration of five elevators in the vertical traffic core. Three elevators (1) are intended for passengers, patients, staff and visitors, and two elevators (2) are service elevators used for transfer of food containers, medical and service supplies, beds and corpses. In emergency cases these elevators can be used for transfer of patients in beds. The passenger elevators face the floor elevators lobby (6). From the lobby there is a direct entrance to family rooms (4), to two inpatient wards (3). The entrances to the wards are near the nurse's station. The service elevators open to the service corridor of the wards (5), along which are located the service and treatment rooms of these wards. A different concept can be seen at the Carmel Hospital where there is a separation between visitors traffic and internal hospital traffic, including staff and patients from inpatient wards to the medical services.

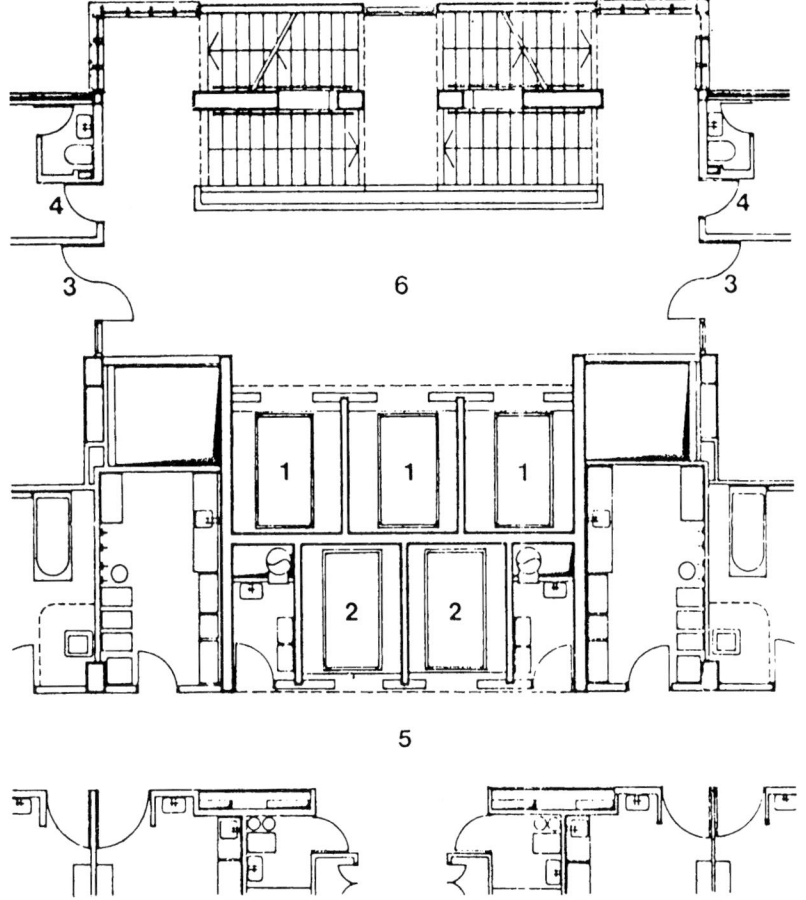

The target is the minimum general area for a given programme of patients' rooms and service rooms within the ward. The smaller the area, without affecting the function of the ward, the lower the construction and maintenance costs of the hospital. The following table shows a comparison of areas within wards.

Combining wards on a typical floor

In the foregoing paragraphs, the elements affecting the planning of the standard ward have been described. The use of the wards by the different departments need not be taken into account in planning. The location of the departments may well change from time to time over the years, and there is therefore no point in regarding the division into departments as a factor for consideration while planning the wards or the overall ward structure. The exceptions to this rule are, perhaps, the obstetrics department and the children's department. In the case of the children's department, there is an advantage in a ground floor location. The structure of its plan differs in certain respects from that of the typical hospital ward. The particular requirements of the obstetrics department, such as accommodation for the infants, connection with the delivery rooms, etc., generally dictate its location and plan. But if we consider the standardization of planning of wards in general and the fact that the changes occurring in the wards over the years are small in comparison with the changes required in the medical services, the structure which houses the wards may be regarded as the "static" part of the entire hospital structure. The standardization of the wards makes it possible to locate them one above the other. If we therefore locate two wards on a floor served by one vertical traffic core, we obtain a five- or six-storey building for a hospital of 400–500 beds. This is quite a considerable block. It is usually planned as a construction block rising above the medical and ancillary services, and it presents the decisive element for the appearance of the building. The manner in which the wards are combined within the typical floor determines not only the shape of the hospital, but also the traffic routes leading to the wards and their connection with the medical and ancillary services.

A comparison chart is given here for the areas of inpatient departments in 5 hospitals. Definition of zones is according to the schematic plans found on pages 43–45. This chart shows that the downstairs area in the inpatient floors is approx. 30 m² in hospitals that include the accepted services in inpatient departments in Israel today. The downstairs area of the hospital depends on the extent of the medical services, administrative services, etc., but as general data, the downstairs area in a 400–500 bed hospital will be about 100 sqm. per bed. I.e. about one third of the area is in the inpatient services and about two thirds in the medical, administrative and other services.

Hospital	No. of beds per ward	Patients' rooms (m²)	Service and treatment rooms (m²)	Dr. and Staff rooms (m²)	Passages, walls, free areas etc. (m²)	Total ward area (m²)	Area per bed (m²)
Meir	39	300	150	75	420	945	24.2
Safed	36	284	200	76	500	1060	29.4
Carmel	36	350	130	112	470	1062	29.5
Dimona	36	290	210	80	410	990	27.5
Sheba	36	300	200	150	550	1200	33.3

4. Health Facilities in Israel

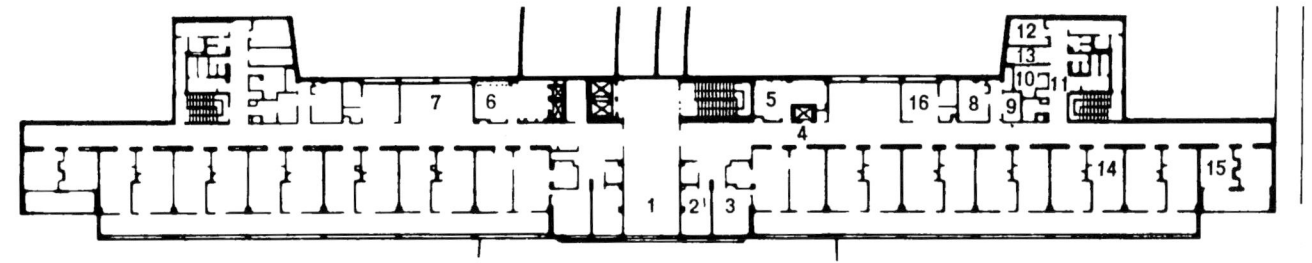

Meir Hospital
Typical ward floor plan

1. Waiting room for families
2. Departmental head's room
3. Doctors room
4. Service lifts
5-6. Kitchenette
7. Day room and dining room
8. Dirty utility/sluice room
9. Store room
10. Clean utility room
11. Service corridor
12. Assisted bathroom
13. General storeroom
14. 3-bedded room
15. 1-bedded room
16. Nurses' station

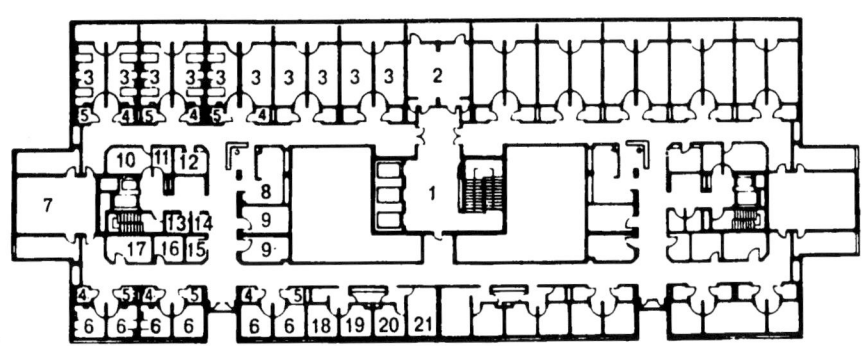

Safed Hospital
Typical ward floor plan

1. Lifts
2. Waiting room for families
3. 3-bedded room
4. Shower
5. Toilet
6. 1-bedded room
7. Day room
8. Nurses' workroom
9. Treatment room
10. Kitchenette
11. Patients' clothing storeroom
12. Sluice room
13. Soiled linen laundry
14. Cleaners' cupboard
15. Linen store
16. General storeroom
17. Bathroom
18. Senior nurse's room
19. Departmental head's room
20. Doctors' room
21. Doctors' room

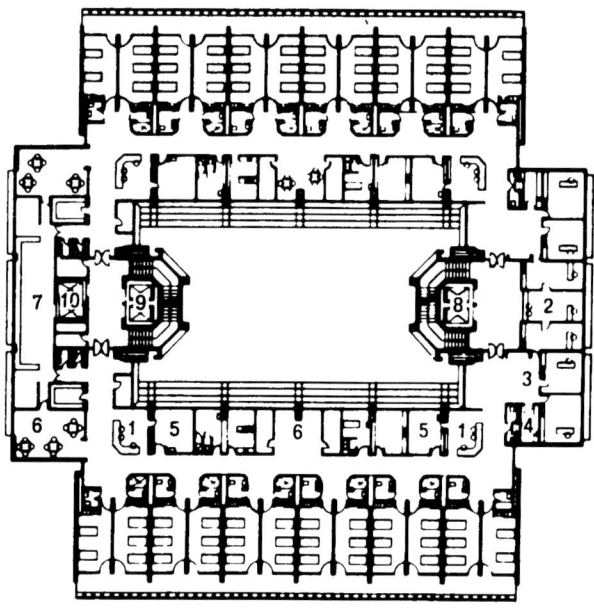

Carmel Hospital
Typical ward floor plan
1. Nurses' station
2. Medical secretary's room
3. Doctors' room
4. Laboratory
5. Examination and treatment rooms
6. Day room
7. Kitchen
8. Visitors' lifts
9. Patients' lifts
10. Food and service lifts

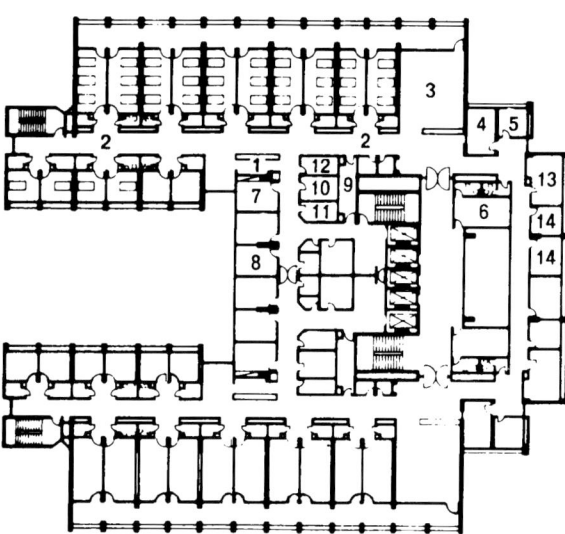

Dimona Hospital
Typical ward floor plan
1. Nurses' station
2. Wards
3. Day room
4. Senior nurses' room
5. Laboratory
6. Waiting room for families
7. Nurses' workroom
8. Treatment room
9. Kitchen
10. Bathroom
11. Utility room
12. Linen storeroom
13. Doctors' room
14. Examination and treatment rooms

4. Health Facilities in Israel

Sheba Medical Centre
Typical ward floor plan

1. Main staircase and lifts
2. Entrance
3. Waiting room
   for families
4. Day room and
   dining room
5. 3 one-bedded rooms
6. Nurses' utility and
   treatment rooms
7. Doctors' rooms
   and offices
8. Store rooms
9. Seminar room

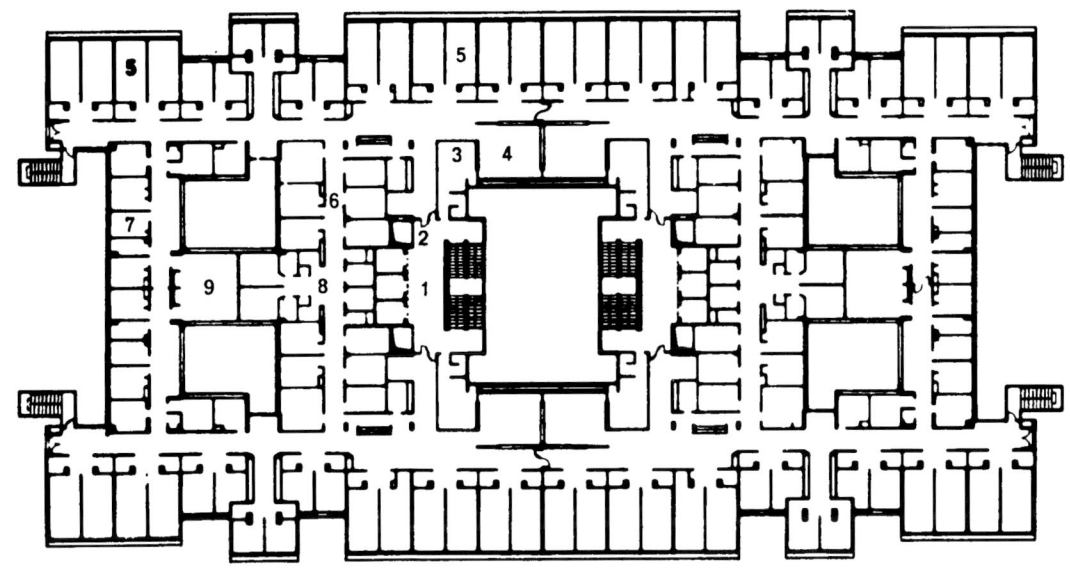

Kaplan Hospital
Typical ward floor plan

1. Ward
2. Kitchen
3. Day room
4. Nurses' station
5. Doctors' rooms
6. Students' rooms
7. Reception
8. Treatment room
9. Nurses' tea kitchen
10. Sluice room
11. Bathroom

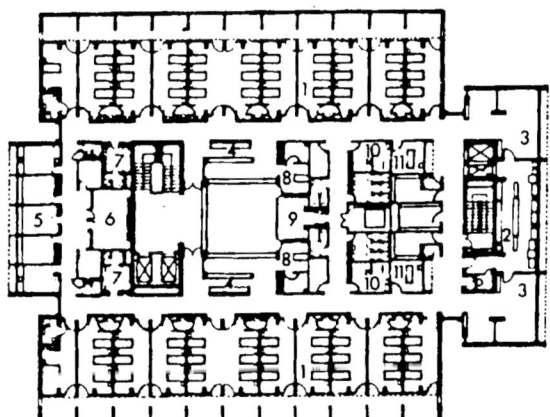

It follows that the considerations which guide the planning of the ward are fairly complex. In addition, every location presents its special data which affect the planning. General concepts of hospital planning also influence the design of the ward. In planning the ward, all these elements must be properly balanced and combined. Generally, no one plan will be able to achieve all the objectives, and it will be necessary to try for the optimum in respect to the special conditions presented by a given site.

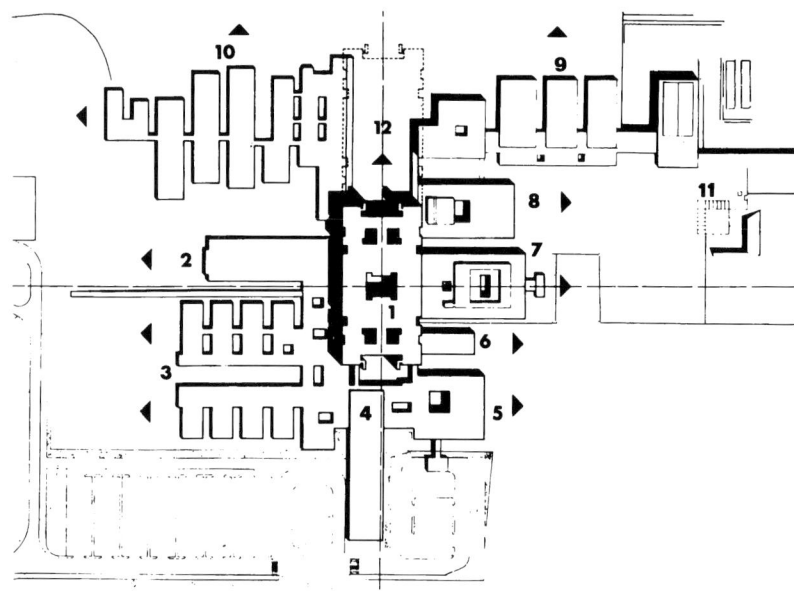

Adding wards

Adding wards once the hospital has been built is a problem for which there is no easy solution. From the viewpoint of the overall hospital plan, adding floors would seem to be a simple answer. The connection with the medical and ancillary services continues to be providing by the same vertical traffic core, so that the traffic problem of the new wards is solved automatically. But practice has shown that building additional floors means much troublesome interference with the normal life of the hospital while the building goes on.

Moreover, building additional floors involves many technical problems, such as the need for a building calculated to bear additional floors, the necessity of extending the lift shaft, etc. Another possibility is the construction of an additional wing. From the operative viewpoint, this is easy, but the possibility must have been taken into account in the original plan.

On the opposite page there are schemes for comparison of typical inpatient floors in six hospitals. The schemes include the following concepts: the "long floor", the "double passage", the "inner courtyard", the "compact" and the "four-ward" concepts. The following zones were marked off for distinction in the scheme: inpatient rooms, service rooms, work and treatment rooms, doctors' rooms and location of nurses' station. The area of zones in the total inpatient department area is given in the comparison chart in the section – Area of ward.

Sheba Medical Centre
Expansion plan
1. Main building – wards
2. Extension area for X-ray department
3. Extension area for outpatient department
4. Entrance wing
5. Extension area for casualty department
6. Extension area for nephrology department
7. Extension area for operating theatres block
8. Extension area for library
9. Extension area for central storerooms and Maintenance service block
10. Extension area for research and clinical laboratories
11. Mortuary
12. Extension area for ward block

4. Health Facilities in Israel

One of the principles used in planning the Sheba Medical Centre was that of "the Growing Campus". This means preliminary planning based on axis of movement and building elements which enable addition to the various wings, to sub-wings, or additional new wings – all this without disrupting the internal or external movement and without harming the shape of the building at any stage. The "changing" status of the campus guided and dictated the shape of the building from the beginning, and the architecture is based on this principle.

The principle is achieved through the layout of the campus. The general layout of the hospital is composed of a main east-west axis (the spine) which is the axis of the ward block, with a secondary axis (the ribs), which is the axis of the medical and supply service wings.

According to the principle, an area is localized (12) for an additional wing of inpatient departments. This wing doubles the number of inpatient departments and can be built in stages. At each stage it forms an organic addition to the campus and is integrated in the axis of movement.

The long floor

For many years, it was customary to plan the wards in a long block, with the traffic core in the middle and wards on both sides. With this structure we obtain a ward constructed along a corridor, usually with the patients' rooms on one side and the other groups of rooms on the opposite side. The result is that the entrance to the ward lies at the end of its main passage; no satisfactory solution can be found for rooms which two wards have in common; there is no way of establishing continuity between two groups of rooms with the same function belonging to two wards (auxiliary rooms, doctors' rooms, etc.); and, for reasons already stated, it is therefore more difficult to divide a ward into sub-units, as is necessary in the case of smaller wards such as ENT.

When the view prevailed in Israel – in the wake of similar tendencies abroad – that medical services should be located on the same level as the ward related to them (e.g. operating theatre on the same level as the surgical ward), this construction of the typical floor in the form of two units with a traffic core between them had its technical advantages: under these conditions it was easy to link another wing with the traffic core in order to accommodate the appropriate medical services. This was, in fact, the standard pattern of the T- or H-shaped building, which was customary for many years. But now the time of this pattern is past; the advantage no longer seems meaningful.

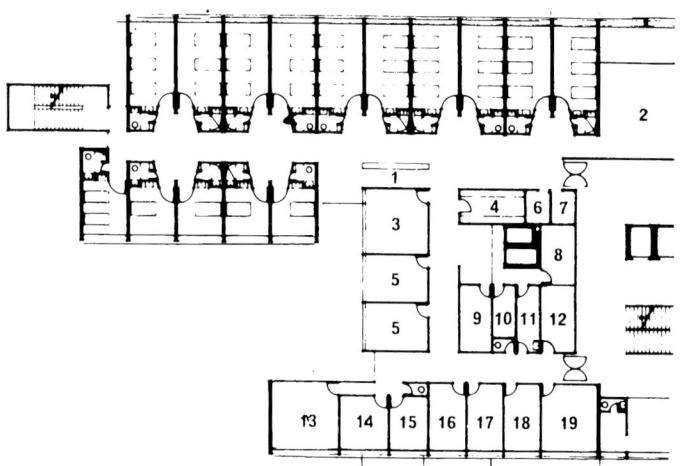

Tel-Giborim Hospital – Project A
Typical ward floor plan

1. Nurses' station
2. Day room and dining hall
3. Nurses' clean utility room
4. Kitchenette
5. Treatment room
6. Soiled linen laundry
7. Cubicle for stretchers and wheel chairs
8. Storeroom for various equipment
9. Dirty utility / sluice room
10. Linen storeroom
11. Storeroom
12. Bathroom
13. Doctors' room
14. Departmental head's room
15. Doctors' room
16. Laboratory
17. Nurses' room
18. Staff rest room
19. Seminar room

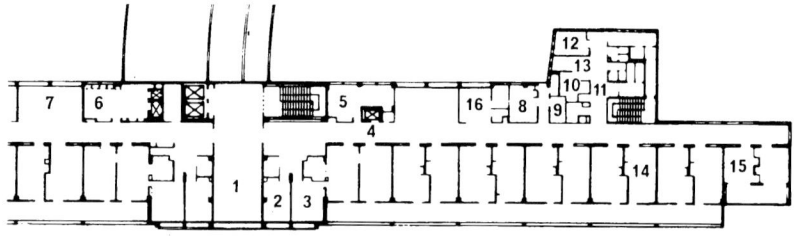

Meir Hospital
Typical ward floor plan

1. Waiting room for families
2. Departmental head's room
3. Doctors' room
4. Service lifts
5. Kitchenette
6. Kitchenette
7. Day room and dining room
8. Dirty utility / sluice room
9. Storeroom
10. Clean utility room
11. Service corridor
12. Assisted bathroom
13. General storeroom
14. 4-bedded room
15. 1-bedded room
16. Nurses' station

4. Health Facilities in Israel

Safed Hospital
Typical ward floor plan

1. Lifts
2. Waiting room for families
3. 3-bedded room
4. Shower
5. Toilet
6. 1-bedded room
7. Day room
8. Nurses' workroom
9. Treatment room
10. Kitchenette
11. Patients' clothing storeroom
12. Sluice room
13. Soiled linen laundry
14. Cleaners' cupboard
15. Linen storeroom
16. General storeroom
17. Bathroom
18. Senior nurses' room
19. Departmental head's room
20. Doctors' room
21. Doctors' room

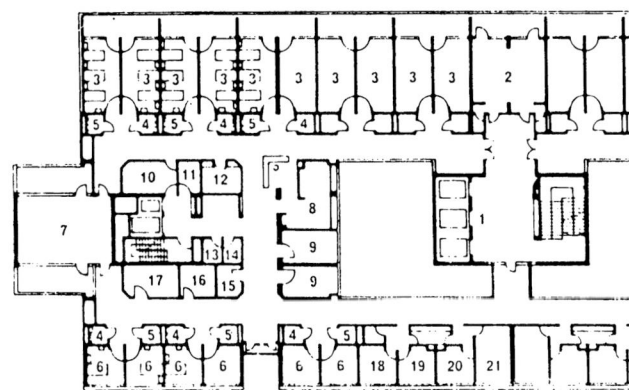

It should be noted that this arrangement of the floor has the advantage of allowing cross ventilation, which is important in the case of a hospital, not only for the comfort of the patients and the staff, but also from the medical viewpoint of preventing infection.

The Meir Hospital provides an example of this concept; cross ventilation has been taken into account by leaving spaces in the arrangement of the service rooms opposite the patients' rooms.

The double passage

Another possibility of combining wards on the typical floor may be seen in the floor plan of the Safed Hospital. The standard ward is planned on the principle of two parallel passages, with the auxiliary rooms laying between two rows of rooms with an occasional area of open floor space, In this case, the traffic core for patients, staff and visitors lies in the middle of the floor, with auxiliary traffic centres for services in the middle of the ward. For the price of a second traffic core, quiet and adequate organization of traffic inside the ward is assured, Other advantages are the continuity of the patients' rooms and of the doctors' rooms. The length of the ward is far less than in the long floor concept, and the general shape of the buildings is far more compact, without sacrificing the possibility of through-ventilation.

These facts were decisive in planning the wards of the Safed Hospital, in adjusting the building to the particular topographical conditions, and in integrating the building within the landscape.

In Plan A for Tel Giborim, one may see the double passage concept of ward planning, with patients' rooms kept together in one passage.

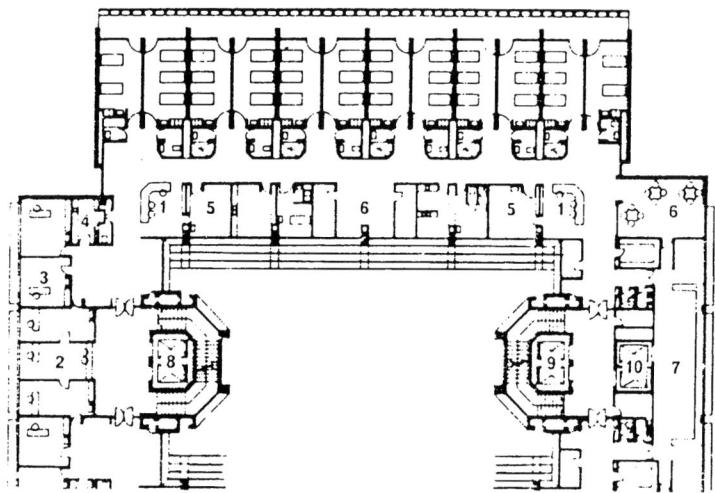

The inner courtyard

Another possibility is to arrange the wards around an inner courtyard, with two traffic cores between the wards, as can be seen in the Carmel Hospital in Haifa and in Plan B of Tel Giborim. In this concept, one traffic core must be reserved for visitors and outpatients, and the other for internal hospital traffic, connections between patients and staff and the medical services, and between the wards and the supply services. The shape of the typical floor plan will be approximately square, with patients' rooms having first claim to the north-south direction. The auxiliary rooms mostly face east, west or onto the inner courtyard. The advantages here are the continuity of doctors' rooms and the concentration of the day and dining rooms near one single kitchen for the entire floor. On the other hand, there is no continuity of the wards, patients' rooms and service rooms.

When we consider the requirements for better supervision of the patients' rooms and shorter walking distances, the best place for the nurses' station is in the centre of the ward. But as we have seen, there are other considerations as well: the nurses' control of the entrance to the ward, proximity of the ward's auxiliary and service rooms, etc. The inner courtyard concept provides no easy answer to the question of a location for the nurses' station which satisfies a maximum of these requirements. It may have its advantages if the ward is to be subdivided.

4. Health Facilities in Israel

Kaplan Hospital
Typical ward floor plan

1. Ward
2. Kitchen
3. Day room
4. Nurses' station
5. Doctors' rooms
6. Students' room
7. Reception room
8. Treatment rooms
9. Nurses' tea kitchen
10. Sluice room
11. Bathroom

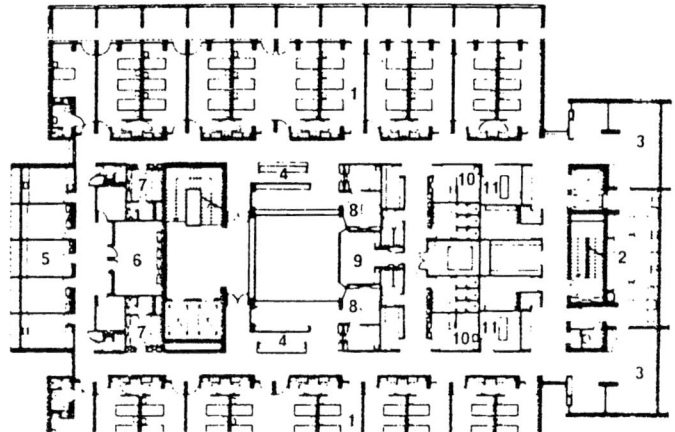

Dimona Hospital
Typical ward floor plan

1. Nurses' station
2. Wards
3. Day room
4. Senior nurse's room
5. Laboratory
6. Waiting room for families
7. Nurses' workroom
8. Treatment room
9. Kitchen
10. Bathroom
11. Utility room
12. Linen storeroom
13. Doctors' room

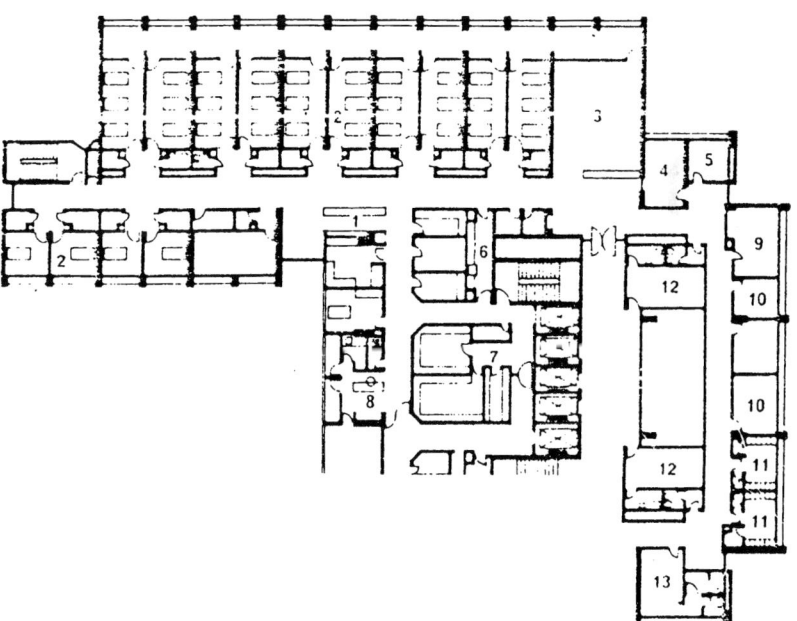

The compact floor

The compact type of floor is possible only on the basis of full air conditioning. The nurses' station is in the centre of the unit and near its entrance. One floor kitchen serves both wards. Doctors' and service rooms are continuous.

Continuous service rooms

An example of a concept in which continuity of doctors' rooms, auxiliary rooms and service rooms of the ward is obtained, and where there is, moreover, a vertical traffic core concentrated in one place with separation of visitor, staff and patient traffic, with supply services traffic according to wards, may be seen at the Dimona Hospital. The location of the nurses' station allows effective control of the patients' rooms and ward entrance and shortened the nurses walking distance.

Four ward floor

An example of a typical floor plan with four wards per floor can be seen in the plan of the Sheba Hospital. The plan provides two vertical traffic cores, each serving two wards, and achieves continuity of patients', doctors' and service rooms. The nurses' station is located in the centre of the ward and near the entrance. All rooms have natural light. The possibility of adding wards in an additional wing has been taken into account.

Sheba Medical Centre
Typical care-unit plan
1. Waiting room for families
2. 3-bedded room
3. 1-bedded room
4. Assisted bathroom
5. Dirty utility / sluice room
6. Nurses' station
7. Clean utility room
8. Treatment room
9. Kitchenette
10. Day room and dining hall
11. Nurses' room
12. Superintendent's room
13. Departmental head's room
14. Secretaries' room
15. Doctors' room
16. Doctors' room
17. Laboratory
18. Seminar room
19. Patients' clothing store
20. Storeroom for various equipment
21. Soiled linen laundry
22. Stretcher cubicles
23. Patients' clothes
24. Cleaners' cupboard
25. Staff rest room
26. Refuse room
27. Emergency staircase

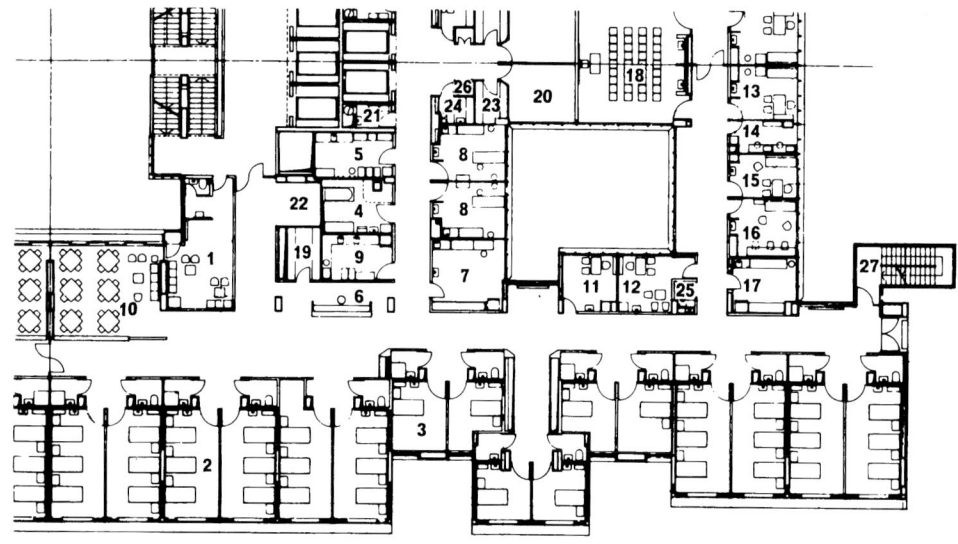

4. Health Facilities in Israel

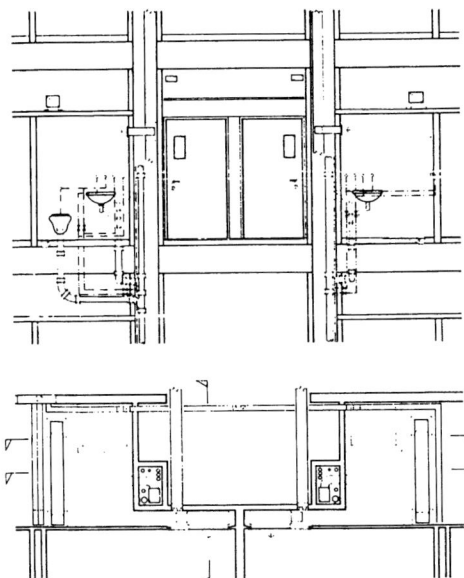

Sheba Medical Centre
Mechanical system of the conveniences

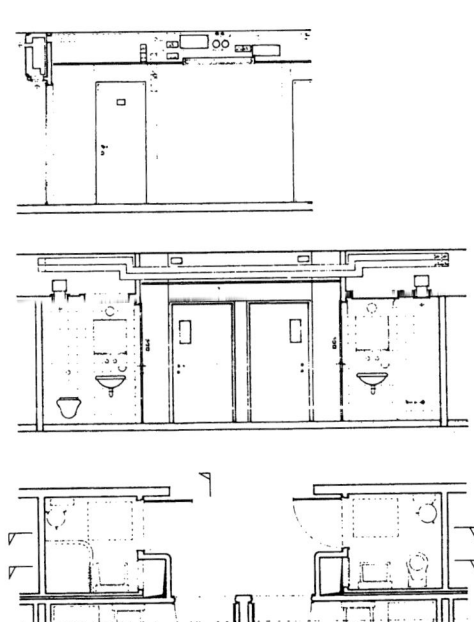

Sheba Medical Centre
A double set of conveniences serving six patients

Electromechanical systems

In most hospitals, rooms are planned in pairs, and each pair of rooms is provided with a double set of conveniences serving six patients. The conveniences are usually located between the patients' rooms and the ward's passage. This means that the nurse cannot keep her eye on the patients' beds. The alternative of conveniences adjoining the outer wall is not acceptable, because it means that the cleaners must pass through the patients' room to reach them. The arrangement of the rooms in the ward is connected with the planning of the electromechanical systems. It should be designed in such a manner that in- and outgoing systems are easy to service and maintain.

Maintenance is of course essential, but is also a nuisance factor which interferes seriously with the orderly course of life in the ward. In wards with service rooms adjacent to patients' rooms and with air conditioning, the problem of maintenance of electromechanical systems is a weighty factor in planning.

Apart from the regular system, the possibility of future additions of new supplies to the patients' rooms must be taken into account. This possibility depends on leaving suitable ducts open for supply lines, and also on the method of supplying the patients' rooms. Supply "strips" make it possible to add lines without requiring building operations, but are more expensive to install initially.

In the ward building, a technical floor should be planned between the ward floors and the floor below. Outflow lines from the wards, air-conditioning equipment and other equipment for the ward floors and the lower floors can be installed on this floor. A technical floor also allows easy access to inflow and outflow systems and facilitates their maintenance.

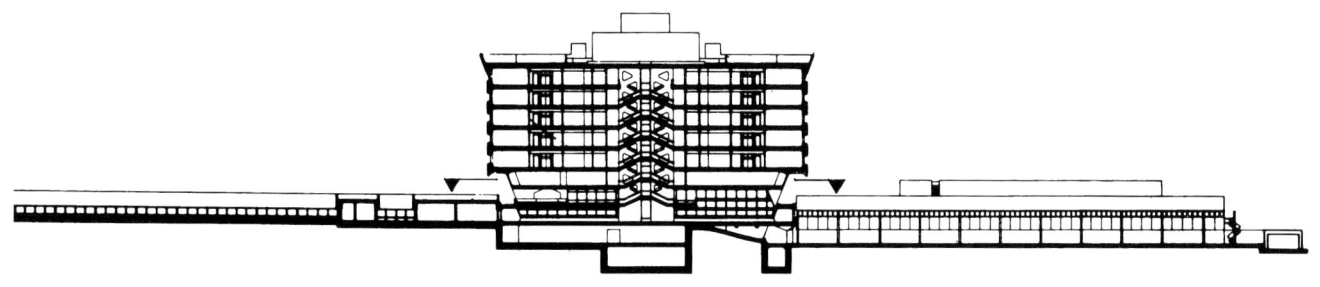

**Sheba Medical Centre
Cross section**

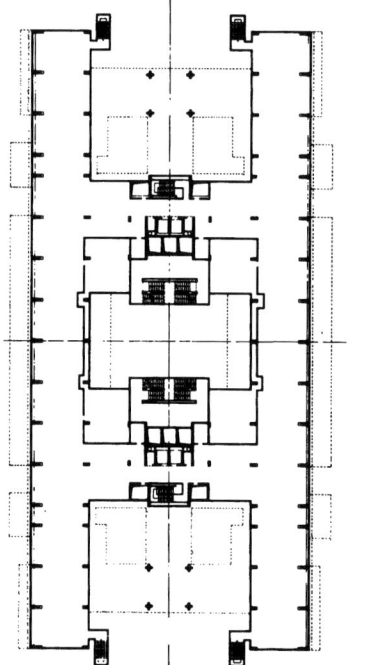

Technical floor

In the Sheba Medical Centre a technical floor
was planned below the wards block. On this floor
there is a concentration of the disposal piping
system, the air-conditioning units, and electromechanical equipment arranged in a manner
that allows for proper upkeep and maintenance.

4. Health Facilities in Israel

Reception and Admission Department

Functions of Admission Department

Under the influence of local conditions, an Israeli concept of the admission and reception department has gradually developed. Its structure and function are different from those of such a department abroad. The department is, by virtue of its function, open day and night. Its approach is roofed and suitable for ambulance traffic and the unloading of patients on stretchers. All emergency cases arrive at this department, and all patients are admitted through it.

From the entrance hall, which also serves as a waiting room for patients and those accompanying them, there is direct access to the admission department. The admission hall is designed as a large hall divided into compartments by means of curtains. Each compartment or cubicle contains an examination couch. In the compartments, the patients are examined by the interns on duty, who assign them to the appropriate ward.

The admission department contains limited medical services, suitable for treating urgent cases or cases not requiring hospitalization: general treatment rooms, rooms for surgery, plaster rooms, a room for the treatment of severe trauma, etc. and sometimes several rooms for short-term hospitalization (for observation purposes). The required auxiliary services are planned for these rooms. In addition, the admission department contains the administrative services dealing with the admission of patients.

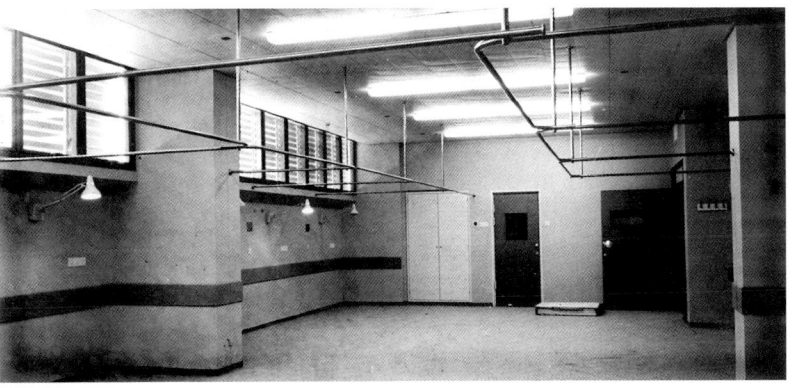

Safed Hospital
Casualty department

The casualty department in the Sheba Medical Centre includes medical, surgical and administrative services. The entrance to the casualty department is covered. Adjoining the entrance (1) there is a storage recess for wheelchairs and stretchers. From the waiting room (2) the patient is brought to the stretchers' ward (6) which is divided into examination cubicles. Children have a separate stretchers' ward (5). The Doctors' rooms (7) are close to the stretchers' ward. If necessary, the treatment rooms (11) can serve the casualty department for minor surgery. There is a special department for patients remaining for observation (12) which adjoins the casualty department. The waiting hall (2) has a direct link to the waiting area in the admission department (15). Called admission (16) is possible not through the casualty department. The location of the casualty department in the total hospital complex enables direct connection at the same level with the operating rooms wing, radiology and the rest of the services. A corridor (17) connects the department with the inpatient wards.

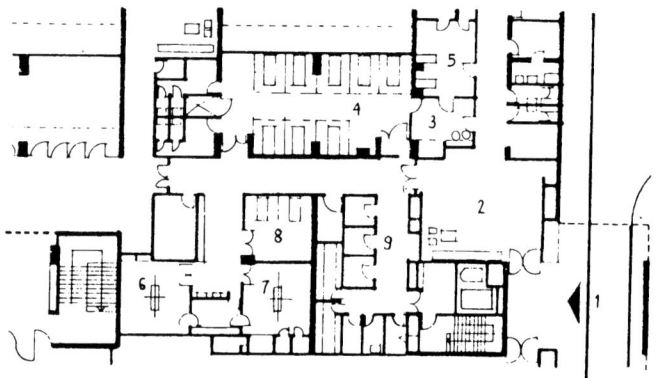

Safed Hospital
Casualty department

1. Covered entrance to casualty department
2. Casualty department's entrance hall
3. Nurses' utility room
4. Stretcher ward
5. Children's casualty ward
6. Plaster room
7. General treatment room
8. Preparation and post-operative room
9. Ancillary rooms

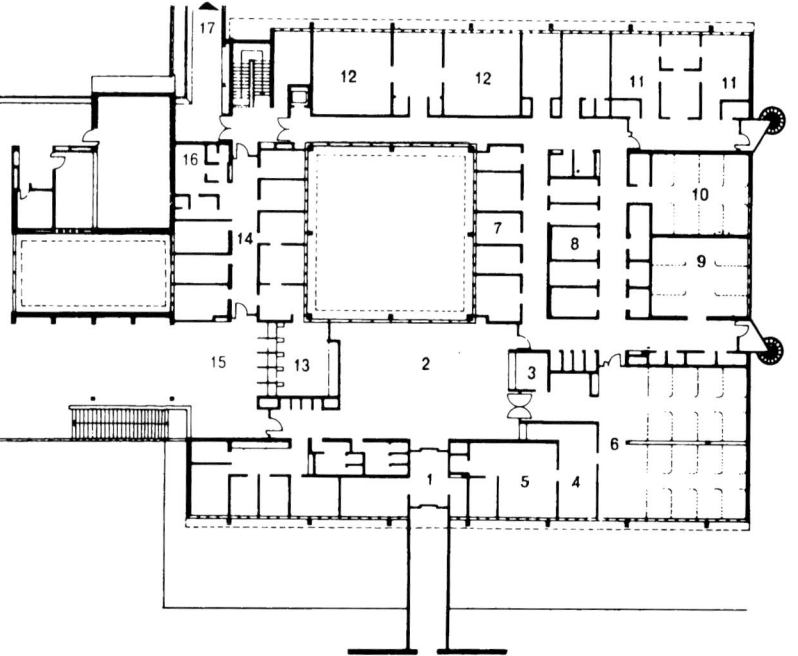

Sheba Medical Centre
Casualty department

1. Entrance
2. Waiting
3. Office
4. Nurses' room
5. Casualty ward for children and nurses' utility room
6. Stretcher ward
7. Medical examination and doctors' rooms
8. Sluice room, kitchenette and storerooms
9. Severe trauma treatment room
10. Preparation and post-operative recovery room
11. General treatment rooms
12. Observation rooms
13. Patient admitting office
14. Clerical staff room
15. Admissions unit for patients
16. Admissions for elective patients
17. Corridor to inpatient wards

Operating Theatres Wing

Of all the medical services wings, the operating theatres wing is one of the most complex. Its planning entails team work; misunderstanding among the planners can lead to poor results, even when all parties are well-intentioned.

The following description relates to the planning of operating theatres in Israeli hospitals, as it has emerged over the course of years, in accordance with accepted local routines for the running of such wings. The principle data supplied by the programmer is the number and type of operating theatres, other information includes data on auxiliary rooms related to the operating theatres and other rooms peculiar to the wing being planned.

The ratio accepted in Israeli hospitals is one operating theatre to 30 surgical beds.

The layout of the rooms is dictated by the overriding consideration for the prevention of infection. Incorrect planning of traffic routes within the wing may be a cause of infection, as may wrongly-placed accesses to the rooms, defects in electromechanical systems, etc.; and all this is without going into other sources of infection such as the patient himself, the staff or the methods of treatment. The prevention of infection affects the arrangement of rooms, their functions, specifications, electromechanical systems: in short – almost the entire planning of the wing. The layout of the rooms – in other words the arrangement and

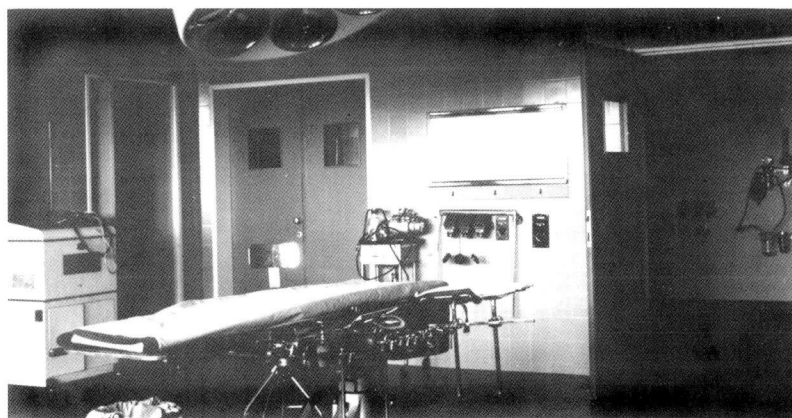

Meir Hospital
Operating theatres

location of the rooms for correct accessibility – depends on the modus operandi and on an analysis of the activities pursued in the wing in question. The problem can be outlined as follows: (1) the main activity is in the operation zone (a); this zone is usually located in the centre of the operating theatre. Adjacent to this zone are rooms whose activity is related to what is happening in the operating theatre, such as preparation of patients, surgeons' scrubbing rooms, changing rooms, etc.; the zone in which these activities take place will be classified as (b). In addition to what has already been mentioned. there exists a further series of activities linked with the operating theatre. These activities take place in zones adjacent to zones (a) and (b). We shall classify them as (c). These zones together constitute the "clean zone." Between the "clean zone" which forms a subsidiary wing and the other zones of the wing, a physical barrier is planned. In the outer ring are, located the other rooms of the wing, forming the "non-clean" zone, (d). There exist yet other activities, which are not to be classed with this wing and they belong to the category of the hospital corridor; we shall classify them as zone (e). Activity in operating theatres sufficiently secured from the risk of infection cannot be, imagined without this zoning. On the other hand, to minute a zoning is a hindrance and an encumbrance to work processes. If the restrictions imposed on the staff are such that they cannot be observed in reality, the outcome will be the opposite of what was intended.

In the given scheme, which includes division into zones, traffic routes and meeting points in the operating theatres, the wing is divided into three zones: clean, non-clean and hospital zone.

The clean zone is divided into the operation zone, operating theatres zone and other zones. The routes (paths) were classified according to route, patient, personnel, sterile material, anaesthetic equipment, general equipment, X-ray equipment, clean linen, cleaning equipment and waste disposal.

The meeting points that require special planning, in the transfer of various traffic routes from a zone of one category to a cleaner zone, are indicated.

Traffic routes

Traffic routes are divided as follows: patient route, staff route, equipment and materials route, electromechanical systems, operation and maintenance staff routes. The layout of the rooms depends on the organization of the traffic circuits.

4. Health Facilities in Israel

Operating theatres
Zoning diagram
1. Patients
2. Staff
3. Sterile material
4. Anaesthetic equipment
5. Equipment
6. Mobile X-ray equipment
7. Clean linen
8. Cleaning equipment
9. Duty disposal

Clean area
a. Operation area
b. Operating theatres zone
c. Other areas in clean zone

Unclean area
d. Non-clean area
e. Hospital zone

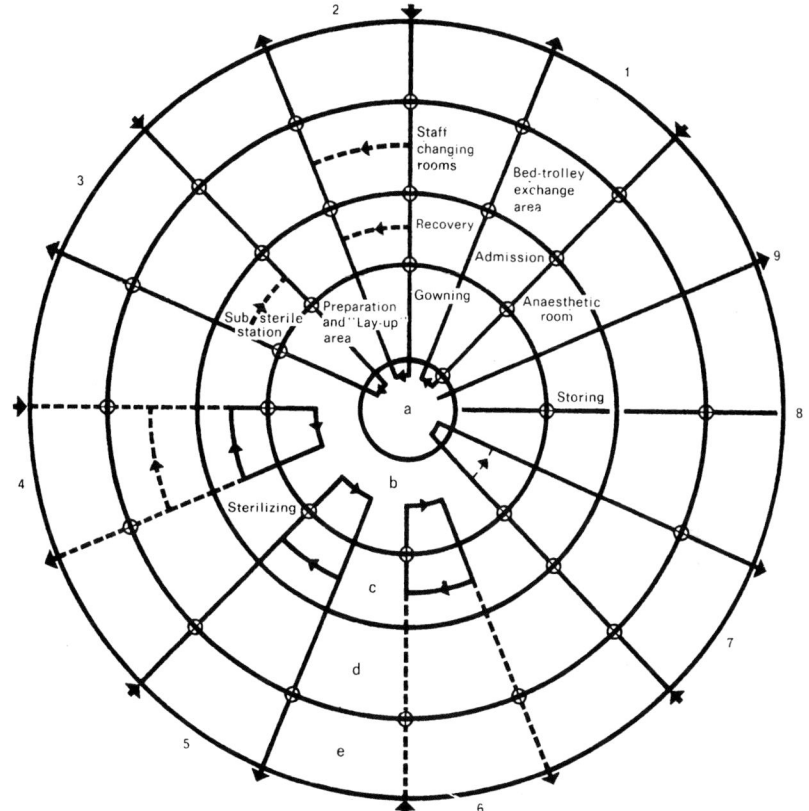

Patient traffic route

The patient is brought to the operating theatre wing on the ward bed or on a hospital trolley. In emergency cases, the patient arrives from the reception department on a hospital stretcher. In the "bed exchange" zone, the patient is transferred from the bed to the operating theatre wing trolley. The trolley does not leave the wing and moves around a closed circuit restricted to the clean area of the wing. The patient's first station is the reception room, where he is given preliminary treatment. In some hospitals preliminary treatment is given in the ward. From the reception room the patient is wheeled into the anaesthetic room (if such a room has been planned) where he is anaesthetized. From here, the patient is taken, under narcosis, into the operating theatre and is transferred from the trolley of the wing onto the operating table (if use is made of trolleys constituting part of the operating table, this action is avoided). After the operation the patient is again moved onto

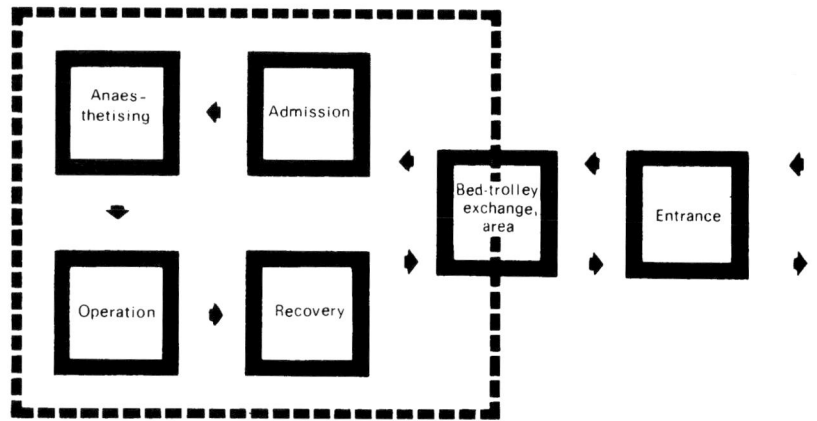

the wing trolley and wheeled into the recovery room. After recovery, in the "bed exchange" zone, the patient is returned to a hospital bed and taken out of the wing. A detailed follow-up of the actions and a study of the moves involved will dictate the spaces required for performance of the above activities. The moving of the patient requires a great deal of attention. The patient sees the rooms from a recumbent position, during that part of the circuit when he is awake. Ceiling design takes on a different significance from this vantage paint. In that stretch of the circuit, where the patient is being moved under narcosis, special pains should be taken to avoid sharp and needless turns because of the danger to the patient while in that condition.

Staff traffic route

Staff members enter the wing through the main entrance and turn to the changing rooms located on the "border" between the clean and the non-clean zones.

The distribution and arrangement of the changing rooms is a problem in itself. In the changing rooms the staff has to discard street or hospital clothes and assume operating wing garb. Changing rooms are divided for men and women and sometimes subdivided according to function, e.g. doctor, cleaners, etc. Experience has shown this division of the rooms to be a weak point, since the numerical ratio of the sexes can never be foreseen. Even the number of staff members to be catered to is sometimes uncertain. It has therefore been found that small, standard changing rooms, in sufficient number, assigned by sex as immediate need dictates, best suit the purpose.

4. **Health Facilities in Israel**

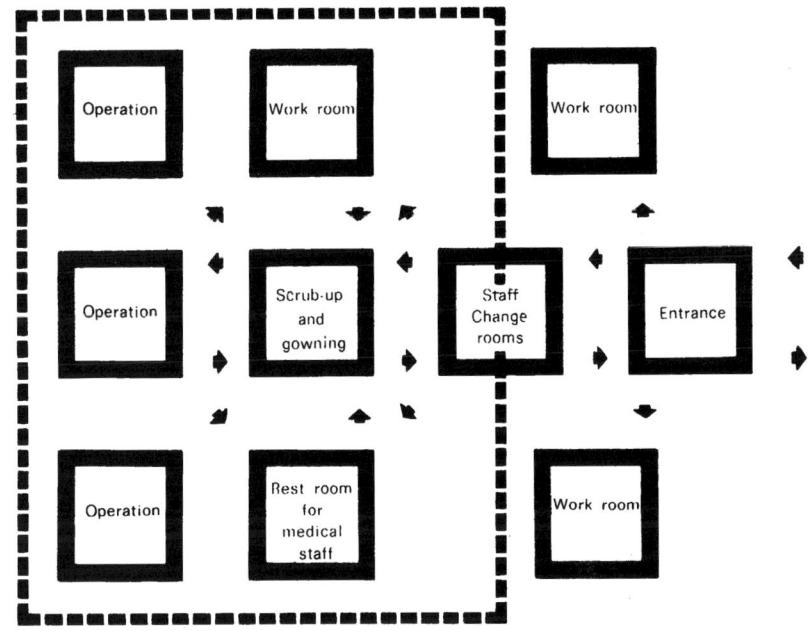

Another problem is the manner in which the changing rooms are to function. Some favour double cubicles with a cross barrier, while others do not believe in this type of changing room. In changing rooms with double cubicles, the staff member enters from the outside, discards his street clothes, which are put into a special cupboard, "sits" on the cross bench and brings his legs over into the "clean" side, puts on galoshes and robes him in the costume of the wing. In reality this is a cumbersome process and one, which the staff in the operating theatres wing cannot be expected to adhere to. For this reason, the accepted arrangement is one of rooms having an entry on one side and an exit on the other. In this method, the border between "clean" and "non-clean" is not clearly delineated. The other alternative is a corridor, along which the dressing rooms are arranged. In this set-up there is a cubicle at the beginning or entrance end of the corridor for putting on the galoshes belonging to the wing, so that the floor of the changing rooms' corridor will not be contaminated by the staffs' shoes. This arrangement simplifies the changing process. From the changing rooms, the staff disperses each to his own job. A distinction must be made between the staff directly involved in the operation and the staff which is not directly involved. The surgeons and the operating theatre

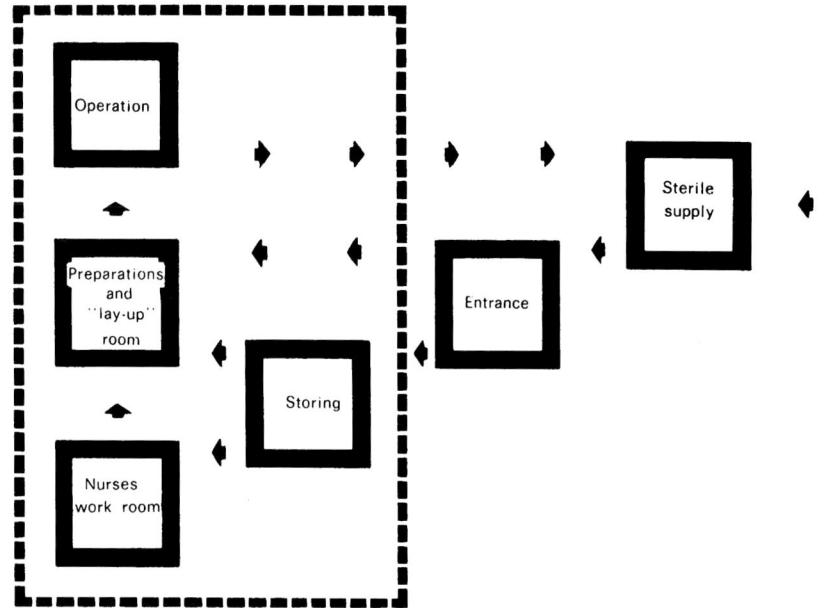

staff arrive in the operating theatres after scrubbing in the rooms or recesses adjacent to the operating theatres. After scrubbing and before entering the operating theatre, surgical gowns and gloves are donned. In most hospitals, the "clean side" has lounge rooms for the staff, for resting between operations. Similarly, in especially large wings, there exist additional rooms for staff seminars, etc. The staff leaves the wing via the changing rooms, where they put on their hospital uniforms or street dress.

Materials traffic route

The main problem in materials supply is to provide the operating theatres with sterile supplies. Under the accepted method, sub sterilization rooms are located between two operating theatres.

Supplies arrive at the storeroom of the wing from an outside source or from central supplies, a pharmacy or other source. The plan provides for a nurses' workroom close to the storeroom. Instrument washing and parceling is done in rooms situated between the operating theatres. Sterilization of the instrument parcels is concentrated at the central sterile supplies. The advantage of this method is in the relative lack, of dependence of the operating theatres wing on the supply of materials. The staff needed to work under this system must be

4. Health Facilities in Israel

first-rate and highly trained. Such a staff is not easy to find or to retain. Another system that has recently been developed is based on the preparation of sterile supplies needed for the operating theatres in the central sterile supply branch of the hospital. Under this system the trays and parcels are prepared in a special area of the sterile supplies wing. By means of this centralization, work can proceed along "industrial" lines and a team can be trained to function within given limits. The materials are supplied to the operating theatres wing in sufficient quantity and diversity. They are delivered to the lay-up rooms located between operating theatres (in place of the sterilization rooms included under the previous system), in the preparation room, trays are prepared on the instrument trolleys and are wheeled into the operating theatres. In a wing planned under this method there should be a small nurses' workroom and one or two wall recesses per wing, to be used only in special cases for special equipment, or for rapid sterilization of instruments that have been dropped. Under this method the preparation room is a "clean" room, whereas under the first method there exists the complicated problem of operating the sterilization room and dividing it into "clean" and "non-clean" zones, and of maintaining an appropriate work regimen.

Removal of waste from the operating theatres wing is different for solids and liquids. Liquid waste material is removed via the removal system through a waste tub located in the "exit room" leading out of the operating theatre, or in the "non-clean" zone of the sterilization room, if the wing plan is in accordance with the first method. For the removal of solids, a lift or chute, usually installed in the sluice room, is used. The planning of space and the various apparatuses connected with the traffic of material's requires a minute study of the details of performance of the above-mentioned operations.

Integration of the various traffic routes
Once the method of planning a given wing is determined and the dimensions of the various spaces required for performance of operations under the suggested plan have been processed, the traffic routes of patients, staff and materials must be integrated in such a way that points of encounter will be in the correct places and that there will be no undesirable crossings of sterile and non-sterile materials. Improper planning of paints of encounter could lead to creation of a dangerous source of infection.

Whenever a wing of the building is being planned, traffic can be made conspicuous or inconspicuous. In the planning of an operating theatres wing, it is essential that traffic be inconspicuous. This requirement will affect the choice of the desirable arrangement of the wing within the plan.

Critical dimensions of rooms Operating theatres
In the planning of a new wing of operating theatres for any hospital, the issue of the dimensions of the operating theatres always arises. The accepted size is 6.0 x 6.0 m. These dimensions suffice for the performance of most operations. The placing of entrances, exits and apertures (vents) is also a determinant factor regarding the dimensions of the operating theatre, but practical experience shows that within the said measurements, all data can be marshaled in the proper proportions. A different situation occurs in operating theatres designed for special jobs such as neurosurgery or heart operations. In rooms of this type a great deal of space must be assigned for equipment, but some prefer to have the equipment and the control apparatus outside the operating theatre, in adjacent rooms. These rooms are, not infrequently, of dimensions as large as the operating theatre itself.

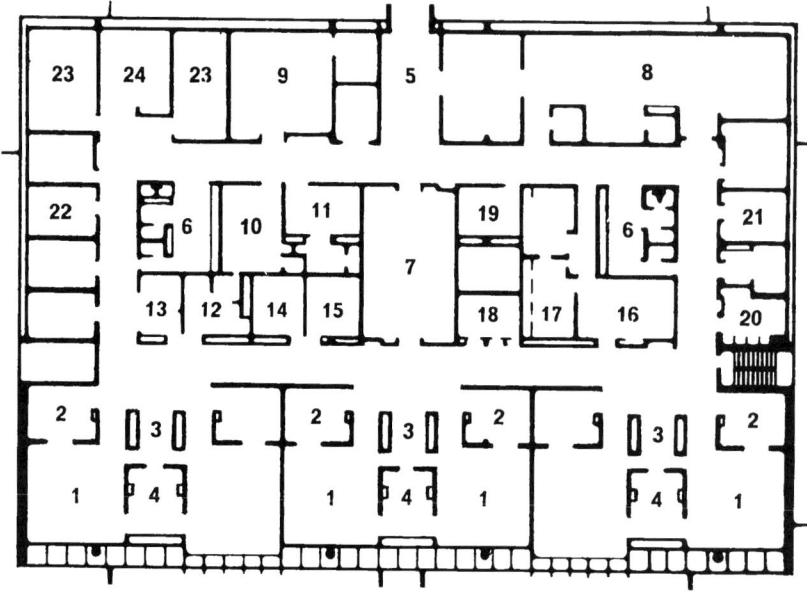

Meir Hospital
Operating theatres block plan
1. Operating theatre
2. Anaesthetic room
3. Scrub-up room
4. Sub-sterilizing room
5. Entrance hall
6. Medical staff changing room
7. Admission and reception
8. Recovery room (short stay)
9. Plaster room including storerooms
    for materials and equipment
10. Endoscopy room
11. Cystoscopy room
12. Darkroom
13. Small specimen and frozen section lab.
14. Storeroom
15. Dirty utility / sluice room
16. Nurses' workroom
17. Sterile storeroom
18. Nurses' station
19. Cleaner
20. Anaesthetic equipment room
21. Chief anaesthetist's room
22. Surgeons' room
23. Staff rest room
24. Kitchenette

4. Health Facilities in Israel

Anaesthetic rooms

Anaesthetic rooms have a definite functional plan. They are designed as ordinary rooms, insofar as is possible, having neither equipment nor apparatus which could produce wakefulness in the patient. The dimensions of these rooms are determined on the basis of what is required to anaesthetize a patient lying on the operating' theatres wing trolley. The usual size of the room is 18 to 20 sqm. Special attention should be given to the process of wheeling the anaesthetized
patient from the anaesthetic room into the operating theatre. Needless turns and complications in this process should be avoided.

Admission (reception) and preparation room

The dimensions of this room are determined in accordance with the number of stretchers the room is to contain and their arrangement within the room. The accepted arrangement provides for 2 m. between the axes of the stretchers. Under the single-row method, a room of about 5 m widths is sufficient.

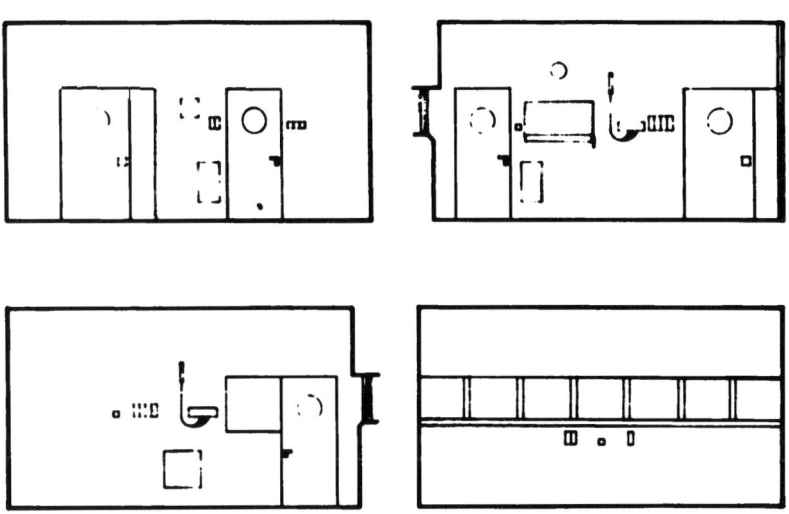

Sheba Medical Centre
Operating theatre detail

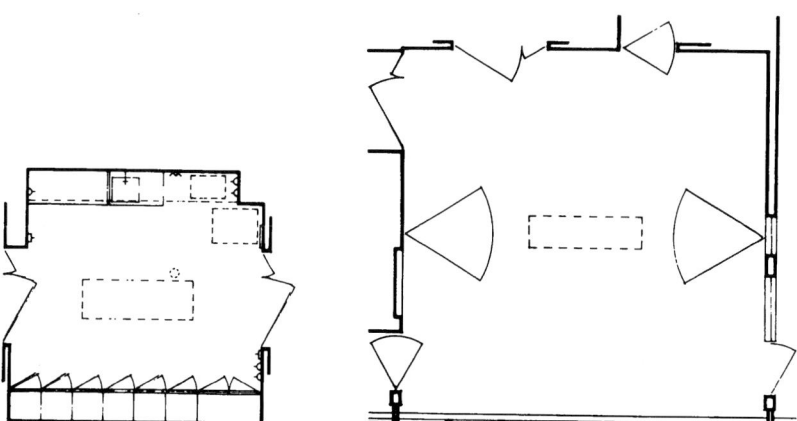

Sheba Medical Centre
Anaesthetic room detail

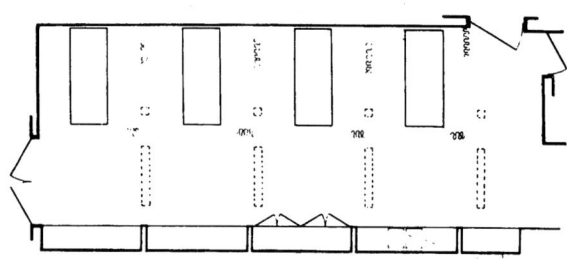

Safed Hospital
Admission room detail

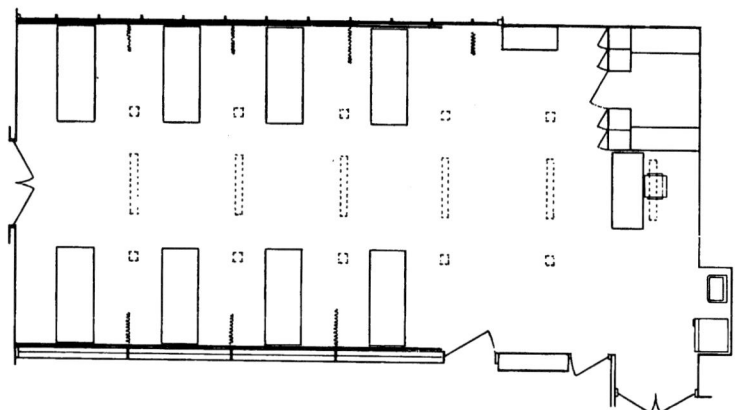

Safed Hospital
Recovery room detail

4. Health Facilities in Israel

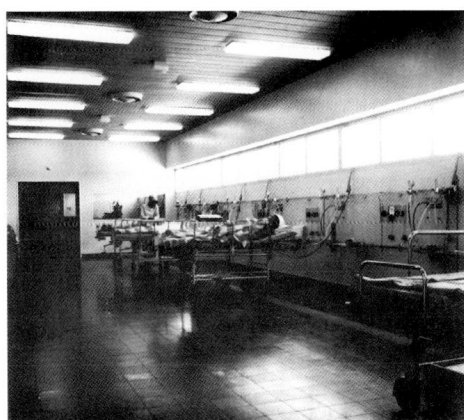

Meir Hospital
Recovery room

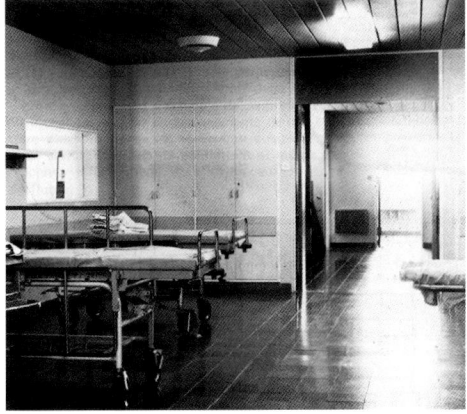

Meir Hospital
Admission room

Recovery room

The dimensions of the recovery rooms also depend on the number of stretchers and the way they are arranged in the room. But here more space is required as it is frequently necessary to bring into this room various equipment for treatment of the patients, and sufficient room must be left to move. The stretchers should be arranged so as to facilitate supervision from the nurses' station in the recovery room. 12 sqm. per stretcher are generally found to be needed in this room. One-and-a-half beds in the recovery room are usually assigned per operating theatre.

Location of the operating theatres wing within the hospital

An important element is the location of the operating theatres wing in the general complex of the hospital. This is determined by taking into consideration the hospital's traffic routes; in other words, the relation of the traffic route systems within the wing to the general traffic route system of the hospital as a whole. The wing should be boldly and clearly connected to the hospital's traffic core or cores since, as a rule, patients are transported from the wards to the operating wing and back again. There should also be good connection with the reception department, for accident cases or other emergencies, when the patient has to be brought rapidly from the ambulance entrance or the reception hall to the operating theatres wing.

There also exist other, looser connections, which need not be enumerated here. The traffic route system in the operating wing itself is an independent system and, relative to the general system, constitutes a sort of cul-de-sac.

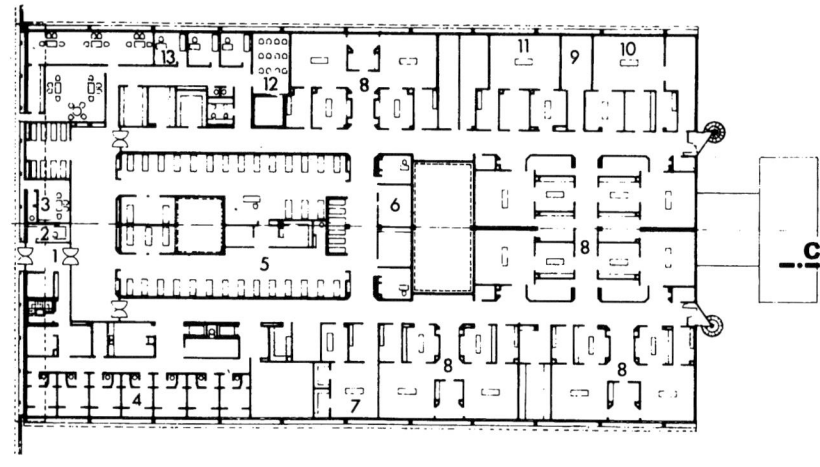

Sheba Medical Centre
Operating theatres
1. Entrance
2. Reception and information
3. Waiting for patients' family
4. Cloakroom – staff
5. Patient admission and preparation
6. Nurses utility rooms
7. Plaster room
8. Standard theatre suite
9. Control room
10. Cardiac theatre
11. Neuro – theatre
12. Seminar room
13. Surgeons' offices
14. Laboratories
15. Recovery room
16. Returning equipment lift
17. Sterile supply lift
18. Restrooms – staff

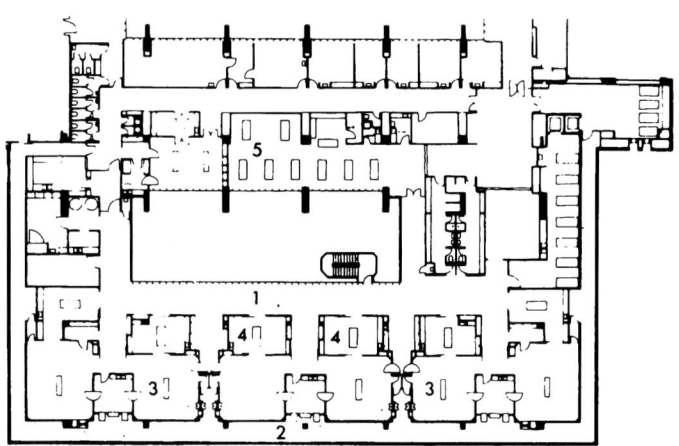

Carmel Hospital
Operating theatres block floor plan
1. "Clean" corridor
2. "Non-clean" corridor
3. Operating theatres
4. Anaesthetic room
5. Recovery room

Traffic routes within the wing are divided in accordance with the areas they serve. The main breakdown is into "clean" and "non-clean" corridors. The former serve zones (a)–(c) and the latter zones (d)–(e) (see diagram). For hospital personnel, the changing rooms form the "border" or passage from one area to another. For patients entering the wing the reception room is the "border", and for patients leaving the wing the "border" is the recovery room. In planning the traffic system within the wing, every effort should be made to minimize unnecessary movement and to guide the flow of traffic of patients, staff, materials, waste, etc., in such a way that the encounters will be at the proper places and the movement routes as clear and as simple as possible.

4. Health Facilities in Israel

Kaplan Hospital
Operating theatres block floor plan

1. Operating theatre
2. Endoscopy room
3. Plaster room
4. Induction room
5. Recovery
6. "Non-clean" corridor
7. Nurses' room
8. Bed storeroom
9. Cloakroom
10. Scrub-up area
11. Sterile storeroom
12. Preparation room
13. Rest room

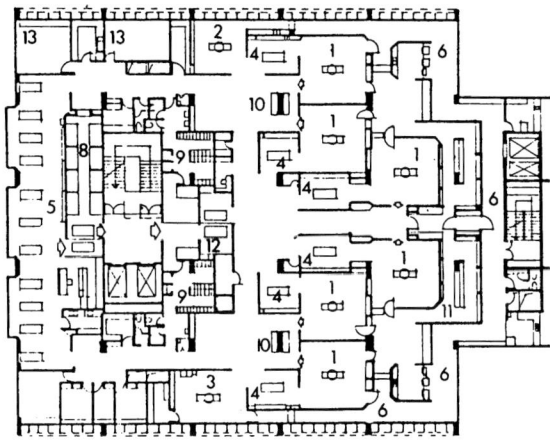

Safed Hospital
Operating theatres block floor plan

1. "Clean" corridor
2. Entrance hall
3. Admission and reception
4. Anaesthetic room
5. Operating theatres
6. Lay-up room
7. Scrub-up room
8. Exit bay
9. Recovery room (short stay)
10. Staff changing room
11. Surgeons' lounge
12. Nurses' lounge
13. Chief nurse's room
14. Chief anaesthetist's room
15. Waiting room for families

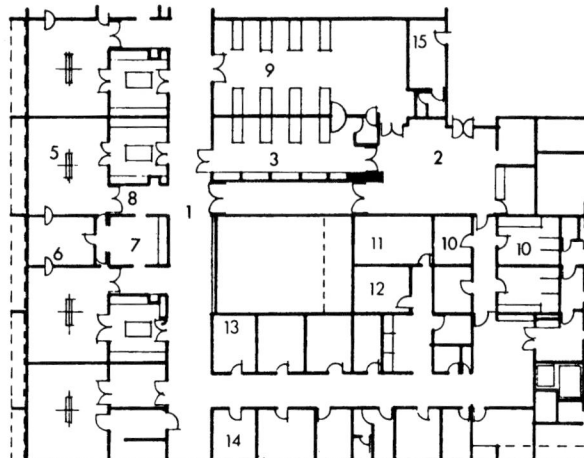

Dimensions and shape of the wing

The dimensions of the operating theatres wing are usually dictated by a large number of data and restrictions. Limitations to the geometric shape of the wing, arising from its location within the entire hospital complex are yet another of the objective difficulties that exist in the planning of this intricate wing.

An operating wing located on one of the floors of the building will acquire the dimensions of a "standard floor". The dimensions of the standard floor are determined by data relating to other departments and other functions. The result will be that planning will take place in an imposed framework, and this will be expressed in the plans. In all hospitals where the operating theatres wings have been designed as part of the main building, examples can be seen of a wing planned within given plan metric-geometric limitations. Another shortcoming in planning operating wings within the main body of the building is that the wing cannot be enlarged at a later date.

An operating wing located on the ground floor level with the ambulance entrance or close to it, can be planned with relative freedom. The dimensions of the wing are determined with reference to the "requirements" of the plan. The problem of traffic route crossings is automatically solved when the entrance to the operating theatres wing is close to the main traffic arteries of the hospital. The enlargement of the wing is in this instance dependent only on the planning of its internal traffic routes. Another advantage of planning this wing independently of the main body of the building is that of greater freedom in the planning of the technical spaces serving the wing, as well as the potential for future enlargement.

Principles of the air-conditioning system and technical spaces

The air-conditioning system in the operating theatres wing should accomplish two tasks: control air cleanliness for the prevention of infection, and provide for the comfort of the patients and staff. Under Israeli climatic conditions, no operating theatres wing can be planned without an air-conditioning system. The desirable temperature for the operating theatres themselves is lower than that considered comfortable in other areas. A temperature range of 18–20 °C is generally considered suitable for the operating theatre. When the temperature stands at 18° or lower, the auxiliary team complains to the chief surgeon. At this temperature, air changes would be effected at the rate of 19 per hour, or one complete air change about every 3 minutes. The size of the air conduits and equipment is governed by the rate of air changes and the temperature. The air-conditioning system must ensure a regular air flow in the various areas of the wing. The rule is that air should flow from the "cleaner area" to the "less clean" area. According to diagrammatic markings pointing from area "A" in the direction of area "E", the flow directions' regimen requirement can be achieved by regulating the quantities of air supplied to and expelled from the various rooms. The air-conditioning system, especially in the operating theatres, is constructed on the principle of supplying fresh air (100%) thus, the air must be filtered. The method of filtering is highly instrumental in determining the degree of air cleanliness. In the operating theatres wing

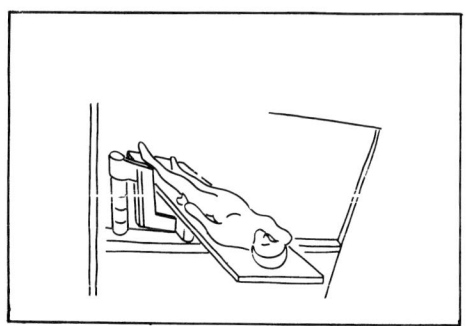

"Maquet Passage" for patient's transfers from bed to operations table

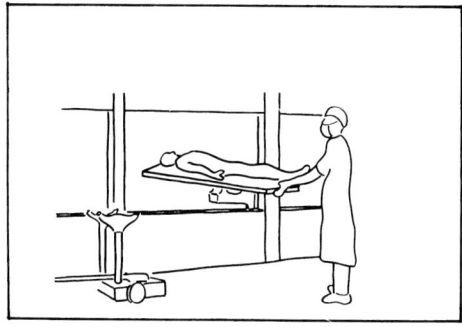

"Maquet Passage", used in some hospitals to transfer a patient from the "unclean zone" to the "clean zone"

Meir Hospital
Plan of air ducts in the technical floor above the operating theatres block

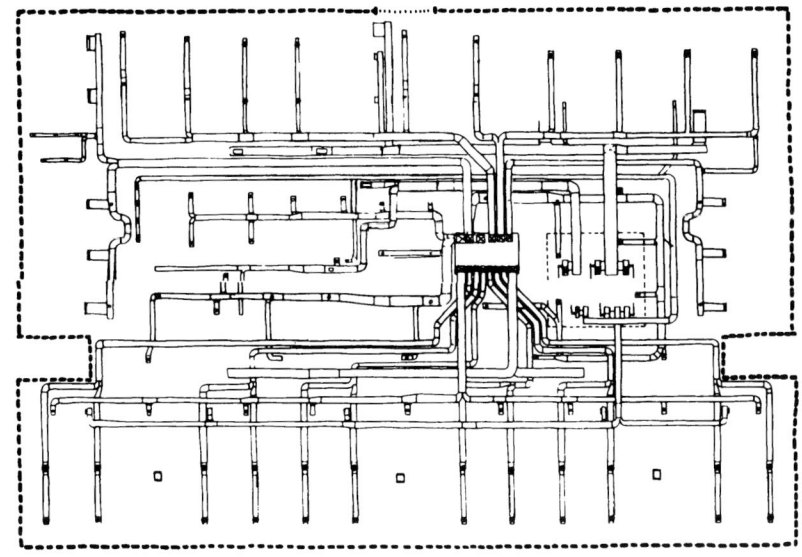

of the Meir Hospital, the air is filtered by a set of 3 filters, arrranged one after another in a row. This system has proved itself in actual use. The first filter is a low-efficiency filter constructed of plates of a special fibrous material (fiberglass) about 5 cm thick. The function of this filter is to remove the visible, coarse-grained dirt such as dust, sand. etc. After it comes a high-efficiency electro-static filter. The air passing through this is drawn through a strong electromagnetic field which endows the dust with an electrical charge, and further along the charged dust is attracted to electrostatic collecting plates. After this there is a high-efficiency mechanical filter which collects the dirt accumulated in the electrostatic filter and also any dust which has managed to get past it. This filter is built in the form of ducts of a delicate filtering substance and operates in the direction of the air flow. Both its efficiency and its dust absorption capacity are very high.

The system described can filter, at over 90% efficiency, particles having a diameter of 1 micron or more. It should be borne in mind that the average size of bacteria-carrying particles against which precautions need to be taken, is about 3 microns, so that the majority of bacteria are unable to pass through the filter.

The supply of air through the ducts should be in accordance with the other apparatus in the room. In general the best rule is for the air supply to be installed in the ceilings, in such a way as to ensure correct distribution, and for it to be expelled from a low area. Air conditioning systems in operating theatres are of fairly large dimensions. Since

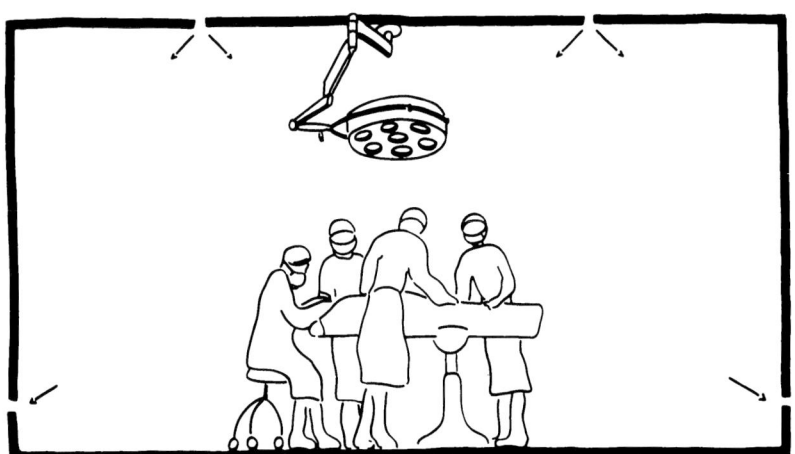

there must be free access to the conduits, filters, air conditioners, etc., it is necessary to make provision for technical spaces, which will occupy a considerable portion of the built-up area. It is best, if possible, to preserve the continuity of the technical spaces so as to eliminate the necessity for maintenance staff to enter work areas in the wing.

Greater security against explosions

Because of the occasional use of flammable substances in the operating theatres, especially for anaesthesizing, the air-conditioning systems of the anaesthetic rooms must be kept separate from those of the operating theatres. Thus, air from the anaesthetic rooms should not penetrate the operating theatres; if there is any flow, it should be from the operating theatres into the anaesthetic rooms. This can be achieved by supplying air to the anaesthetic room and expelling it from that room, creating a small deficiency of air in circulation. Then, if air is supplied to the operating theatres and not retaken directly from there, the flow of air will always be from the operating theatre to the anaesthetic room. In addition, care should be taken that the air-conditioning regulator system be devoid of electrical contacts liable to cause sparks while in operation.

Humidity control

The air-conditioning system affords the possibility of humidity control in the operating theatres. Relative humidity should be in the range of 55–60%, so as to avoid formation of static electricity in clothing etc. as a result of friction created in the dry air.

4. Health Facilities in Israel

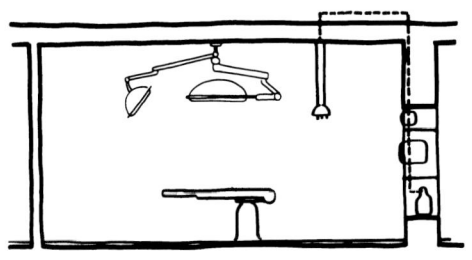

Ceiling-mounted "supply arm"

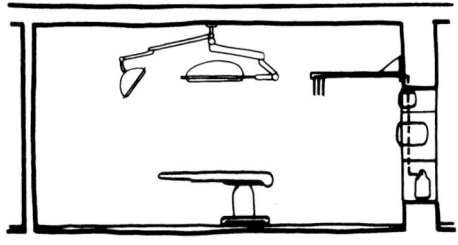

Wall-mounted "supply arm"

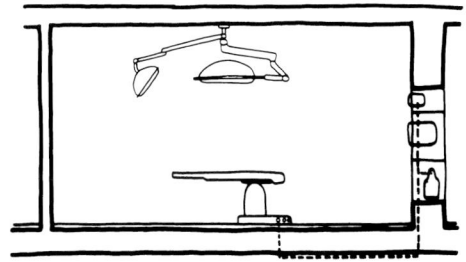

Floor supply in the base of the operating table

Type of operating tables

Various operating wings in hospitals in Israel use different types of operating tables. Surgeons have reached no consensus of opinion on this point. Operating tables are not manufactured in Israel and it is thus easier to experiment with tables imported from other sources. At any rate, it is possible to find movable tables, fixed tables with supplies in the leg, or fixed legs with movable upper panels.

Naturally, the choice of the type of table to be used will have a far-reaching effect on the planning of the wing and the electromechanical systems. Moreover, the choice of the type of table is also connected with the choice of supply system: – from the ceiling, from the floor, or through a system of moving arms, etc.

Use of materials and colours

Terrazzo tiles are widely used in most areas of the wing, except for the operating theatres and anaesthetic rooms. In these rooms use is recently being made of P.V.C. floors which have conductive properties suitable for preventing the danger of explosion due to an accumulation of static electricity. The walls are oil-painted except in the operating theatres and other sensitive rooms in which it is the practice to use ceramic wall tiles. All corners are rounded and the materials used are designed to withstand constant cleaning. In view of the function of the operating theatres wing, the colours in use are quiet colours: light green, blue, beige, grey, etc., in light shades so as to give sufficient reflection of light rays.

Planning for diverse activities

It should be borne in mind that in the practice of medicine, methods of treatment are frequently updated, and planning should not, therefore, be rigid, or done in such a way as to meet only those requirements stipulated at the time at planning. The wing should be regarded as an arena of activity of the medical service, allowing for the comfortable performance of medical motions, in accordance with methods both prearranged and those changing with time. It should be remembered that activities cannot be performed if the physical environment hampers performance.

Planning should, therefore, allow for the performance of activities of a diverse nature and also for future change and growth. Good planning and even good equipment are no substitute for a capable surgeon, but they allow and even contribute to good operative performance and can save the patient unnecessary suffering.

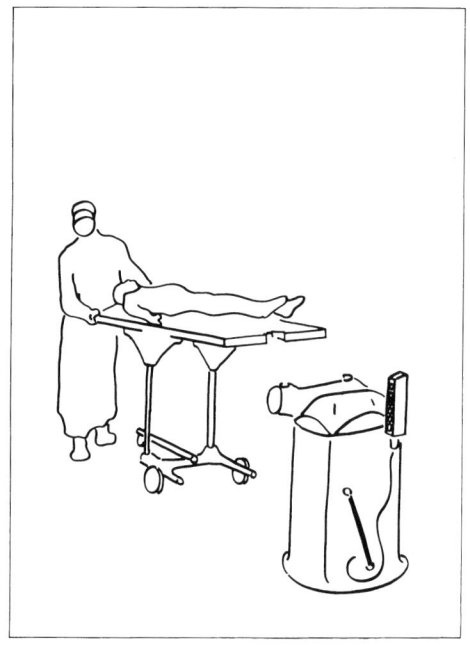

Operating table
Fixed leg movable upper panel

Radiology Department

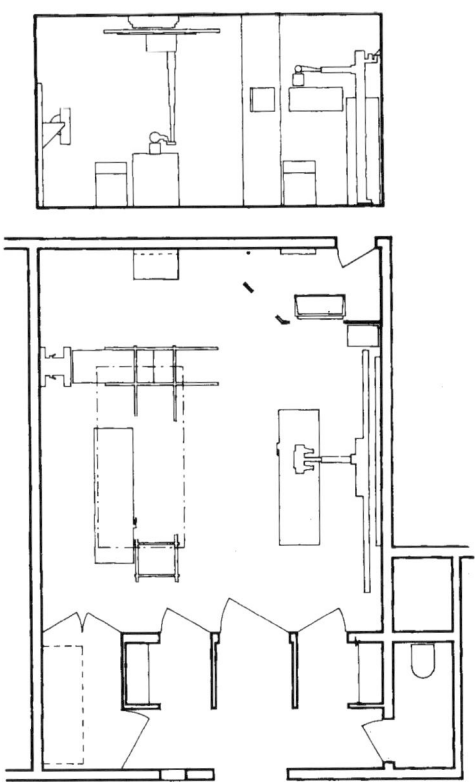

**Sheba Medical Centre
Diagnostic radiology workroom**

Functions of radiology department

The radiology department deals with general radiology, tomography, neurology, uroradiology, angiography, fluoroscopy, etc. Research in pathological, histopathological and comparative radiological fields may be carried out in the radiology department, the pathology department, or the animal house, as the case may be.

The department serves in- and outpatients. Particularly large departments may give treatment in addition to their diagnostic functions. The size of the department is determined by the estimated number of operations to be provided by it. The figure of 20 operations per day per "table" is realistic. Generally, one may assume that in a general hospital with 500 beds, the radiology department will consist of about 10 workrooms.

Location of radiology department

The location of the radiology department within the hospital is of great importance. The department serves the inpatient wards, the surgical department, the admission department and the outpatient clinics. Inpatients are wheeled in by a nurse or, if their condition allows, reach the department by themselves, usually according to a predetermined timetable. In special cases, particularly in the case of accidents or emergencies, the patient is brought to the radiology department from the admission department before he is taken to the operating theatre. While most surgical departments have mobile X-ray equipment, its performance is limited. Many outpatients arrive at the radiology department for diagnosis or treatment from the clinics.

If the plan of the hospital provides no possibility for efficient connections with anyone of the departments mentioned, it becomes necessary to establish an additional radiology room in that department, far from the main radiology section. Since radiological equipment is expensive and staff scarce, any unnecessary duplication of equipment or staff results in high acquisition and operation costs. Preferably, the radiology department should be established near the vertical traffic core of the wards section, near the admission and surgical departments and in direct traffic communication with the outpatient clinics.

Also, if possible, it should be located on the same level as these departments.

Grouping of rooms in the radiology department

We distinguish several groups of rooms in this department:

a. Workrooms. These are the rooms in which the radiological equipment is located and where the main work of the department is carried out. As far as possible, one tries to design them as standardized rooms. The accepted dimensions are 25 sqm. by 3.20 m. in height. The entrance to these rooms is from the waiting room through dressing cubicles, where the patient leaves his clothes and changes into a hospital gown. The waiting rooms should be of ample size and, unlike the workrooms, should preferably look out on a garden or on the landscape outside, so as to make the patients feel comfortable. The workrooms are planned in groups of four to six. Each group is served by a developing room (darkroom). Modern developing rooms have automatic developing equipment. Next to the developing room lie sorting rooms which serves for a first examination of the films by the staff. All these rooms are interconnected and form one complex of work, dressing, developing and waiting rooms.

b. Staff rooms. These rooms form a continuous group of rooms which should be located near the workrooms, without requiring the staff to pass through the areas used by the patients. Most staff rooms have an area of 12–16 sqm., with the exception of the demonstration room, which serves the medical staff of the hospital and where films are projected by means of special equipment (alternator). The size of the demonstration room depends on the number of doctors which it serves: in hospitals with 400–600 beds it will be about 50 sqm. In certain cases an additional entrance to the radiology department is planned, which leads to these rooms and serves the staff.

c. Files and archive. The radiology archive, which contains the patients' files, is planned near the reception office. The office looks out on the entrance to the department, and preferably also on the waiting areas. Next to the file stack, an office working area for registration and typing is planned. The problem of the file stack or area for storing patients' files is not an easy one. Using photographs of reduced size involves technical difficulties. Consequently, the area needed for

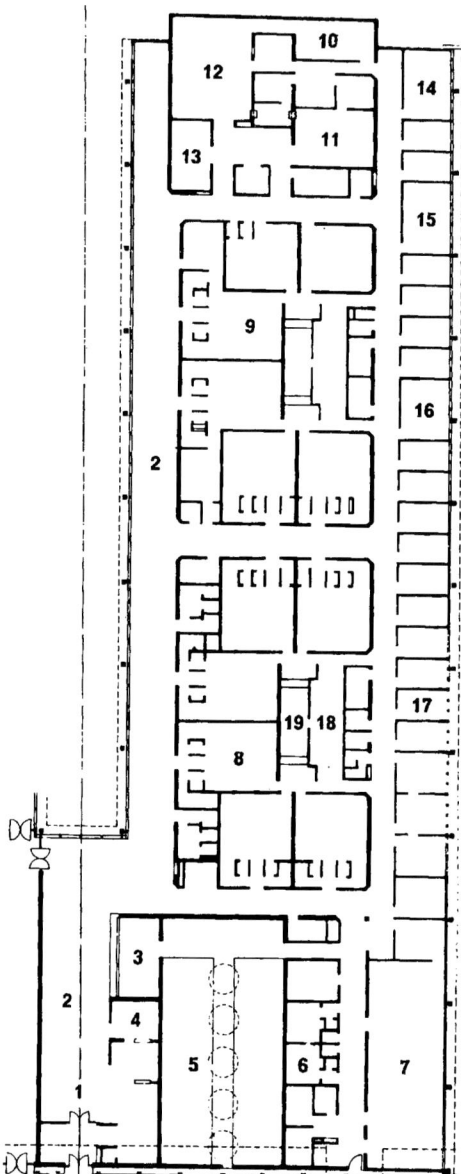

4. Health Facilities in Israel

Sheba Medical Centre
Diagnostic radiology department plan
1. Entrance
2. Waiting area
3. Reception
4. Nurses' room
5. Filing and film archives
6. Staff cloakroom
7. Demonstration / conference room
8. X-ray rooms – general purpose
9. X-ray rooms – specialized investigation suite
10. Gas analysis laboratory
11. Neuro- and peripheral angiography
12. Cardio- and abdominal angiography
13 Patient preparation, anaesthetic and recovery room
14. Histological research laboratory
15. Seminar room / library
16. Staff rest room
17. Radiologists' and X-ray technicians' rooms, including radiography school
18. Immediate viewing and sorting room
19. Processing room

Meir Hospital
Diagnostic radiology department plan
1. Waiting
2. Reception
3. Filing and film archives
4. Angiography room
5. X-ray photography room
6. General purpose radio diagnostic room
7. Processing room
8. Immediate viewing and sorting room
9. Departmental head's room
10. Senior radiologists' room
11. Demonstration room
12. Technicians' room
13. Storeroom

file storage increases yearly, and it is practically impossible to allocate large enough areas where they would be needed. Generally, some temporary solution is found, such as assigning old files to part of the hospital's general storage areas.

As the patient is registered for examination and sent to a given workroom, his form is sent along with him and returned together with a film. This process of sending files and returning them to the file stack dictates the communications and routes between the file stack and the workrooms. A waiting space is provided in front of the reception office. A separate space is reserved for bedridden patients under the supervision of a nurse.

Dimensions and shape of the radiology department

The contacts between the different rooms and the grouping of rooms as described above determine the parameters by which the planning is limited. A further limitation is imposed by the location of the department and by whether or not another department is planned above or below it. A given system of pillars, windows, etc. restricts the planning and makes it difficult to find the optimum solution for the interaction of the rooms. If feasible, the department should therefore be given a place within the general hospital layout which allows it to be planned without unnecessary restrictions and which permits a geometric shape suitable for the needs of the department.

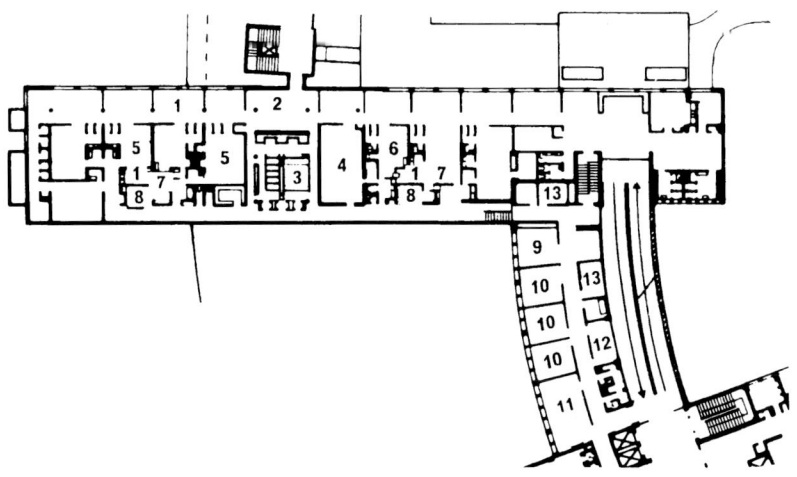

Institutes

A concept unique to the Israeli hospital is that of the "institute". The so-called institutes, which are part of the hospital's medical services, include the Cardiology Institute, Gastroenterology Institute, Lung Function Institute, Electroencephalography Institute etc. In recent years, these services have developed into departments of large dimensions. Institutes which used to occupy one or two rooms have grown to the size of sub-departments. The trend toward specialization (in medical practice and medical equipment) has turned the institutes into consultant facilities serving all hospital departments. Unlike medical service departments abroad, the Israeli institutes serve both in- and outpatients, and must be located accordingly.

The Cardiology Institute, for instance, has become the center for services which used to be located in different parts of the hospital, and now operates as a central service. Heart patients continue to be treated in the different clinical departments, but the central cardiology service acts in a consultant capacity for all hospital units. It is provided with equipment for special electrocardiographic and heart function tests. It is assisted by other hospital units such as radiology, radioactive isotopes and different laboratories. In large Cardiology Institutes, there is a special sub-department for cardiac catheterization.

The nature of the institutes requires, in addition to lines of communication as indicated above, locations which permit growth and expansion independently of other parts of the hospital. The problem becomes particularly complicated if an attempt is made to allow for the differential growth and development of each institute without reference to the others.

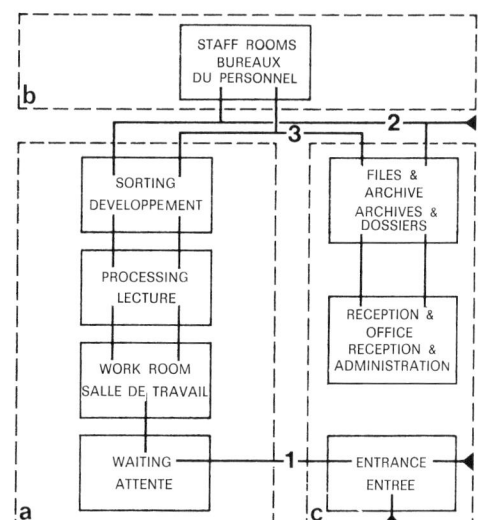

Route diagram
in diagnostic radiology department
a. Workrooms group
b. Staff rooms group
c. Staff and archives room
1. Patient route
2. Staff route
3. File route

Meir Hospital
Angiography workroom

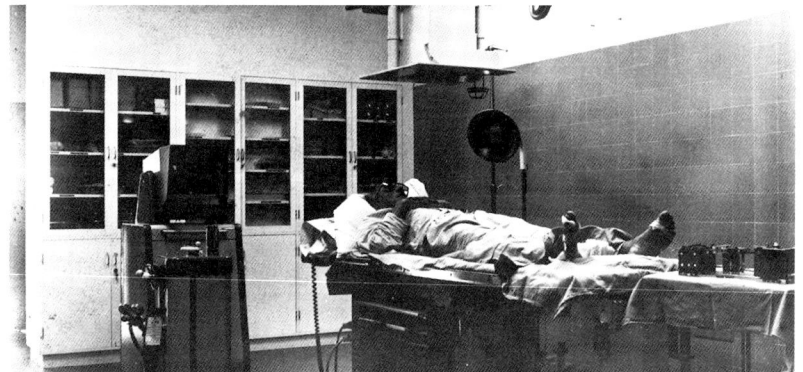

Meir Hospital
Diagnostic radiology workroom

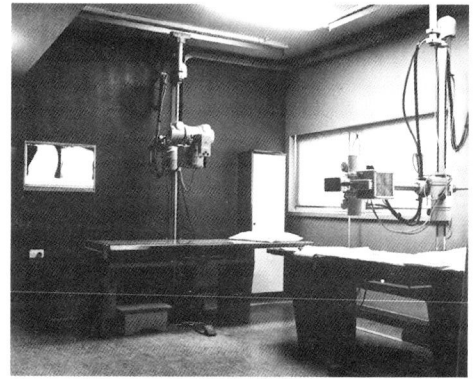

4. Health Facilities in Israel

Laboratory Department

Functions of the laboratory department

Hospital laboratories deal with a wide range of tests in the fields of bio-chemistry, bacteriology, parasitology, serology, virology, haematology, immunology, cytology, cytogenetics, etc. In most hospitals in Israel, routine work on samples taken from patients and research work are carried on side-by-side. According to some opinions, it is not desirable to separate routine work from research. For the planner at any rate, there is no difference between the shape of routine and research laboratories. The area required for routine laboratory work depends mainly on the volume of work, which is a function of the number of beds and outpatient clinics in the hospital. The research laboratory area depends entirely on the extent of the research carries out at the hospital. In recent years, the relative size of the laboratory department within the overall area of the hospital has increased. Our experience shows, that it would be a mistake to plan a laboratory department without allowing for its increase. The laboratory department must be able to be enlarged without reference to other hospital departments. In addition to the routine and research laboratories, in some hospitals there is a sub-department for radioactive isotopes and radiation services for therapeutic purposes. Also an animal house is sometimes attached to the laboratory department, for tests and experimental surgery.

Uniform planning of entire laboratory area

Working methods in the laboratories depend on the development of scientific working methods in the world at large. Advances in science and laboratory technology have been considerable and rapid. It is therefore necessary to adapt the laboratory to up-to-date working methods and instrumentation. The division of the laboratory area according to purpose depends on the composition of the staff and the subjects of work and research. These two factors also change from time to time. It is therefore obvious that the laboratory department requires frequent changes. Administrative opposition to change will not prevent the changes from eventually occurring anyway, and is therefore only counter-productive. Our experience indicates, that the solution to the problem of effectively designing the laboratory area should be sought in the form of sophisticated planning which permits changes to be made by the maintenance staff without requiring construction work, or at any rate without basic changes in the structure of the building. Uniform, modular, two-stage planning of the entire area of the laboratory department is a solution of proven effectiveness.

According to this philosophy, the entire area of the laboratory should be planned uniformly, without regard to purpose. The exceptions to the rule are such specific areas as radioactive isotopes, glassware washing and other services common to all the laboratories. The planning is based on a fixed, standardized laboratory module. First-stage planning includes the construction and main supply systems, without reference to divisions according to purpose. In this stage, all the invariant planning components are laid down. These components include the skeletal system of the building, the system of external openings and sometimes the passages and main internal openings as well. The first stage also includes the main supply and waste disposal systems.

The actual building work can be carried out according to the plans prepared at this stage. The first-stage planning should be undertaken without the cooperation of scientists. In the second stage, the divisions according to purpose, the details of the area, furnishings of the laboratories and the supplies to these furnishings, are planned.

This planning can only be effected with the full cooperation of the scientists. Generally, the second stage of the planning proceeds while the building operations of the first planning stage are being carried out, according to the rule: "Design as you build."

Planning the laboratory department according to this philosophy requires considerable experience, since the first stage must be designed in such a manner, that the second stage can be completed without running into complications. The first-stage plans must take into account most of the data on the uses of the area, and also the methods of supply and waste disposal to and from the laboratories.

Uniform module for working area

The uniform planning of the laboratory areas is, as we have seen, based on a fixed module. This module is determined according to an analysis of the operations to be carried out in the laboratory unit. The width of the modular laboratory is obtained by adding the measurements of the width of the laboratory bench, the working space required at the table, and free passage between the persons working at the benches. The width of the bench is determined by the length of the arm of the

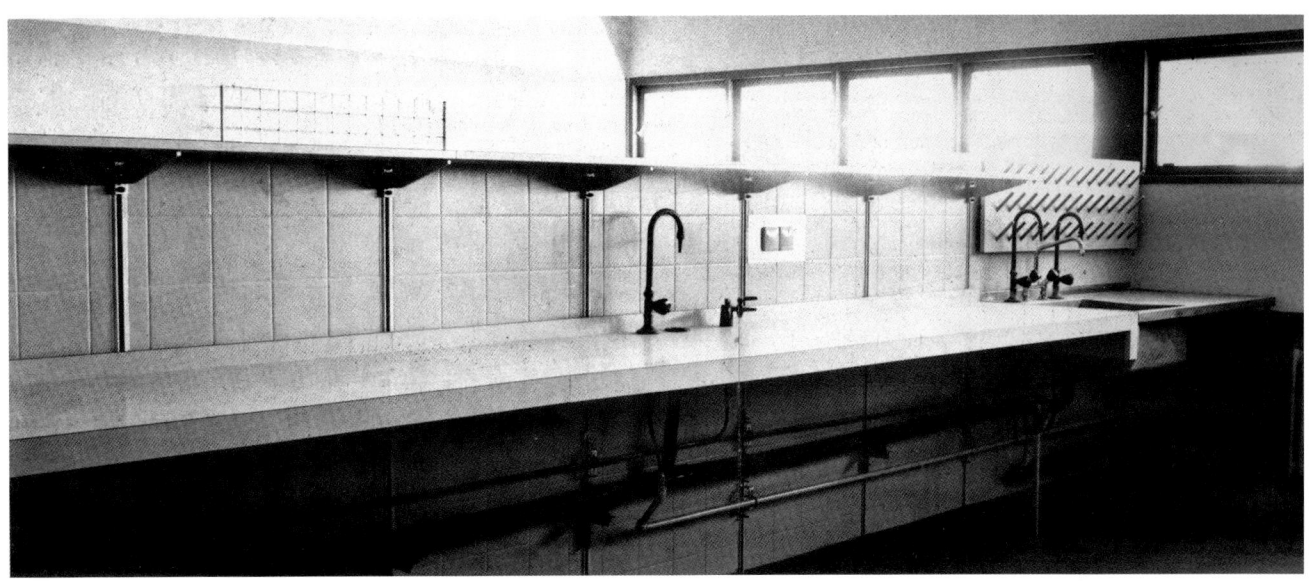

person who works at the bench. In other words, the width of the laboratory is obtained by adding measurements which depend on parts of the human body. These measurements are more or less stable for a given population. In our experience, the axial width obtained from the job analysis concerned is 3.20–3.60 m. This is confirmed by actual working conditions. The "depth" of the modular laboratory is given by the conditions prescribed by the division of the area and by reasonable proportions relating to the movements of the workers in the laboratory unit. Experience shows that in dividing the laboratory areas according to purpose, it is often necessary to provide for areas smaller than the modular unit. These areas which are usually in the order of 10–12 sqm., are assigned for the laboratory office or for small special-purpose laboratories. If the width of the laboratory is 3.20–3.60 m., a depth twice as large will be a reasonable modular measurement. Accordingly, the modular laboratory unit will be 3.60 × 7.20 sqm. The laboratories area will be a multiple of the modular laboratory. In- and outflow systems will relate to the modular laboratory unit. Experience, as well as simple calculation, will show that with these measurements, an optimum ratio of laboratory bench length for the total area of the laboratory department is obtained. The ratio of bench length divided into laboratories area expresses the efficiency of use of the laboratory area and the maximum number of laboratory workers for the given area.

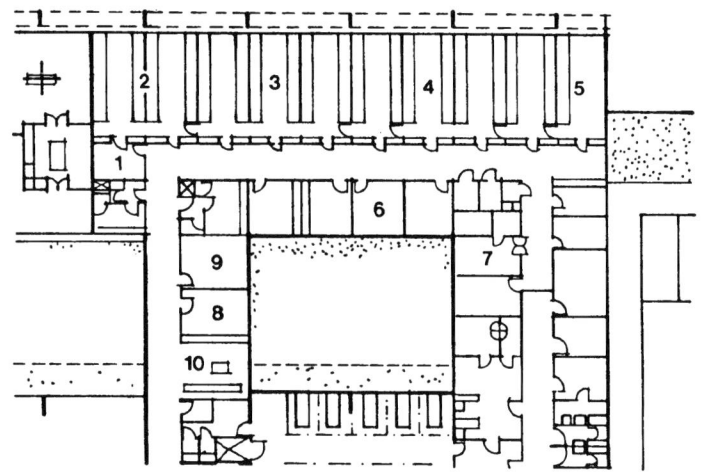

Safed Hospital
Laboratory wing
1. Blood bank
2. Haematology
3. Bacteriology
4. Virology
5. Cytogenetics and cytochemistry
6. Laboratories' offices
7. Laboratories' kitchen
8. Patients' and specimen reception
9. Specimen-taking and examination room
10. Waiting area

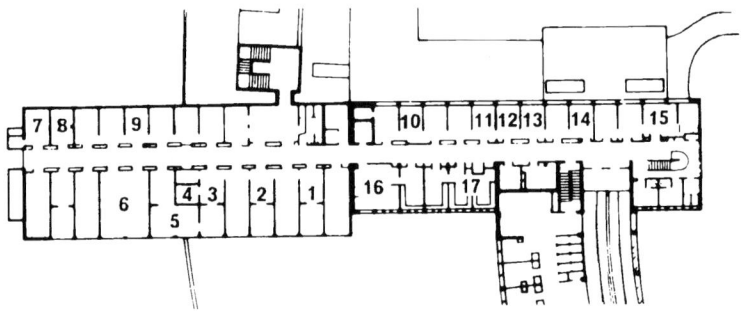

Meir Hospital
Laboratory wing
1. Specimen-taking and examination room
2. Haematology
3. Cytogenetics and cytochemistry
4. Processing room
5. Departmental head's room
6. Seminar room
7. P.B.I. room
8. Chromatography
9. General laboratory space
10. Bacteriology
11. Culture room
12. Serology
13. Parasitology
14. Clean room
15. Radioisotope diagnostic laboratory
16. General storeroom

Joint facilities

In large laboratory departments which contain several sections, such as virology, bacteriology etc., there is a tendency for section heads to concentrate the equipment needed for their work in their own departments. This trend is particularly marked in research laboratories. We refer, of course, to expensive equipment, not to standard laboratory equipment. Such equipment can generally be used by several sections or even the entire laboratory department. The concentration and installation of such equipment in a manner enabling it to serve all the sections which need it, results in a working system and a distribution of areas according to purpose, based on the "joint services" principle.

4. Health Facilities in Israel

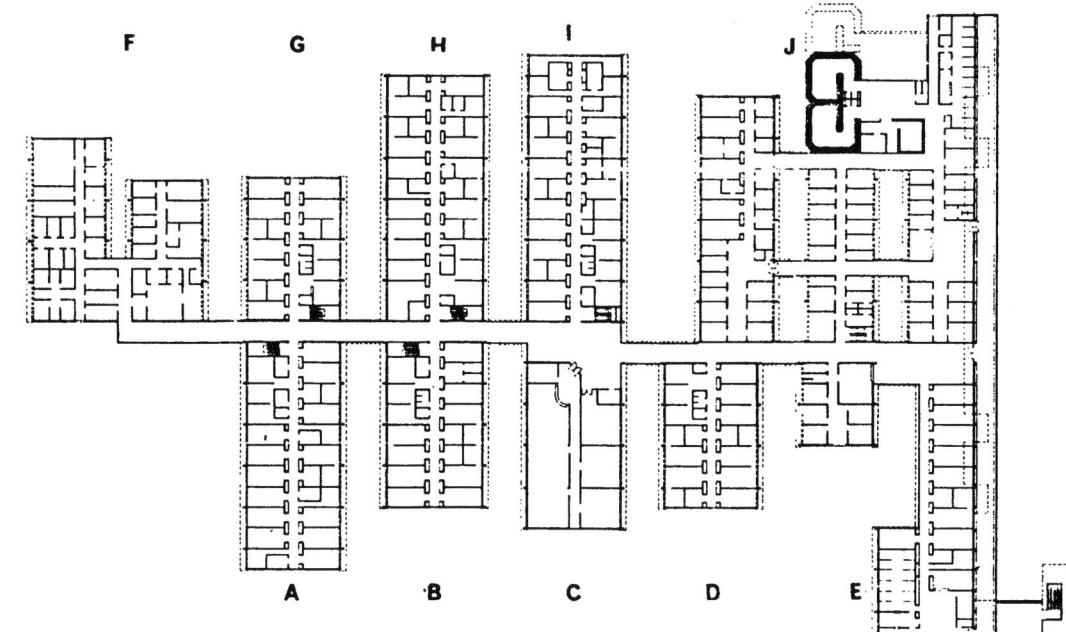

Sheba Medical Centre
Laboratory wing

A. Bacteriology
B. Cytogenetics and cytochemistry
C. Shared laboratory services
D. Haematology
E. Patient reception area and blood bank
F. Animal house
G. Clinical research laboratories
H. Biochemistry
I. Histology and electron microscopy
J. Radiotherapy and radioisotopes

The "joint service" may be of a pure service nature, like washing and sterilizing of glassware, or of such a sophisticated nature as electron microscopy. The planning of the department's work according to this principle occasionally meets with resistance on the scientists. The designer of the department must take the possibility of centralized services into account, even if the scientists do not agree to it to begin with. Scientific equipment becomes more expensive and more complicated each year. Work in a laboratory department which is not based on centralized services results in duplication of equipment and inadequate use of the equipment acquired. Without any doubt, the day will come when it will be practically impossible to supply expensive laboratory equipment to each separate section. Moreover, there is the question of specialization in the use and maintenance of such equipment. Centralization of equipment makes it possible to specialize in its operation and maintenance.

Planning the work of the laboratory department according to the "joint services" principle permits each scientist to make the maximum use of the equipment available to the department; experience shows that this is not the case in departments where the expensive equipment is kept by the different sections and the section heads are in charge of it.

Supply and waste disposal methods

Decisions as to the type of supply and waste removal systems to be used are extremely important. For all practical purposes, these decisions will determine most of the data characterizing the laboratory department, especially with regard to the division of the laboratory area according to purpose. It may be said that these initial decisions lay down the "rules of the game" for planning the laboratory area. There are several methods of supply and waste removal; each has its own advantages and disadvantages. The choice of a given method depends on different aspects of the project in question, although any method employed is subject to the following conditions:

a. Planning and execution of the main and sub-main systems independently from the division of the laboratory areas according to purpose.

b. Provision of standard supply and waste removal facilities for all laboratories in a modular manner and in accordance with a uniform plan for the laboratory areas, adjusted to the architectural design. According to this "philosophy," standard supply lines are determined for the entire area. Generally the list of facilities to be supplied includes ordinary water, hot water, gas, pressurized water, one or two reserve lines, a "uniform 4" run-off system and a 220 V. electrical supply. Decisions about "standard" supplies often involve tiresome arguments with scientists. Any additions to the list make the system more complicated and more expensive.

It is desirable to determine the method of supply to the laboratory benches at this stage as well. Planning of the laboratory benches themselves will take place in the second stage. The method used to connect supply and waste disposal lines with the secondary system should be uniform for the entire laboratories area.

4. Health Facilities in Israel

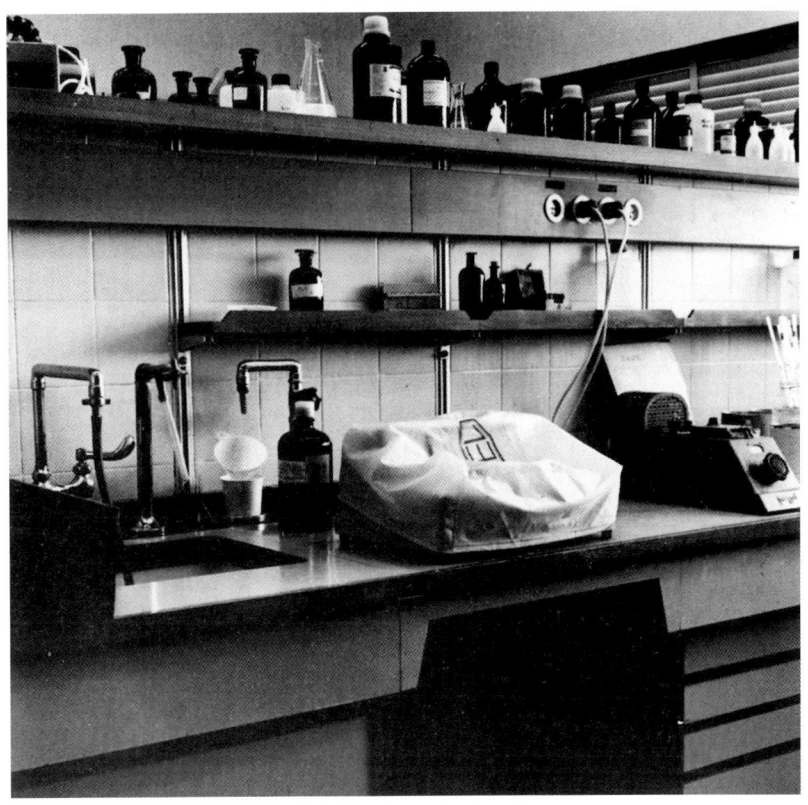

All the methods of supply and waste removal described below are based on the same philosophy and follow the same planning principles:

1. Horizontal main supply in the area of the central corridor and vertical sub-main supply. In this method, the main system is planned in the centre of the department, below or above the corridor area. From this main system, a secondary system ascends (or descends) through the area between the corridor and the area assigned to the laboratories, generally on both sides of the door of the fixed module. The secondary system has standard branching points at a suitable height. The laboratory bench system is connected to these branch paints.

This is usually the least expensive method of supply. However, its use places certain limitations on the planning and maintenance of the department. The choice of a "descending" secondary supply system means that the waste removal system, which works by gravity, must be planned separately. A low level horizontal main supply system with "ascending" secondary supply requires the planning of a service tunnel under the first floor of the laboratory department – not always possible in view of the overall plan of the hospital. Since the branch lines to the laboratory benches come from vertical secondary supply lines, a system cannot be cut off by a section or floor of the laboratory department. Often in- and outflow by floor or department is prescribed as a condition of the design, and in such a case, use of this method is ruled out. Moreover, employment of this method requires that the department be divided by the corridor, making it impossible to plan a section across the entire width of the floor. This is rarely a requirement in routine laboratories, but rather in research laboratories.

2. Vertical main supply at the end of the department and horizontal sub-main supply above the corridors: According to this method, the secondary supply lines run along the corridors, above the level of the doors. The space available for supply lines is limited. Since air-conditioning ducts must sometimes be accommodated in the same space, very careful planning is required. In order to adhere to our philosophy (leaving open possibilities for changes in purpose) it is necessary to install an exhauster in each laboratory module or at least one for each two laboratory modules. In the method described here, such an exhauster would be a "deviation". Since it is desirable to expel the air from each exhauster separately and release it in the roof region, the use of vertical exhaust lines appears to be the more logical method.
The vertical supply method allows every module to be planned with a suitable passage for an exhaust channel. Generally, this system is feasible in a building with three or four laboratory floors, while the system based on horizontal secondary supply lines leaves no practical possibility open for the installation of a horizontal exhaust channel. Vertical placement, however, cancels out a considerable part of the advantages of this method.
According to this method, the waste disposal system lies in the corridor region of the floor below the one served by it.

3. Vertical main supplies and horizontal peri metrical sub-main supply lines near the outside walls. In this system, the main supply lines run vertically through shafts located in the corners of the laboratory wing or in other places. The secondary lines run along the outside walls, usually below the windows, with secondary branching points to the laboratory benches in each modular laboratory unit. With this method however, the length of the secondary supply lines is limited by

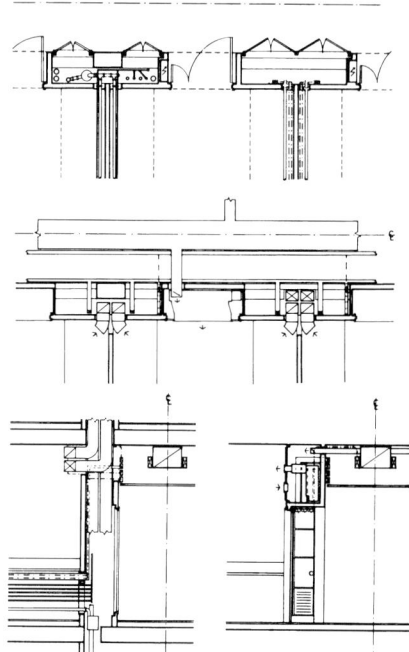

Mechanical system in standard laboratory module

the inclination of the waste disposal lines. A further difficulty arises if the possibility of passage from one laboratory to another via doors near the outside walls is insisted upon, since if outflow lines are not located in the floor space below the labs, they will be hard to accommodate elsewhere.

The question of doors between the laboratories is always a complicated one, regardless of which supply method is used. In most cases, the installation of doors near the outer walls of the corridors is made possible by manoeuvering the supply lines to some extent. For reasons of safety, doors near the outer walls are to be preferred.

4. Horizontal main supplies and vertical secondary supplies near the outside walls. This method has the same disadvantage as method 1; the system cannot be divided according to department or floor. Moreover, providing vertical secondary supply lines on the outside wall (which contains the windows of the laboratories), makes it difficult to use the dividing walls to sub-divide the area according to purpose.

As we have seen, the entire area is divided into standard units or fixed modules. The fixed module is about 24 sqm. (net), (obtained by multiplying the width of the laboratory by its "depth"). This module may be subdivided into two smaller laboratories of 12 sqm. each, but that does not mean that the laboratory programme can be composed exclusively of 12 sqm. in. units. There will always be requirements for larger or smaller units (darkrooms, cold rooms, special storerooms or larger laboratories for specific instruments), and therefore the planning solution is to divide the standard laboratory into smaller units. This means that it must be theoretically possible to build dividing walls on each division line. If the laboratory is 3.60 m. wide, it can be divided into four areas resulting in a possible laboratory width of a multiple of 90 cm. In order to make such a division possible, the placement of windows in the outside wall will have to be planned accordingly.

All the methods discussed present the difficulty of coordinating the modularity of the supply lines with the division according to purpose. Experience shows that the problem can be dealt with by suitable manoeuvering of the supply lines to the laboratory benches; but in the case of method 4, the difficulty is greater than in the other methods.

5. Intermediate floors method: An extreme solution to the supply-line location problem is that of planning a service floor between the laboratory floors. This is too expensive for ordinary hospital laboratories,

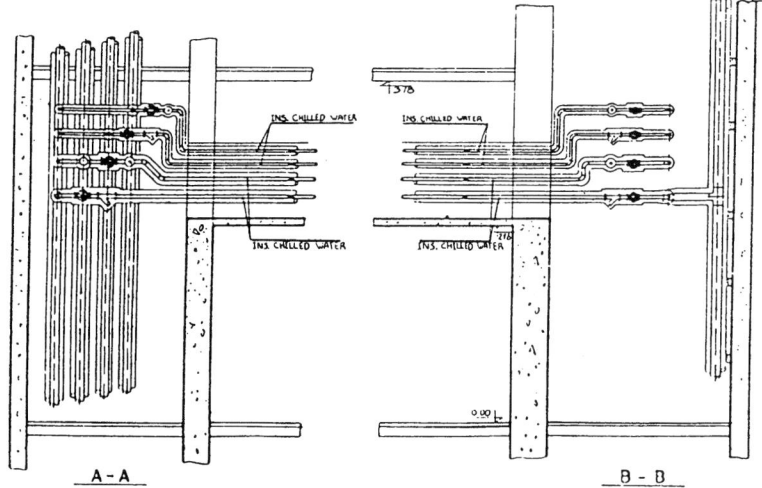

Hebrew University, Jerusalem
Diagram of supply sub-mains in the Life Sciences
Building

but may be justified for special research labs. A possible compromise
is to run the pipes under the ceiling of the floor below the one served by
these pipelines. When a single laboratory floor is located above a floor
in which the laying of pipelines is unrestricted – such as a technical
floor – this method presents an inexpensive and flexible solution with
a maximum of advantages.

Air conditioning for the laboratories department

Given the climatic conditions in Israel, it may be assumed that most
of the laboratory area will be air conditioned. The problems of planning air conditioning for a laboratory differ from those of planning
air conditioning in other areas. If effort has been invested in the planning and building of a laboratory area with flexible possibilities for
sub-division according to purpose, this principle must not be negated
by the installation of an "inflexible" air-conditioning system. Apart
from flexibility, there is also the question of thermic load, which may
vary according to the use in each laboratory of Bunsen burners, ovens,
exhausters, etc. Obviously, the aim of the air-conditioning consultant
must be to plan a system which will not limit division according to
purpose and which will adjust itself automatically to the conditions
prevailing in any laboratory.

Several sophisticated systems developed abroad have been tried in
Israel and have been in use long enough to allow some conclusions to
be drawn. As in the case of other types of systems, the methods which
may work well elsewhere cannot simply be copied here. Differences in

4. Health Facilities in Israel

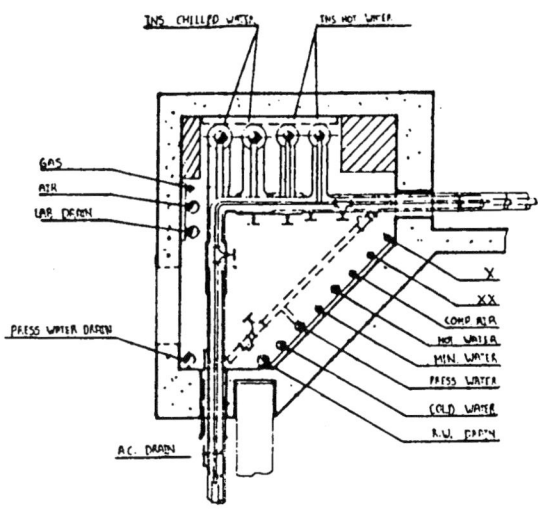

climatic conditions and working habits, maintenance difficulties, and cost of installation and operation, all make it imperative to use methods and systems suitable for local conditions. The air-conditioning, ventilation and exhaust systems must be adjusted to and integrated into the planning of the laboratory department. Generally, the main machine rooms lie outside the laboratory department and do not concern us in this context. We shall therefore discuss only those components of the system which belong specifically to this department.

As mentioned above, certain conditions must be met when choosing the air-conditioning system for the laboratories wing. The most important of these are: flexible possibilities for sub-division according to purpose, preservation of constant climatic conditions in each laboratory unit by automatic adjustment of the air-conditioning system to the changing laboratory conditions and prevention of contamination from one laboratory unit to another.

A method known as the reheat method is inexpensive to install while still meeting the above requirements. With this method, the air flows to the laboratories through a duct system at temperatures lower than required. An electric coil located in the air outlet to the laboratory space is regulated by a thermostat located within the laboratory itself. This method, however, consumes a great deal of electricity, which is very expensive in Israel. Therefore, because of the high maintenance costs involved, the reheat method is not really acceptable for general use. Another system which meets the above-mentioned conditions is based on the fan & coil method. In this system, the fan & coil units are installed in the laboratory spaces, near the outer wall, above or below the window, or near the corridor wall, usually above door height. Air is circulated in the laboratory space by the units' fan. The air passes through the heated or cooled coil, whichever is necessary. Temperature of the coil is regulated by a thermostat located in the laboratory space. A piping system connected to the heating/refrigeration centre of the hospital feeds the unit's coils.

When the fan & coil method is employed, part of the circulated air must be exchanged for "fresh" air. This is accomplished either by pumping in air from outside (when the unit is located near an external wall), or by flowing pre-treated air in ducts to the fan & coil units. The fan & coil method is used in many laboratory wings in Israel. The main drawbacks are expensive installation and high maintenance costs.

Still another method acceptable for use in Israel is the double ducts method. In this method the air flows into the laboratory spaces through a system of two ducts. The air moving through one duct is much colder than that in the other. "Mixing boxes" are installed at the air outlets of the laboratory units, and contain a regulating system controlled by a thermostat located within the laboratory space. This regulating system determines the "mixing", i.e. the quantity of air flowing from each duct to the laboratory space, and thus regulates the temperature of the flowing air.

The double duct method is expensive to install and takes up the spaces needed for passing the ducts (these spaces are smaller than the spaces required in a regular system because a high velocity system is usually used). The main advantage of this method, however, is its inexpensive maintenance and reliable functioning.

Other systems exist of course, as do variations of the systems described. In any case, a system must be chosen according to the architectural concept of the laboratory wing. An unfortunate condition is created when there is no coordination between the planning of the air-conditioning system and the architectural plan for the laboratory wing.

Outpatient Clinics

Functions of the outpatient clinics

The description given here relates to outpatient clinics which are attached to the hospital and whose function is to provide specialist consultation and follow-up for patients who have been discharged from the hospital. Outpatient clinics deal with most branches of medicine and include general examination rooms; treatment rooms; and departments for ophthalmology, skin diseases, psychiatry, audiology, gynaecology, obstetrics, pediatrics, surgery, orthopedics, etc. A number of hospitals have clinics which in addition to these functions, serve as polyclinics for the population of the district. The most familiar is the widespread network of polyclinics belonging to the Labour Federation Sick Fund.

Location of the outpatient clinics

The outpatient clinics make use of the hospital's medical service departments, including the various institutes, the laboratories etc. Patients reaching the clinics are, according to need, sent to the Radiology Institute, the Lung Function Institute, the Cardiology Institute, and so forth. The outpatient clinics must therefore be located within the general plan of the hospital, in such a way that these services can be provided.

Since the medical staff of the hospital also serves in the clinics, internal lines of communication must therefore provide the staff with adequate access to the clinics.

The hospital's different supply services (supply of pharmaceuticals, sterile supplies, etc.) must also be available to the clinics. Supply routes connecting these services with the clinics are therefore planned.

Outpatients reach the clinics through the main entrance of the hospital or through a special entrance. Outpatients may be brought to certain medical services, such as the Radioisotope Institute, the Radiotherapy Institute, the Physiotherapy Institute, etc., on stretchers. Traffic connections thus dictate the location of the department within the general hospital plan. An effort is made to locate the department so that it is not necessary for the public to pass through other sections in order to reach the outpatient clinics, and so that regular hospital traffic is not interfered with.

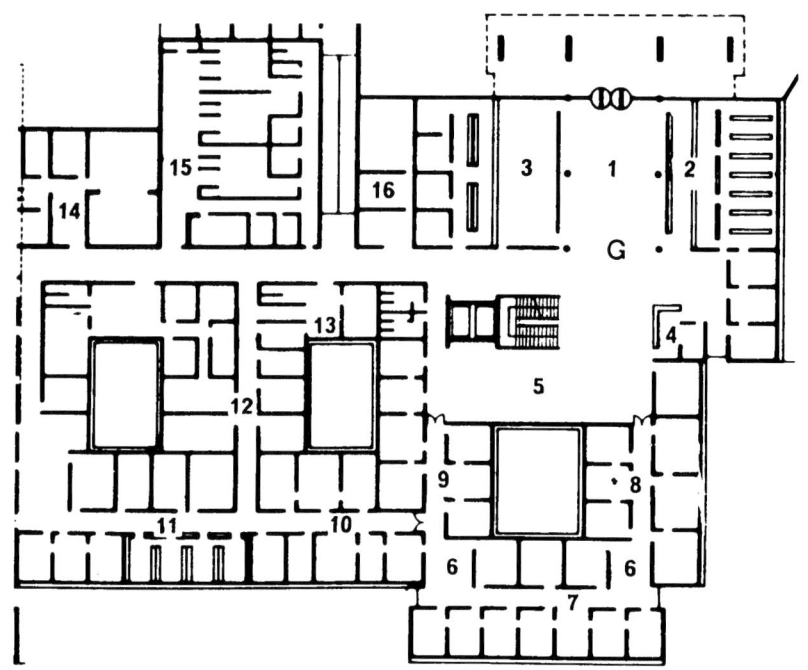

Meir Hospital
Outpatient department
Entrance floor

1. Entrance hall
2. Reception and archives
3. Cafeteria
4. Information
5. Floor waiting area
6. Local waiting areas
7. Internal medicine
8. Cardiology
9. Immunology
10. Pulmonary function
11. Radioisotope unit
12. Laboratories
13. Blood bank
14. Occupational therapy
15. X-ray department
16. Pharmacy

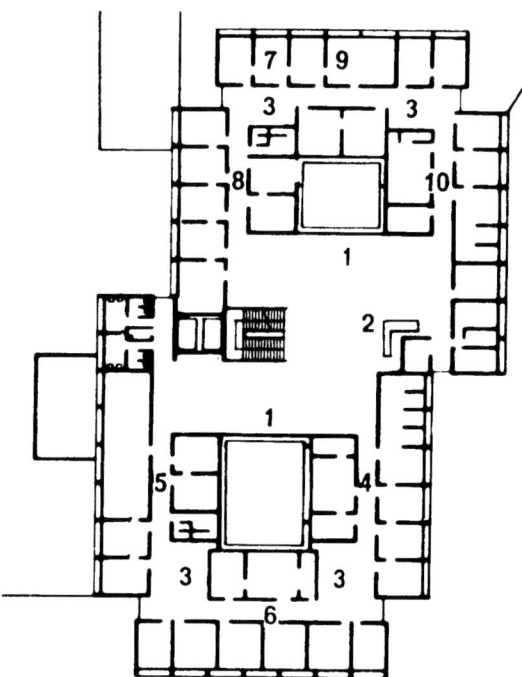

First floor plan

1. Floor waiting area
2. Information
3. Local waiting areas
4. Orthopedics
5. Surgical treatment
6. Minor surgery
7. Oncology
8. Gynaecology
9. Electroencephalography
10. Urology

4. Health Facilities in Israel

Lower ground floor plan
1. O.P.D. lower ground floor
2. Future extension of O.P.D.
3. Machine room
4. Staff lockers
5. E.N.T.
6. Opthalmology
7. Floor waiting area
8. Information
9. Local waiting areas

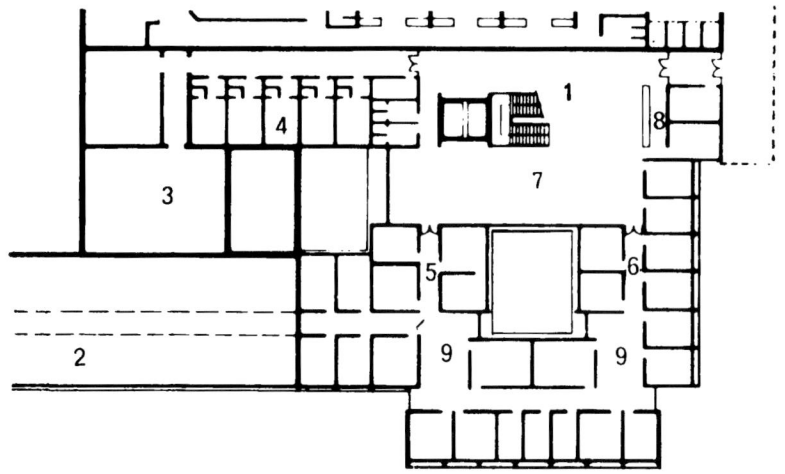

It is not always possible to provide a system of internal and external routes which take into account all of the required communications. In some cases, duplication of services is difficult to avoid, and this results in greater building, procurement and maintenance costs. Moreover, a larger hospital staff is then required to operate the duplicated services. These services should be administratively answerable to the central hospital services but, human nature being what it is, they occasionally tend to develop independently, entailing an increase in expenditure beyond what is necessary and essential. Hence, choosing the right location for the outpatient clinics is extremely important.

Waiting facilities for patients
The main problem in planning the outpatient clinics is that of providing adequate waiting facilities for the patients. Several methods of allotting time and directing patients to the appropriate rooms for examination and treatment are in use, but no method can ensure that the waiting time will be short, that there will be no time gap between the patient's examination and treatment, and that the staff's workload will be even and continuous. There are many reasons for this.
Since the population of patients attending the outpatient clinics is far from homogeneous, their conduct is not easy to predict. Some will come before the hour for which they have been summoned, others will

be late. Many patients will not conform to the established waiting procedure, but prefer to wait outside the door of the examination room. Attempts to plan a general waiting room with comfortable waiting facilities, where patients are called by number or name, have not been successful in Israel. Too often the waiting area is empty, while the patients crowd the corridors and stand outside the doors of examination and treatment rooms. Attempts at direction by means of signboards or other devices have not been successful, partly because of the language problem of a multinational public, and sometimes because the habit of following signboards and instructions is not established.

Arrangements for waiting and for directing the public have developed in Israel against the background of these difficulties. The reception desk looks out into the entrance hall, where a general waiting area is located. An information clerk stationed at a clearly visible place in the waiting area directs the patient to the right department or floor.

The patient stays in the waiting area of the floor or department until he is called to the examination room. In order to assure the continuity of visits, a local waiting facility is provided near each group of examination or treatment rooms. Sometimes the waiting facility of the floor and the local waiting facility are combined and a waiting area is provided outside the examination and treatment rooms. An attempt is made to plan the traffic routes for the patients as clearly and simply as possible and to keep walking distances short. Attempts are made to make the waiting areas attractive and pleasant for the patients.

This system of entrance half with general waiting area, waiting facilities on each floor, and local waiting facilities results in a flexibility which allows the outpatient clinics' administration to direct and regulate the movements of the public as required at any given time. Forecasts of the number and type of patients to be dealt with by each department serve as the basis for planning the waiting areas.

Typical group of rooms and typical examination room
The examination rooms are planned as interchangeable standard rooms. Great effort is invested in the planning of the typical examination room so that it will be serviceable for most departments. Examination rooms are grouped so as to provide internal access for the staff without requiring them to pass through the waiting rooms. The typical examination room includes a dressing corner for the patient, an examination couch, an "office" corner for the examining doctor and of course, all the accessories required by the function of the room.

4. Health Facilities in Israel

Sheba Medical Centre
Outpatient department

A. Reception and waiting
1. Entrance
2. Waiting
3. Information and registration

B. Ophtalmology
4. Combined consultation and examination rooms
5. Darkroom
6. Darkroom for refraction and retinoscopy

C. General
7. General purpose combined consulting and examination rooms

D. Dermatology
8. Examination room and laboratory
9. Nurses

E. Psychiatry
10. Treatment room
11. Examination room

F. Audiology
12. Audiometry room
13. Doctors' room

G. E.N.T. and jaw
14. Consultation and treatment rooms
15. Waiting
16. Recovery room
(Shared by general treatment)

H. General treatment
17. Cystoscopy
18. Nurses' and treatment rooms
19. Plaster room

I. Cardiology – dept. A and B
20. Entrance
21. Waiting
22. Departmental head's room, reception and Records
23. Dept. A
Phono- and vector-cardiography rooms
Dept. B
Functional evaluation laboratories, exam., doctors' rooms
24. Consultation / examination rooms
25. Specimen laboratories – dye dilution; clinical laboratory and instant blood examination; histology laboratory
26. Doctors' rooms

K. Epidemiology research unit
27. Office and reception
28. Examination rooms

L. Pace-maker department
29. Pace-maker
30. Doctors' room and patient preparation area
31. Control room
32. Laboratory

M. Gastroenterology
33. Gastroscopy
34. Laboratories
35. Doctors' rooms

N. Pulmonary function and e.E.G
36. Pulmonary function examination Rooms
37. Electromiography and neurology
38. Examination rooms
39. Patient preparation room

O. Records department
40. Head librarian; medical secretaries; Statistics and microfilms
41. Offices
42. Records and filing office
43. Computer units
44. Files

P. Physiotherapy
45. Reception
46. Gymnasium and hydrotherapy
47. Examination and treatment

Q. Medical photography department
48. Office
49. Photocopying and photomicrography
50. Medical photography

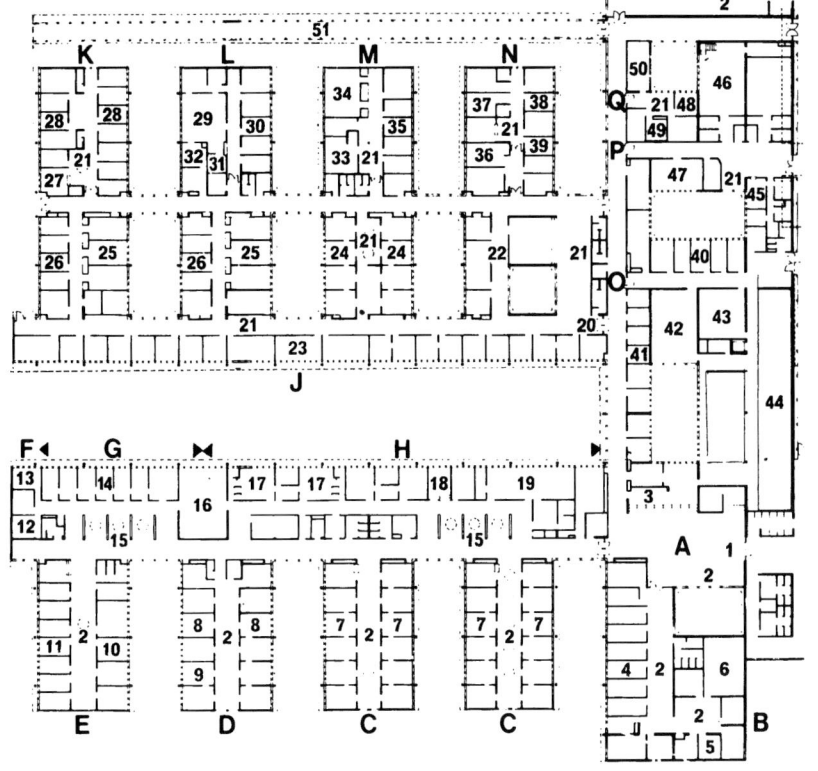

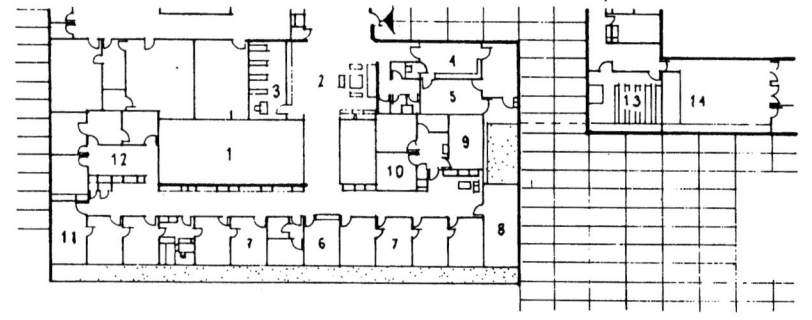

Safed Hospital
Outpatient department
1. Patio
2. General waiting area
3. Information and registration
4. Children's waiting room
5. Consultation and examination room
6. Nurses' room
7. Combined consultation and examination room
8. Plaster room
9. General treatment room
10. Cystoscopy room
11. Gynaecology room
12. Ophthalmology room
13. Synagogue
14. Circumcision hall

Examination and consultation rooms account for the bulk of the outpatient clinics. The treatment rooms are also grouped by department. Treatment rooms are provided with local waiting facilities in the manner already described, and include general treatment rooms, plaster rooms, cystoscopy rooms, etc.

This set-up of standard examination rooms and treatment rooms is unsuitable for certain departments, for instance, the ophthalmology department which requires special arrangements. The clinics are therefore divided by department, according to the different branches of medicine, and each department includes the special facilities it requires. At the same time, however, uniformity of planning is attempted, so that different branches may be able to use the same rooms on different days of the week.

Next to the entrance to the clinics, space is provided for a reception room and medical records office. Near the space used for storing the medical records, an area for office work is planned. The space needed for storing records is calculated for 8–10 years, based on current needs. Microfilms can be made for long-term storage beyond this period. Obviously, facilities for storing and projecting microfilms and for making such prints as are required must also be planned.

The medical records may be used as a source of data for medical statistics, epidemiological research and other medical research projects. To this end, space for a computer has been planned recently, near the medical records section in several hospitals. Mention must be made of the tendency of departmental heads to keep records of their own. The battle with directors for the concentration of all medical records in one area is a story which repeats itself in most outpatient clinics.

Safed Hospital
Typical consultation and examination room

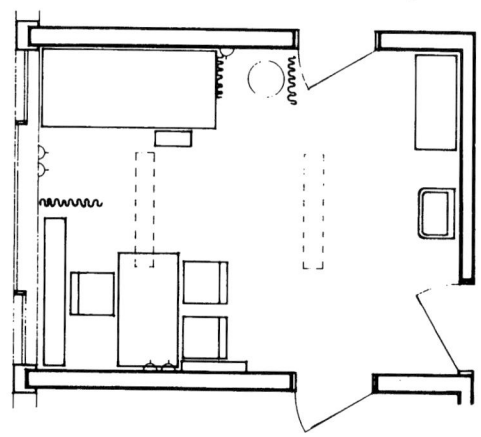

4. Health Facilities in Israel

Conclusion

The aim of the preceding descriptions has been to shed light on some of the intricate problems encountered in the planning of hospital wards and medical services. These descriptions have been included in order to demonstrate a specific philosophy and to show its application to the layout and design of a building. The development of basic planning ideas for hospital design will result in more efficient medical and supply services as well as savings in manpower.

Hospital equipment is often technologically sophisticated and also extremely expensive. Finding suitable staff to operate such equipment is a perpetual problem, particularly in developing countries. It is therefore necessary for cooperation to exist among the various departments within the hospital, as well as among the rooms within the departments themselves. Certain medical services may be shared by in- and outpatients, resulting in savings in equipment and staff. Available equipment must be utilized to the maximum. Such cooperation thus influences the general layout of the hospital.

Such cooperation (the "joint services" concept) has proved to be an important key to the problem of making quality medical services available to every member of Israel's society, from cabinet minister to the humblest citizen. The rapid growth of Israel's population, along with constantly improving medical services and care, indicates that without cooperation and efficient arrangement of medical and supply services, it becomes increasingly difficult to provide suitable medical services.

The basic problem with the layout of the medical services is to convince the client that one has to bring the suitable medical personnel to the patient (in the suitable medical service) and not to scatter the patients among different wings which are often built as a result of pressure by a noted medical personality.

The **modus operandi** of the medical and supply services are based on methods acceptable abroad and are, at the same time, influenced by the special conditions of the country, the region and the outlook of the client or operator of the hospital. Very often the doctors, departmental heads, administrators and head nurses have great influence on the size of the department and on its location within the hospital. All these influencing factors are changeable. When there are new advances in methods of supply and service or when staff changes results in changes in operating procedure, changes in the planned hospital structure become inevitable, and even strong administrative opposition is insufficient to prevent such changes and adjustments from being instituted. These changes usually affect the building's physical image, especially in regard to the medical and supply services which comprise about two-thirds of the building's area. From the moment this process begins, there exists a danger of general deterioration up to a complete loss of the building's appearance. Rooms and departments take on functions other than those originally designated. Changes are usually made unprofessionally. The areas being altered tend to take on a temporary and disorderly appearance. Traffic routes, etc. are disrupted. The attitude of the staff, patients and visitors to the building becomes one of disregard. People begin to behave in ways unacceptable under other circumstances. A situation is created that the cleaning staff cannot overcome. Valuable property deteriorates and facilities do not function properly. Danger of contamination increases as does the suffering of the patients and the tension of the medical staff. The end result is the relocation of divisions, so that the shape of the built-up area is altered until it is impossible to recognize the original plan. This process also impairs the medical work, is extremely costly and causes anguish to all those involved.

A follow-up of these developments in various hospitals and medical facilities indicates that nothing was done to prevent this deterioration. Every effort must be made to prevent such a process. However, there is no doubt that the problem is connected with administrative difficulties, the programmatic structure of the medical institutions, and with other problems not discussed here.

We shall deal only with the effect of this problem on the planning of the medical institution. The "life span" of the building is much longer than the reasonable service period of a departmental head and then the duration of a certain working system. Therefore changes in the building cannot be avoided as changes in methods of medical and supply services occur. The planning of any medical institution is based on working methods in use at the time of construction, as well as on the requirements of the clients or the operator at that particular time. When these change, alterations must be made to the building.

Therefore, attention must be given to this problem during the preliminary planning of the medical institution. The basic structure of the plan should form the "skeleton" and foundation of the traffic routes, passages, main supply systems, etc. The basic plan must allow for growth and enlargement. The structure must have dimensions that are acceptable both at the time of the plan's inception and in the foreseeable future. The layout of the departments of the medical institution must allow for additions without harming the main design concept of the institution.

From the preceding discussions it seems that the general guideline for planning a hospital includes two opposing directives. One says: plan each department specifically to suit its function; i.e. plan for specific jobs, as described by experts. But plan so that it will be able to function properly despite changing working methods. We have to mention here that different medical experts very seldom agree with one another. Therefore, a ward or medical service should not be planned to suit one personality. All medical and supply departments should be planned in such a way that options are left open for changes in procedure, etc.

The other directive says: plan as universally as possible so that you will not be "stuck" after a short period (sometimes even before the building has been completed). In other words, plan the wards and the departments with a common denominator dictated by the general concept of the building, so that in each department, changes and extensions can be made independently of the other departments.

Creating a common denominator means: planning based on preferred modules, planning modules, functional modules, structural modules, mechanical modules, etc.; repeated use of facades and openings; "open-end" planning of departments, etc. and a site plan that allows for future growth, based on present principles. Planning principles impose no limitations on design freedom. They encourage order and discipline – they are a good tool and serve as guidelines upon which design can be based and from which architectural creativity can flourish.

Hospital design is both complex and intricate, demanding a mature approach to a problem that is both technical and cultural. The essence of culture is the relationship between man and his fellow man and between man and his environment. The architect is creating an environment in which the patient often undergoes a critical period in his / her life. The patient may be greatly influenced by this environment, which, if it is a positive one, can contribute to the patient's recovery, or at least prevent unnecessary suffering.

Thus, along with mastery of complex functional problems, a principal challenge for the architect is to create an optimum relationship between the physical environment and the patient.

5

The Hospitals and Health Facilities of Zarhy Architects

1. Sheba Medical Center

Tel Hashomer, Ramat Gan

Tel Aviv, 700 Beds, 120,000 sqm, 1967–2010

Planning Principles

In planning, the accent was placed on the following principles:

a) Imparting a human scale on the hospital buildings. This is particularly important in a hospital building, which must "welcome" the patient, and try to eliminate the feeling of being a very small cog in a large machine. The vast scope of this project demanded special awareness of this factor.

b) Creating the character of a medical centre, which besides its main function of hospitalization, would also serve outpatients visiting the clinics and institutes, and engage in medical instruction and research. In a central hospital it is necessary to stress this principle without doing so at the expense of scale.

c) Flexibility of planning, allowing functional changes to be implemented with minimum changes to buildings, and allowing for increasing the size of the various units, independently and possibly at different times, as well as the addition of new departments without affecting the normal working of the hospital.

d) Maximum utilization of medical services, supply, etc., such as the X-Ray unit and the other medical institutes for hospitalized patients and out-patients.

e) The simplest possible traffic routes and flows. Such as circulations of patients, staff, out-patients, visitors, supplies and bodies. Traffic flows were separated from one another where inherent differences in character demanded this.

The General Hospital

Description of the new hospital and its Approaches

The new Tel Hashomer Hospital will be located in the area to the south of the existing Children's Department and the Maternity Hospital.

The main entrance to the Hospital, and to the casualty and admission department, is from the west. Adjoining the entrance is parking space for 600 cars. This will serve the new hospital, the Children's Section and the Maternity Hospital.

Access will be from the main road which will join the intersection of Aluf Sadeh and the Lod Road near the Ramat Pincas junction. From the external access roads are feeder roads to the following sections:

- Service Yard
- Plant rooms
- Funeral court
- Emergency hospital
- Helicopter pad
- Ministry of Health stores
- The area designated for rehabilitation buildings (future)
- Reserve areas and radiation treatment department

The Hospital Buildings

The general composition of the hospital buildings is arranged about a main east-west axis (the spine) which is also the axis of the wards, with secondary axes (the ribs) of the health and maintenance services. The ground floor of the building containing the wards serves as a link between the entrance and its adjoining facilities, the casualty and admittance section and the different health service wings.

This scheme permits the complex to be planned so that each wing can be enlarged separately if necessary, with the added possibility of enlarging the whole complex.

The Various Wings of the Building

The building includes the ward-unit wing (l) (5floors of wards). There are 20 ward units, 4 to each floor. Two circulation cores connect the various floors with the entrance level, maintenance services and supply of materials, and the gallery level. At this level corridors are linking

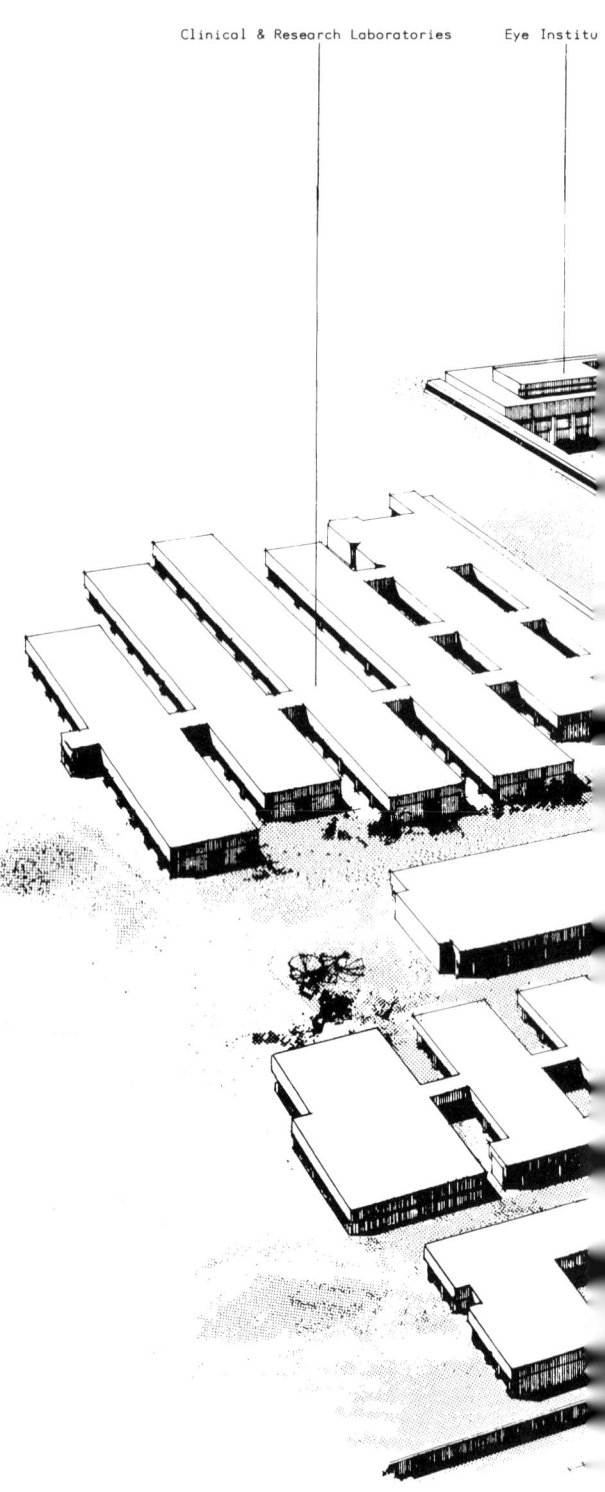

5. The Hospitals and Health Facilities of Zarhy Architects

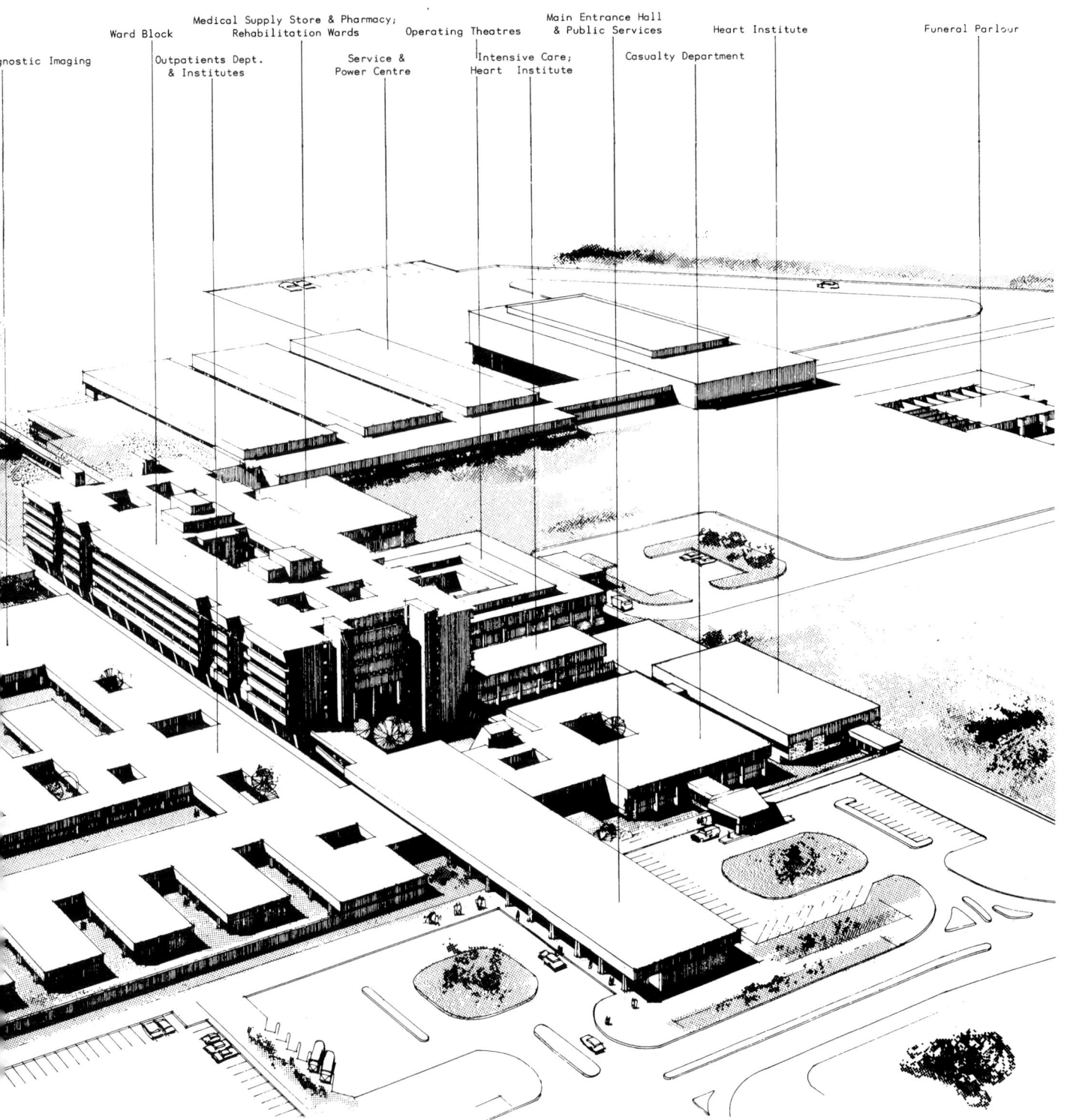

gnostic Imaging

Ward Block

Medical Supply Store & Pharmacy;
Rehabilitation Wards

Outpatients Dept.
& Institutes

Service &
Power Centre

Operating Theatres

Intensive Care;
Heart Institute

Main Entrance Hall
& Public Services

Casualty Department

Heart Institute

Funeral Parlour

the medical services wings with circulation cores of the ward-unit wing. Maintenance and services are at the lower level, below the medical service wings. The remaining wings of the building are one or two-floors in height and include:

Main entrance (4), out-patient clinics, physiotherapy, archive and medical photography, units for cardiology, pulmonary function, electro-encephalography and gastro-entrology (3), radiology (Z), laboratories: (lo), staff dining room and kitchen (9A) General stores, laundry and other services, service yard, garage, workshops (9b) plant rooms (9C):Funeral Parlour (11). The pharmacy is at ground level, with an auditorium and teaching laboratories at first floor level (8). Central sterile supply, locker rooms and the emergency hospital are at ground level with the operating theatres at first floor level (7).

Duty doctors' rooms are at ground level, with nephrology on the first floor (6). Administration is at ground level, casualty and reception on the first floor (5) with direct access at road level.

Circulation

Circulation within the Hospital

The main entrance is for staff, ambulatory patients and visitors. The public will have free access to this entrance hall. From the hall there is convenient access to administration section, and patient reception area. In addition easy and direct access is planned between patient reception area and admission and casualty wing. From the entrance hall there is also free access to the clinic wing. Check points have been strategically located, controlling the entrances to the main hospital corridors connecting the various units of the hospital, except the Reception, Admission and Casualty, Outpatient department and Administration. The admission and casualty wing is connected to the main corridor without crossing the main entrance. A convenient corridor links the clinic wing with the radiology department and laboratory wing. Pedestrian circulation is separated from that of supplies, and likewise the different types of traffic use separate lifts. Thus separate passenger and goods lifts were planned. There is no separation in the passenger lifts between patients, staff and visitors. Sources of supply in the service area are stores, kitchen, pharmacy, medical stores and the central sterile supply section. Goods will be carried in the service lifts to the various sections requiring them, while the same good lifts will be used to return various items to the mechanical units for cleaning and re-use.

5. The Hospitals and Health Facilities of Zarhy Architects

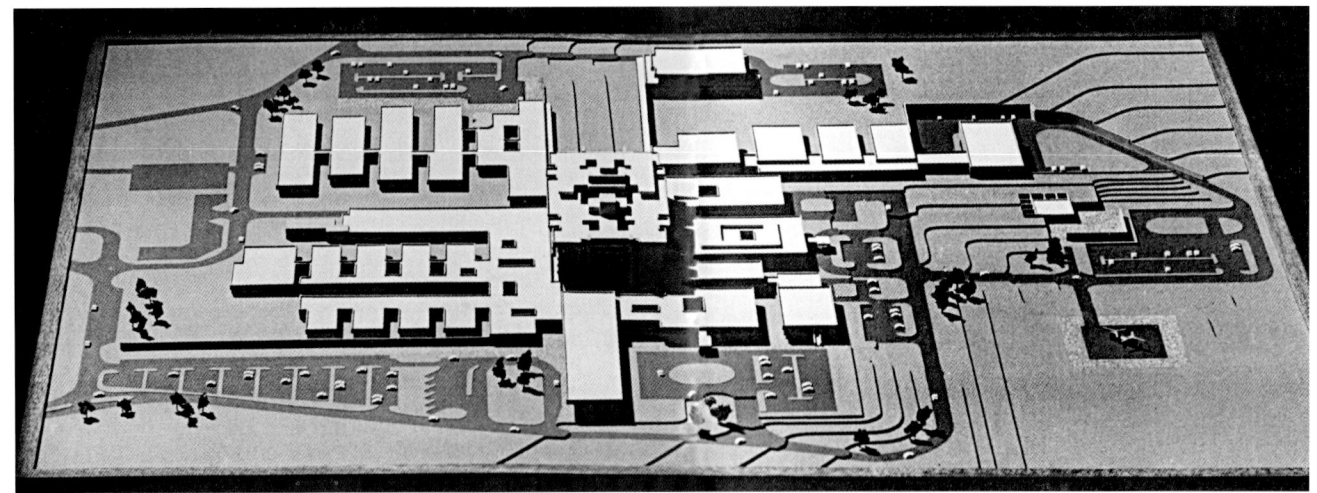

Model of Sheba Medical Center

Responsibility for supplies will fall on workers in the supply section, and not on those who receive them. This relates to general, medical and food supplies. All sterile supply will be from the central sterile supply unit. Bed-pans will be issued from a central unit; each patient receiving his own bed-pan which will be kept at his bedside and returned to the central unit for sterilizing on his discharge from hospital soiled linen will not be counted in the different units. The soiled linen will be placed in soiled linen containers, and only closed bags will be transferred via a special chute. Sterile laundry for the operating theatres will be folded at the laundry service, sterilized in the central sterile supply unit and supplied from there together with the remainder of the sterile material. Internal communication will be by means of automatic telephones. It will be possible to page certain key members of staff by radio, connected to the telephone system. In the general wards there will be an electronic communication system between patients and nurses. The corridor for transferring bodies to the mortuary has no contact with any other circulation.

Circulation of Patients

There is a separate entrance to the admission and casualty section. A link connects the main entrance to the admission and casualty entrance, through the reception wing. There is direct access for patients between this section and all the medical services, all of which are located on the same level, and also the circulation cores of the ward-unit wing by means of a covered passage.

Staff Circulation

From the main entrance hall, staff enters the system of corridors connecting all the medical services and the circulation cores of the ward-unit wing. From this level there are steps down to the building service area. Nurses' locker rooms are located at building services level.

Circulation for Visitors and Outpatients

The main entrance to the building is through the main entrance hall (4). From this hall, visitors will use a ramped corridor to the circulation cores of the ward-unit building. Thus, the public entrance to the lifts and the main steps is one level above that of the medical services. There is a corridor connecting the main entrance to the out-patient clinic entrance (3A). The radiology department (2) is located so that it can also serve the outpatient clinics. A direct link connects the main entrance and the waiting room of the reception department in building (5). From the main entrance there are steps down to the administration wing located in the ground floor (5).

Circulation on the Technical-services Floor

The maintenance section as well as medical supply services are all located on the level below that of the medical services. From the service corridor there is a direct link to the circulation cores of the ward-unit section and the health services. This supply link will be connected by a covered passage to the children and maternity sections.

Special Entrances

a) Emergency hospital – a special protected entrance on the south.
b) For special cases or where patients are brought by helicopter –
   a special entrance from the southern road.
c) To the funeral court and mortuary entrance
   from the perimeter road.
d) To the power centre and the service court –
   entrance from the perimeter road.
e) To the Radiotherapy department –
   entrance from the perimeter road.

5. The Hospitals and Health Facilities of Zarhy Architects

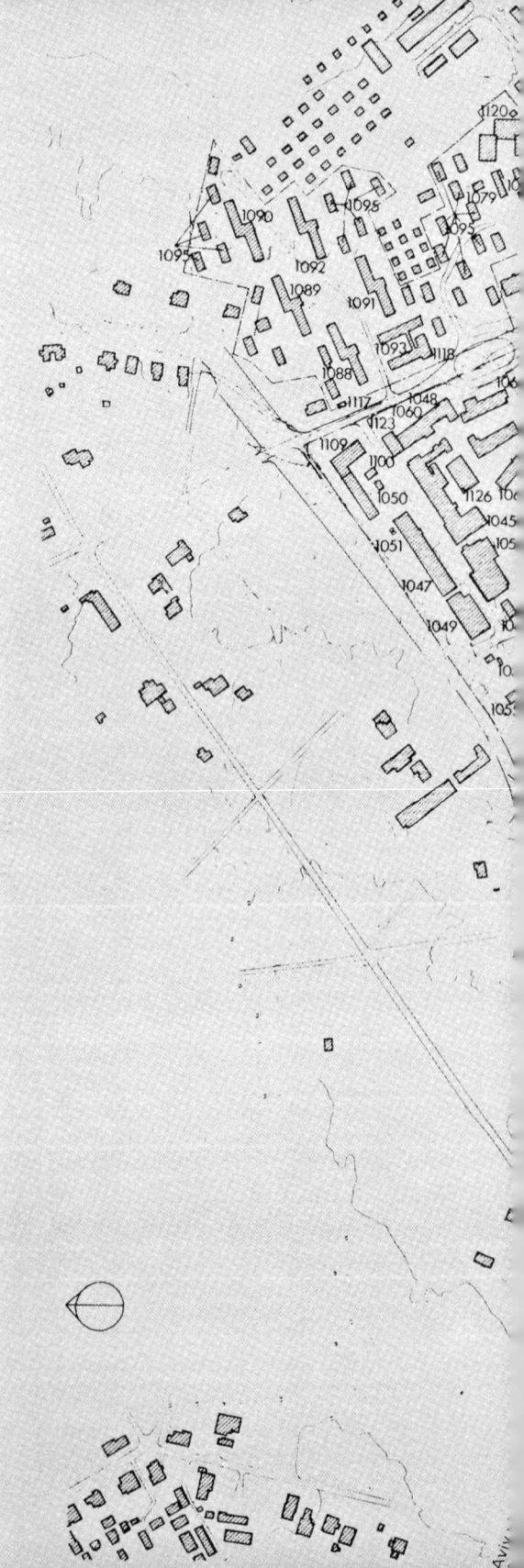

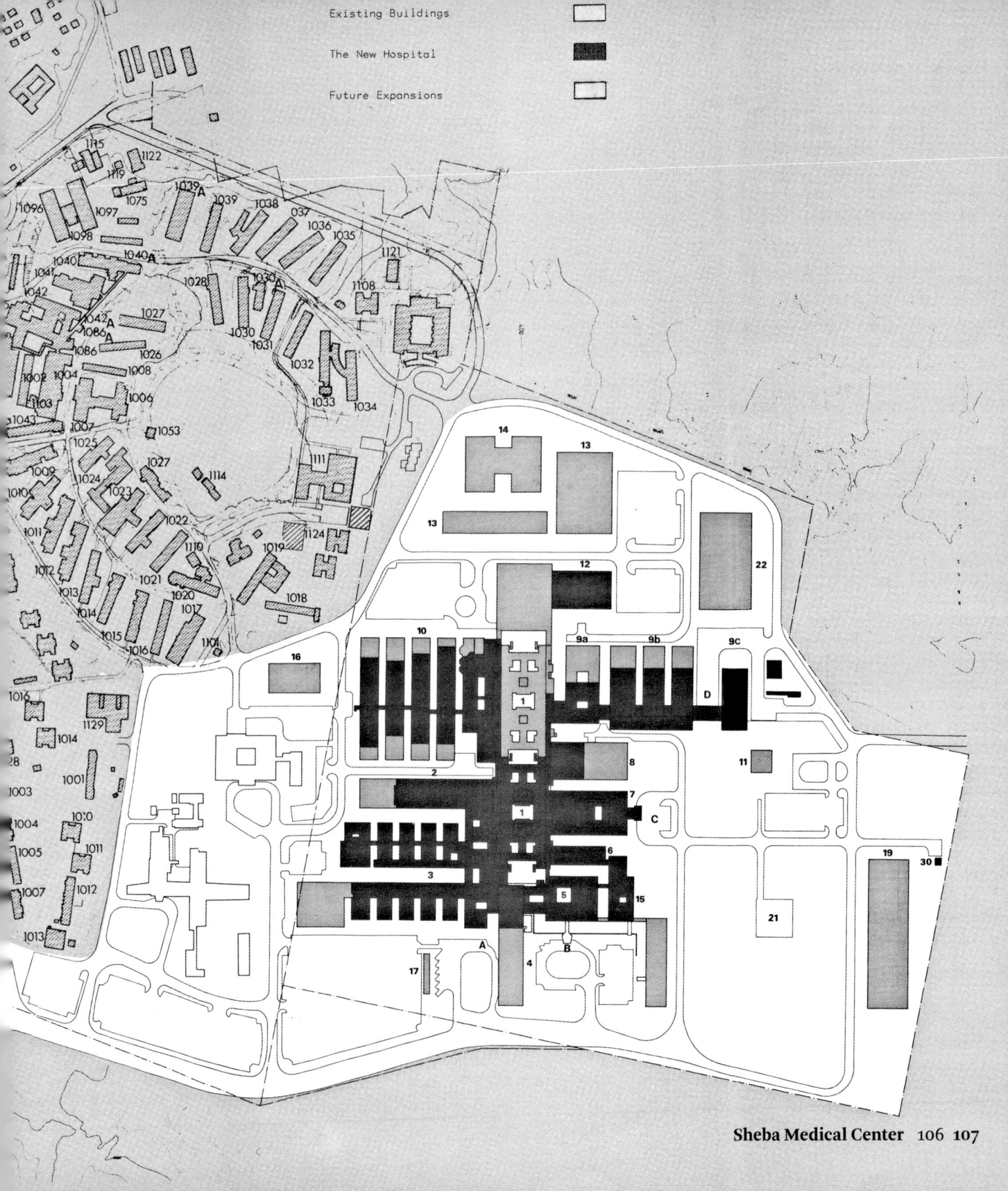

Existing Buildings

The New Hospital

Future Expansions

Departments

General Wards

Standard wards will comprise 36 beds, with intrinsic teaching facilities. Thirty beds are in 3-bed wards, and six in private wards. In certain cases, such as for heart patients, certain modifications will be made. In the first stage, as was stated previously, 20 such units are planned. The basic ward-unit comprises wards, nurses' station, stores, ancillary rooms, treatment rooms, doctors' rooms and rooms for seminars and medical students. The ancillary functions serving each of the 4 ward-units per floor are grouped together. This type of planning allows for flexibility in dividing the departments according to needs.

Casualty and Admission Section

All casualty patients will be brought to this department, and all patients will be received here, except for maternity cases and children. The department therefore contains medical, surgical and administrative services. Attached to the medical and surgical services there will be cubicles, a treatment room for shock, an operating theatre and a plaster-room, overnight beds, and all ancillary facilities. Nearby will be administration facilities for admitting patients to hospital.

Administration

The administration of the general hospital will be concentrated in one wing, located on the ground floor of building (5). The psychiatric hospital will have separate administrative facilities.

Nephrology

This unit will also be centralized. Dialysis facilities are planned for patients with chronic uremia and urgent cases in need of dialysis of the kidneys, as well as for the other departments, such as preparation of patients for kidney transplants. This unit will serve as a central station for the hospital for treatment of this kind.

Duty Doctor's Living Quarters

Twenty rooms for duty-doctors have been planned.

Medical Records and Secretariat

Place has been set aside for storage facilities for about 8 years, for storing microfilms, and for projection. Likewise, there will be data

5. The Hospitals and Health Facilities of Zarhy Architects

Master plan of the new hospital

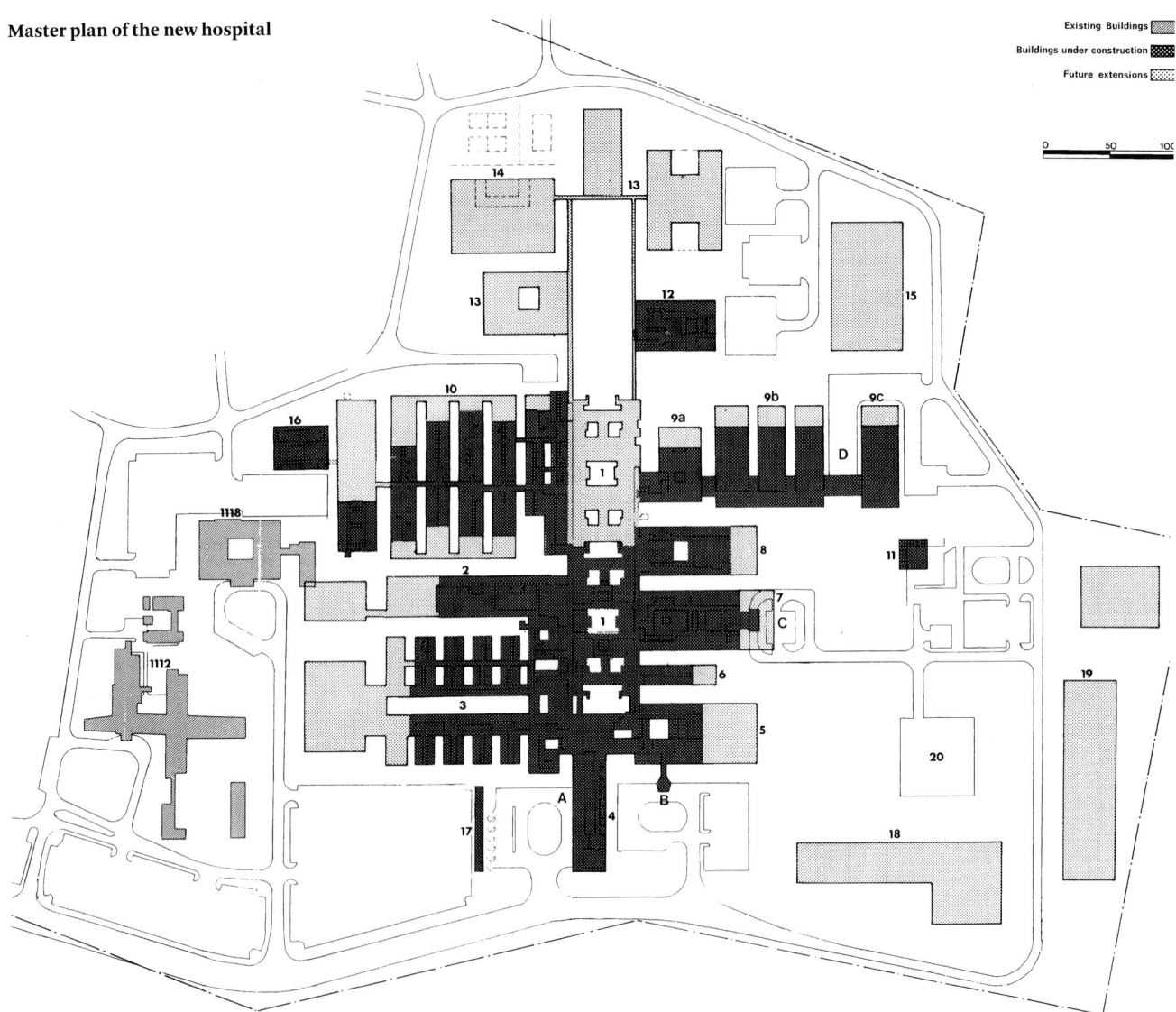

Existing Buildings
Buildings under construction
Future extensions

0   50   100

1. Main building
2. Radiology
3. Outpatient department
4. Entrance hall and public services
5. Casualty and admission
   Ground level – administration
6. Nephrology. Ground level – Night duty
7. Operating theatres
   Ground level – Central cloak rooms
   Central sterile supply dep.
   Underground casualty unit
8. Lecture hall and library
   Ground level – Pharmacy

9. Main dining hall
   Ground level – Service
   maintenance and central
   power supply
10. Clinical and research laboratories
11. Mourners' parlour
12. Eye institute
13. Institutes
14. Recreation centre and occupational
    therapy
15. Service and maintenance building
16. Animal house and
    experimental surgery

17. BUS station
18. Rehabilitation centre
19. General store building
20. Helicopter landing pad

1112. Obstetrics and maternity
1118. Children's hospital

A. Main entrance
B. Entrance to casualty department
C. Entrance to underground
   casualty unit
D. Service entrance

processing facilities for medical statistics, for epidemiological studies, and research projects. In the basement floor reserve space has been set aside for storage of past medical records, and there is space for a computer.

Outpatients' Services

It is intended that these services shall be consultative and follow-up in nature. Facilities will be provided for all the medical and surgical disciplines, apart from obstetrics, gynaecology, pediatrics and psychiatry, which have their own buildings. Outpatients will use the central radiological department and the central medical services.

Physiotherapy and Occupational Therapy

In this field only limited services will be available, as wider facilities exist at the rehabilitation centre.

Medical Photography and Illustration

A central unit is planned for these services, with facilities for photography and clinical screening, for developing and enlarging films of all kinds, mainly micro-films.

Electro-encephalography

This unit will only serve the central hospital. There will be separate facilities for the Psychiatric Hospital.

Central cardiological services

All the existing services will be concentrated in one wing, which will constitute a central service. Heart disease patients will continue to receive treatment in the various clinical departments. The central cardiology service will act in a consultative capacity to all the hospital departments and for out-patients. Specialized electro-cardiography and cardiac function tests will be carried out. In addition to its own special equipment the cardiology centre will also use equipment located in the departments, such as radiology, radio-active isotopes and the various laboratories. It will also be active in teaching and research.

Pulmonary Function

As in the case of the existing unit, the new one will serve both inpatients and outpatients.

5. The Hospitals and Health Facilities of Zarhy Architects

Entrance level, ±0.00.

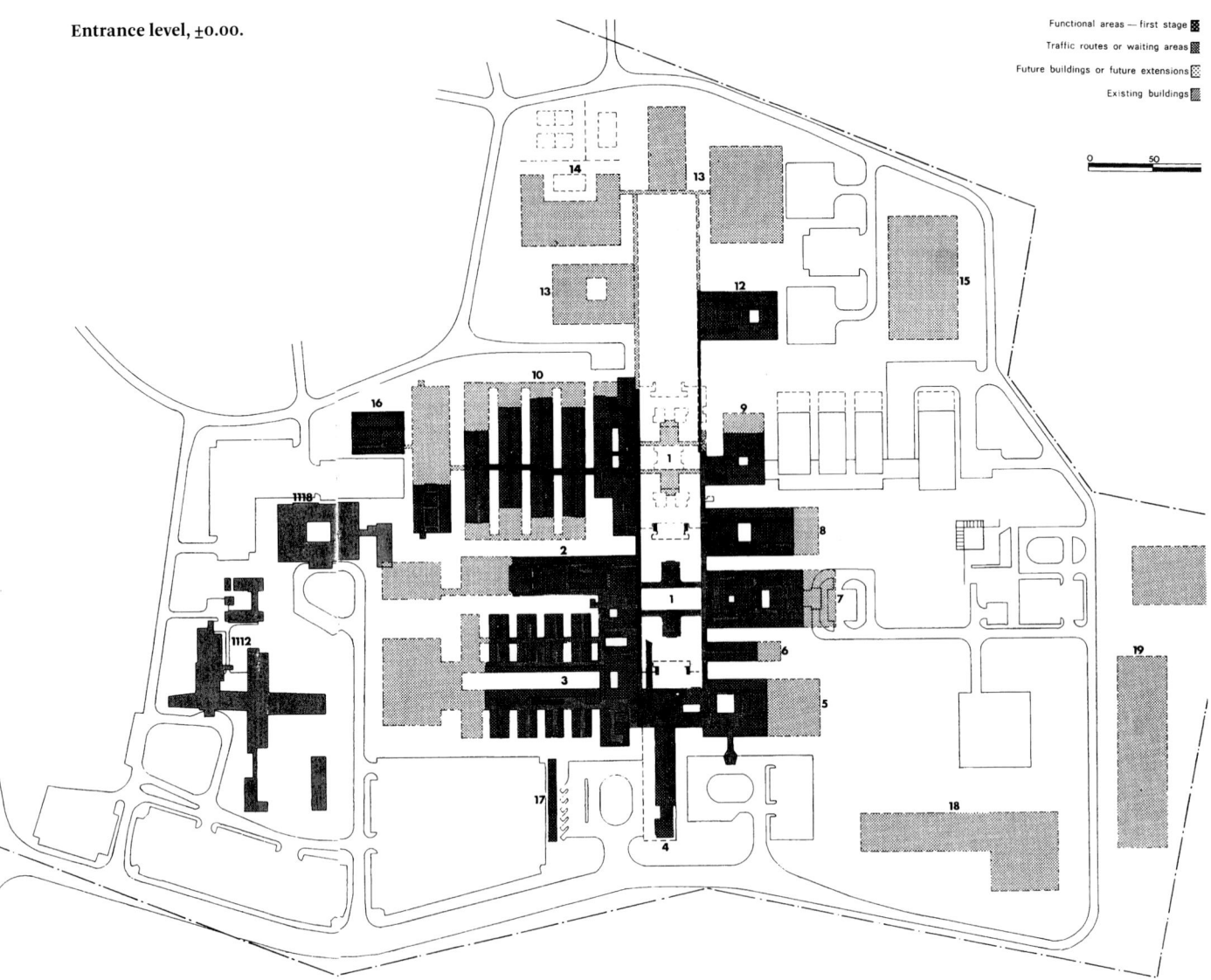

Functional areas — first stage
Traffic routes or waiting areas
Future buildings or future extensions
Existing buildings

0   50

1. Main building – concourse level
2. Radiology
3. Outpatient department
4. Entrance hall and public services
5. Casualty and admission
6. Nephrology
7. Operating theatres
8. Lecture hall library and teaching laboratories
9. Main dining hall
10. Clinical and research laboratories
12. Eye institute

13. Institutes
14. Recreation centre and occupational therapy
15. Service and maintenance building
16. Animal house and Experimental surgery
17. Bus station
18. Rehabilitation centre
19. General store building

1112. Obstetrics and maternity
1118. Children's hospital

Radiology Department

When the new hospital is in operation it is estimated that it will have to carry out approximately 70,000 examinations annually. In this department facilities are planned for general radiography, tomography, neuroradiology, uro-radiology, angiography, in addition to general fluoroscopic facilities, probably consisting of image intensified television fluoroscopy with electronic enlargement and video tape and spot film recording. There will be facilities for demonstration, teaching, research and maintaining records of film, micro-films and video-tapes. This department is planned about two developing centres, besides the angiography department's developing centre. As far as possible, rooms have been standardized to facilitate changes, and to provide flexibility for the examination rooms.

Clinical and Research Laboratories

These laboratories will engage in a wide variety of research in the fields of biochemistry, bacteriology, parasitology, serology, virology, hematology, immunology, biological assays, cytology, cytogenetics, histopathology, histochemistry, and electronic microscopy.

In order to ensure maximum flexibility in their use, the laboratories have been planned on a modular basis with the possibility of differential expansion. The ordinary laboratories and the research laboratories will, to a large extent, share equipment and central services. Attention has been paid to the automation factor and the possibility of adapting micro methods. AII the clinical and search laboratories are located near the ward-units in order not to differentiate between the clinicians, laboratory personnel and research workers.

Blood Bank

It is estimated that about half of the blood requirement of the hospital will be provided by donors in the hospital itself, and the other half from outside sources. The blood bank is located in the vicinity of the hematology laboratory, with an entrance from the main clinical corridor.

Laboratory for Radio-active Isotopes and Radiation Services

These services are planned adjoining one another. Each can be expanded independently.

5. The Hospitals and Health Facilities of Zarhy Architects

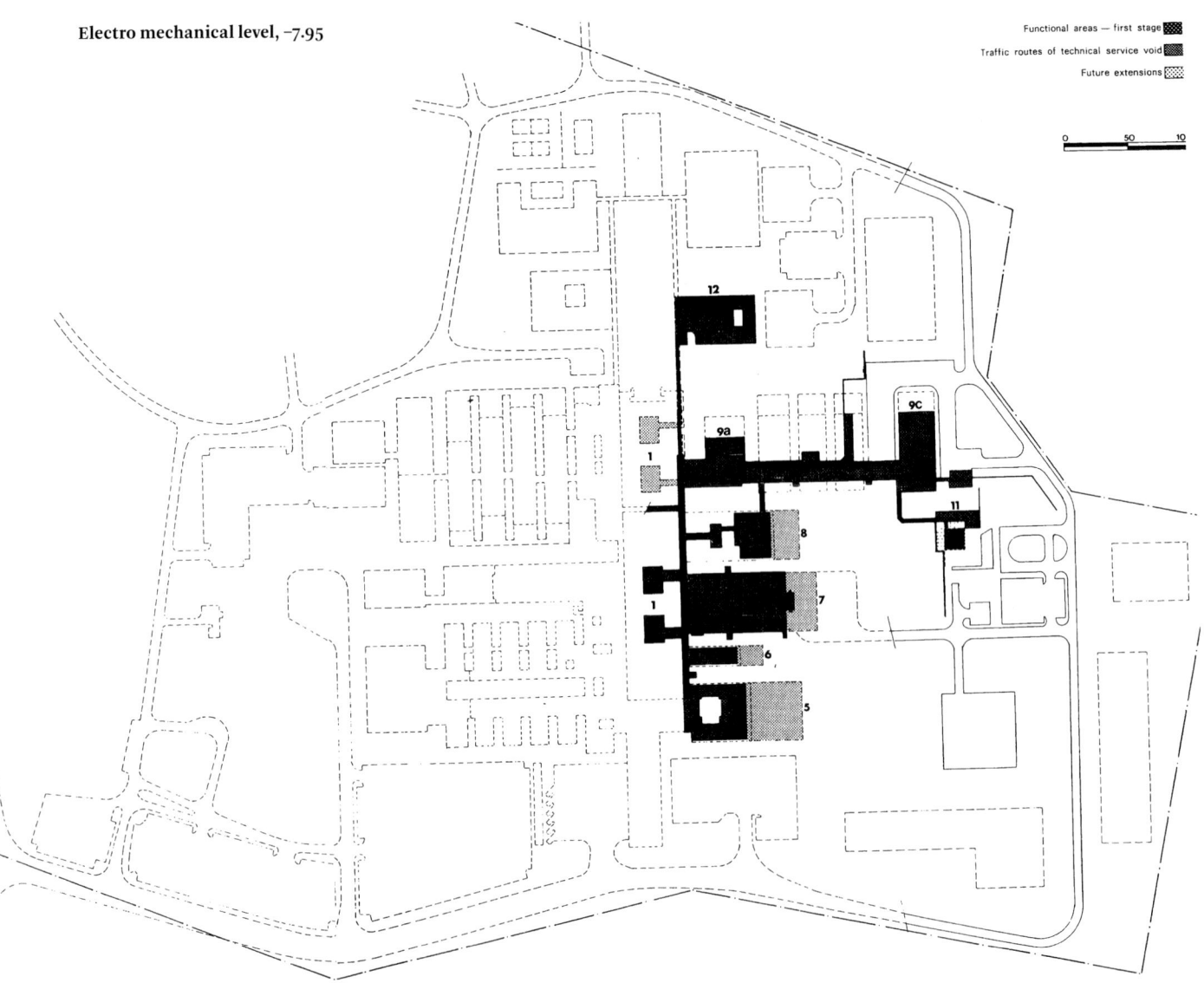

Functional areas — first stage
Traffic routes of technical service void
Future extensions

0   50   10

1. Main building – mechanical level
5. Main telephone switch board
6. Nephrology, technical service void
7. Underground casualty
   unit-machine room
8. Pharmacy – machine room
9a. Main kitchen – machine room
9c. Boiler house and main machine room
11. Mourner's parlour
12. Eye institute – machine room

Animal House

A central building housing animals of various types and sizes is planned. Planning takes into account isolation of newly received animals, cage rooms, equipment for food preparation, for cage and sterilizing, and for carrying out operations.

Library and Reading Rooms

The library serves the permanent staff, the young doctors, and students of medicine during their clinical studies. The library is designed on the open-shelf system. In the library area there is a special research room.

Seminars and Exhibitions

Adjoining the library, a number of rooms, this can be used separately or as a single large apace, have been planned for seminars. There is also a room for exhibitions.

Auditorium

An auditorium for about 300 people has been planned in the same building as the library. There are projection facilities, with television, and facilities for showing operations from the operating theatre wing, and from the radiology department.

Pharmacy

The pharmacy is planned on the ground level of the building containing the library, auditorium and teaching laboratories. It is located at the supply services level. The pharmacy has separate entrances for supplies and for medical staff. Pharmaceutical services include sterilizing facilities, preparation of formulae, a laboratory, a sterile laboratory, and medicine storage on the "compactus" system. Adjoining the medical staff entrance there is a study, and rooms for the pharmacy administration.

Operating Theatre Wing

This comprises a series of operating theatres to deal with all types of surgery. There are reception rooms operating theatres with adjoining, anaesthetic rooms, scrub-up rooms, instrument rooms, a plaster room, special rooms for cardiac and neuro-surgery, a recovery room, intrinsic teaching facilities and other services, a mobile X-Ray unit, a laboratory, staff change rooms and rest rooms, etc.

5. The Hospitals and Health Facilities of Zarhy Architects

12 Operating theatres have been planned, two of which are for special surgery. Sterilizing of instruments has been planned to take place in the central sterile supply, located at ground floor level of the operating theatre wing. Adjoining the wing, with a separate entrance from outside, a family waiting room has been planned. There are separate circulation routes for staff and patients from this wing's entrance hall. Standard toilets and change rooms have been planned for staff for greater flexibility.

Emergency Hospital

As was mentioned earlier, the central sterile supply unit, the hospital's lockers, and the emergency hospital are located at ground level in the operating theatre wing. The lockers are for male and female nurses, and students. Location of these units was determined by the need for direct connection between the central sterile supply, the operating theatre wing and the emergency hospital. The possibility of using part of the lockers for the emergency hospital, and the remainder of the lockers as shelter space in times of emergency, was also taken into account. There is a separate entrance to the emergency hospital, with all ancillary services, a large space for sorting patients, and hospitalization, and 10 operating theatres.

Maintenance and Service Wing

This wing includes the staff dining room, kitchen, central stores, laundry services, work-shops, and power supply. There is direct access from the service court to the central stores, the food stores, laundry services, workshops, the central incinerator, equipment for the removal of refuse, and the hospital garages. This section has been designed so that the various parts can be expanded independently.

Ward Block

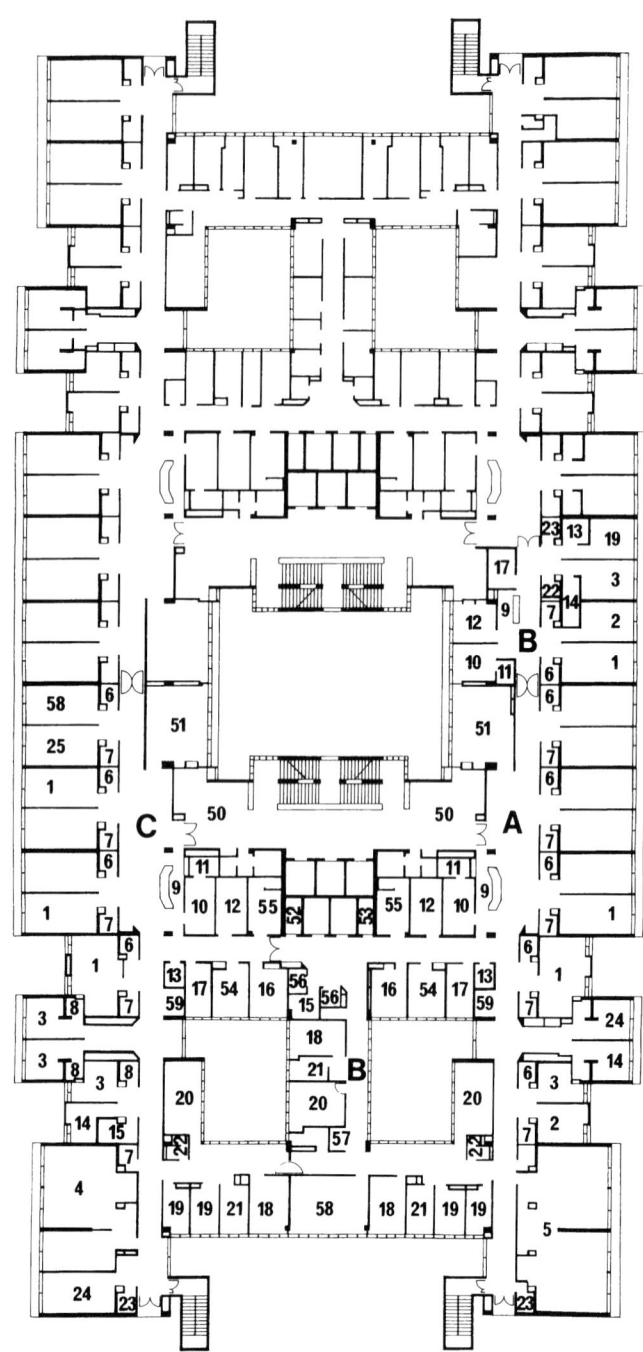

First floor

A. Open heart surgery
2. 1-bed room
5. 8-bed room
6. Shower
7. Toilet
9. Communication and information desk
10. Nurses' room
11. Medicaments
12. Treatment room
13. Linen room
14. Medical equipment storeroom
17. Head nurse
18. Head of dept.
19. Doctors' roam
20. Doctors' room
21. Secretary
22. On duty physician's toilet
23. Staff toilet

B. Thoracic surgery
1. 3-bed room
2. 2-bed room
3. 1-bed room
6. Shower
7. Toilet
9. Communication and information desk
10. Nurses' room
11. Medicaments
12. Treatment room
13. Linen roam
14. Medical equipment storeroom
15. General storeroom
16. Utility room
17. Head nurse
18. Head of dept.
19. Doctors' room
20. Doctors' room
21. Secretary
22. On duty physician's toilet
23. Staff toilet
24. Students' room
52. Family waiting room

53. Day/dining room
54. Kitchenette
55. Bathroom
58. Seminars room
59. Stretcher and wheelchair nook

C. Neurosurgery
1. 3-bed room
3. 1-bed room
4. 6-bed room
6. Shower
7. Toilet
8. Shower and toilet
9. Communication and information desk
10. Nurses' roam
11. Medicaments
12. Treatment room
13. Linen room
14. Medical equipment storeroom
15. General storeroom
16. Utility room
17. Head nurse
18. Head of dept.
19. Doctors' room
20. Doctors' room
21. Secretary
22. On duty physician's toilet
23. Staff toilet
24. Students' room
25. Physiotherapy room
52. Family waiting room
51. Day/dining room
52. Soiled laundry
53. Garbage
54. Kitchenette
55. Bathroom
56. Janitor
57. Mobile X-ray nook
58. Seminars room
59. Stretcher and wheelchair nook

5. The Hospitals and Health Facilities of Zarhy Architects

Second floor

A. General surgery	**B. Vascular surgery**
1. Family waiting room	1. Family waiting room
2. 3-bed room	2. 3-bed room
3. 2-bed room	3. 2-bed room
4. 1-bed room	4. 1-bed room
5. 4-bed room	5. 4-bed room
6. Shower	6. Shower
7. Toilet	7. Toilet
8. Shower and toilet	8. Shower and toilet
9. Communication and information	9. Communication and information
10. Nurses' station	10. Nurses' station
11. Medicaments	11. Medicaments
12. Treatment room	12. Treatment room
14. Day/dining room	13. Examination room
15. Treatment roan	14. Day/dining room
16. Bathroom	15. Kitchenette
17. Utility room	16. Bathroom
18. Linen room	17. Utility room
19. Medical equipment storeroom	18. Linen room
20. General storeroom	19. Medical equipment storeroom
21. Stretcher and wheelchair nook	20. General storeroom
22. Janitor	21. Stretcher and wheel choir nook
23. Head nurse	22. Janitor
24. Head of dept.	23. Head nurse
25. Doctors' room	24. Head of dept.
26. Doctors' room	25. Doctors' room
27. Secretary	26. Doctors' room
28. On duty physician's toilet	27. Secretary
29. Students' room	28. On duty physician's toilet
30. Seminars roam	29. Students' roam
31. Staff toilet	30. Seminars room
50. Soiled laundry	31. Staff toilet
51. Garbage	50. Soiled laundry
52. Laboratory	51. Garbage
53. Mobile X-ray	52. Laboratory
	53. Mobile X-ray nook

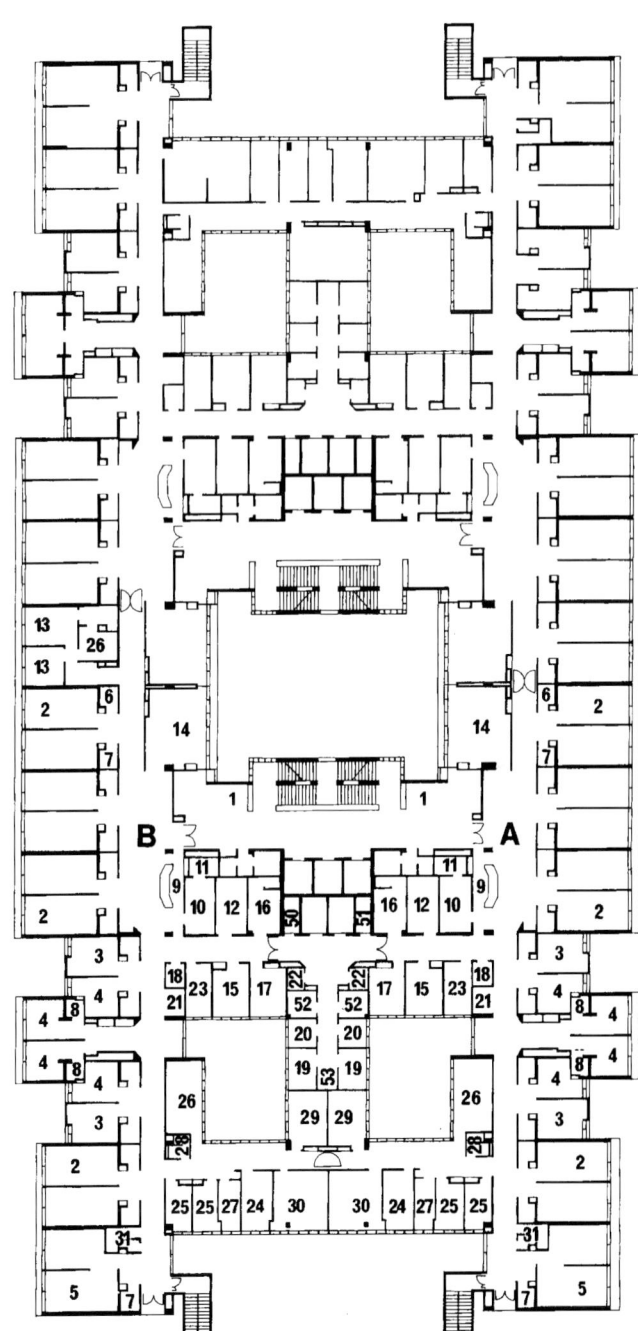

Ward Block

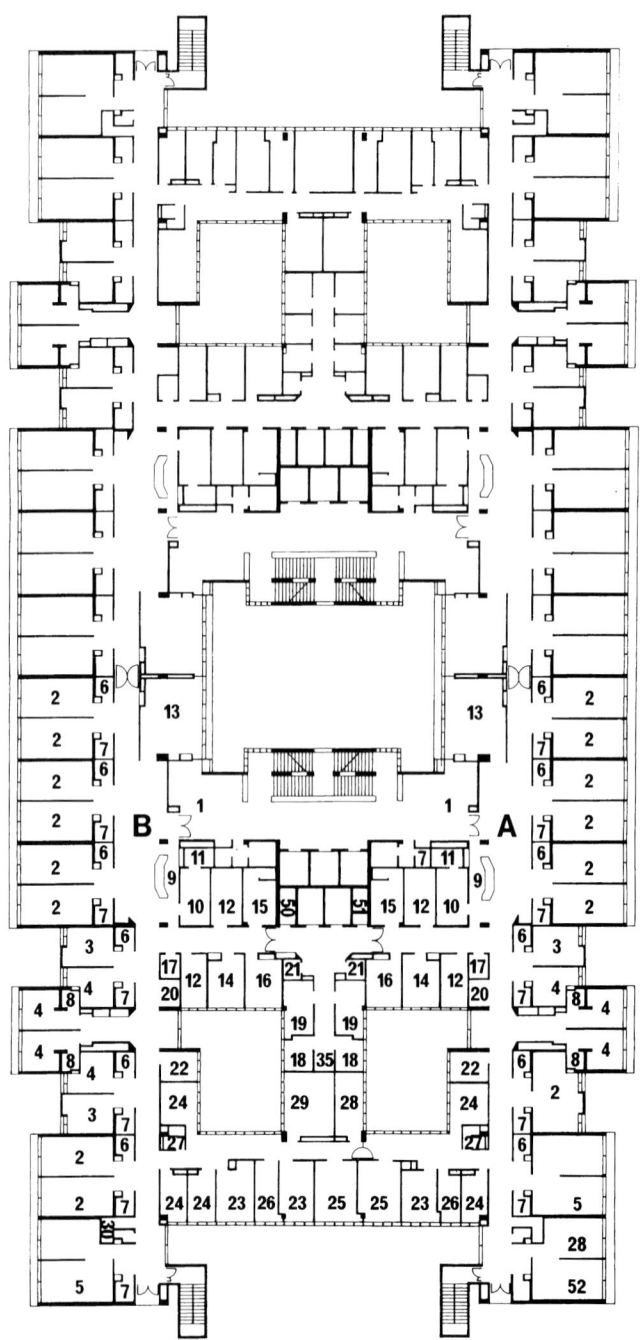

Third floor

A. General orthopedics

1. Family waiting room
2. 3-bed room
3. 2-bed room
4. 1-bed room
5. 4-bed room
6. Shower
7. Toilet
8. Shower and toilet
9. Communication and information desk
10. Nurses' station
11. Medicaments
12. Treatment room
13. Day / dining room
14. Kitchenette
15. Bathroom
16. Utility room
17. Linen room
18. Medical equipment storeroom
19. General storeroom
20. Stretcher and wheelchair nook
21. Janitor
22. Head nurse
23. Head of dept.
24. Doctors' room
25. Doctors' room
26. Secretary
27. On duty toilet
28. Students' room
29. Seminars room
30. Staff toilet
50. Soiled laundry
51. Garbage
52. Physiotherapy
53. Mobile X-ray nook

B. General prthopedics and hand surgery

1. Family waiting room
2. 3-bed room
3. 2-bed room
4. 1-bed room
5. 4-bed room
6. Shower
7. Toilet
8. Shower and toilet
9. Communication and information desk
10. Nurses' station
11. Medicaments
12. Treatment room
13. Day / dining room
14. Kitchenette
15. Bathroom
16. Utility room
17. Linen room
18. Equipment storeroom
19. General storeroom
20. Stretcher and wheelchair nook
21. Janitor
22. Head nurse
23. Head of dept.
24. Doctors' room
25. Doctors' room
26. Secretary
27. On duty physician's toilet
28. Students' room
29. Seminars room
30. Staff toilet
50. Soiled laundry
51. Garbage
52. Physiotherapy
53. Mobile X-ray nook

Fourth floor

A. Internal Medicine "A"	**B. Internal Medicine "B"**
1. Family waiting room	1. Family waiting room
2. 3-bed room	2. 3-bed room
3. 2-bed room	3. 2-bed room
4. 1-bed room	4. 1-bed room
5. 4-bed room	5. 4-bed room
6. Shower	6. Shower
7. Toilet	7. Toilet
8. Shower and toilet	8. Shower and toilet
9. Communication and information desk	9. Communication and information desk
10. Nurses' station	10. Nurses' station
11. Medicaments	11. Medicaments
12. Treatment room	12. Treatment room
13. Laboratory	13. Laboratory
14. day / dining room	14. Day dining room
15. Kitchenette	15. Kitchenette
16. Bathroom	16. Bathroom
17. Utility room	17. Utility room
18. Linen room	18. Linen room
17. Medical equipment storeroom	19. Medical equipment storeroom
20. General storeroom	20. General storeroom
21. Stretcher and wheelchair nook	21. Stretcher and wheel choir nook
22. Janitor	22. Janitor
23. Head nurse	23. Head nurse
24. Head of dept.	24. Head of dept.
25. Doctors' room	25. Doctors' room
26. Doctors' room	26. Doctors' room
27. Secretary	27. Secretary
28. On duty physician's toilet	28. On duty physician's toilet
29. Students' room	29. Students' room
30. Seminars room	30. Seminars room
31. Staff toilet	31. Staff toilet
50. Soiled laundry	50. Soiled Laundry
51. Garbage	51. Garbage
52. Mobile X-ray	52. Mobile X-ray nook

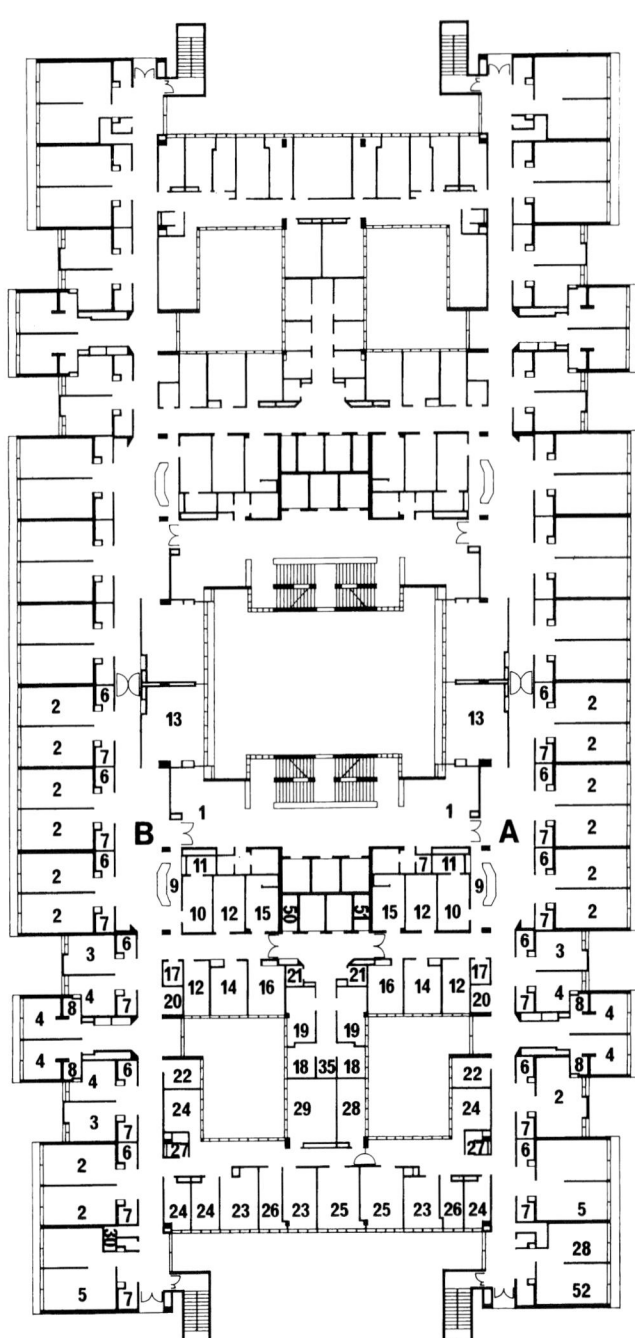

Ward Block

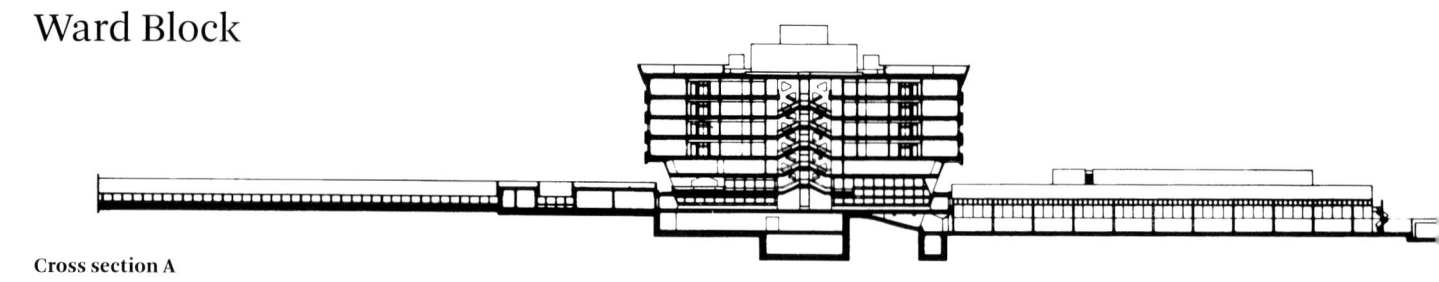

Cross section A

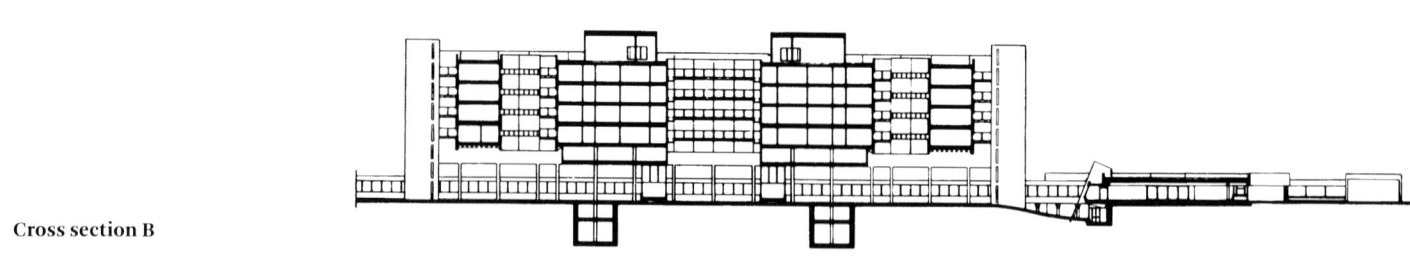

Cross section B

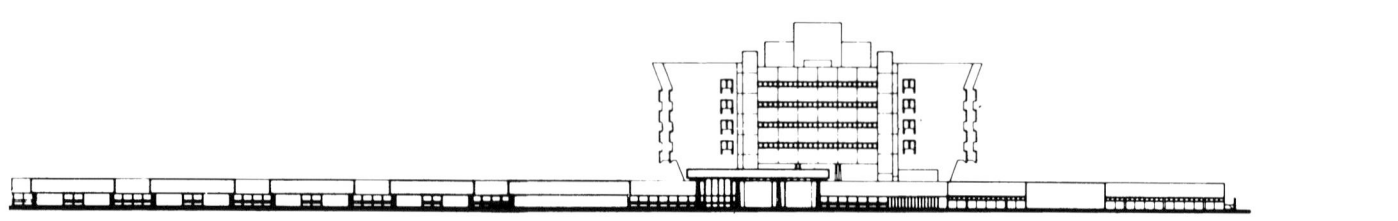

West elevation

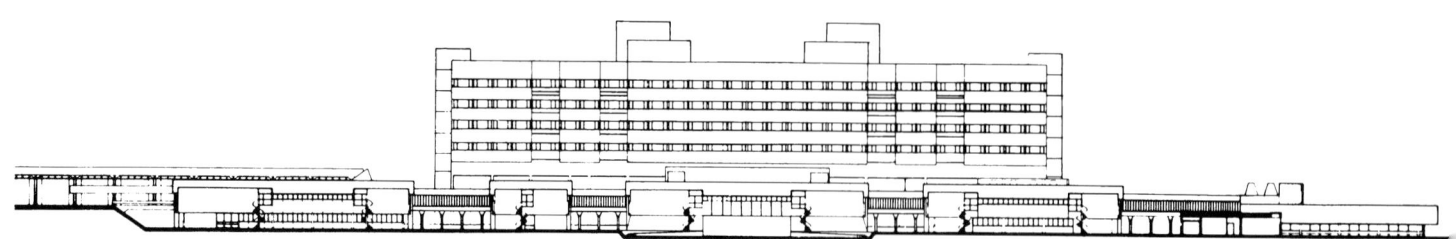

West elevation

5. The Hospitals and Health Facilities of Zarhy Architects

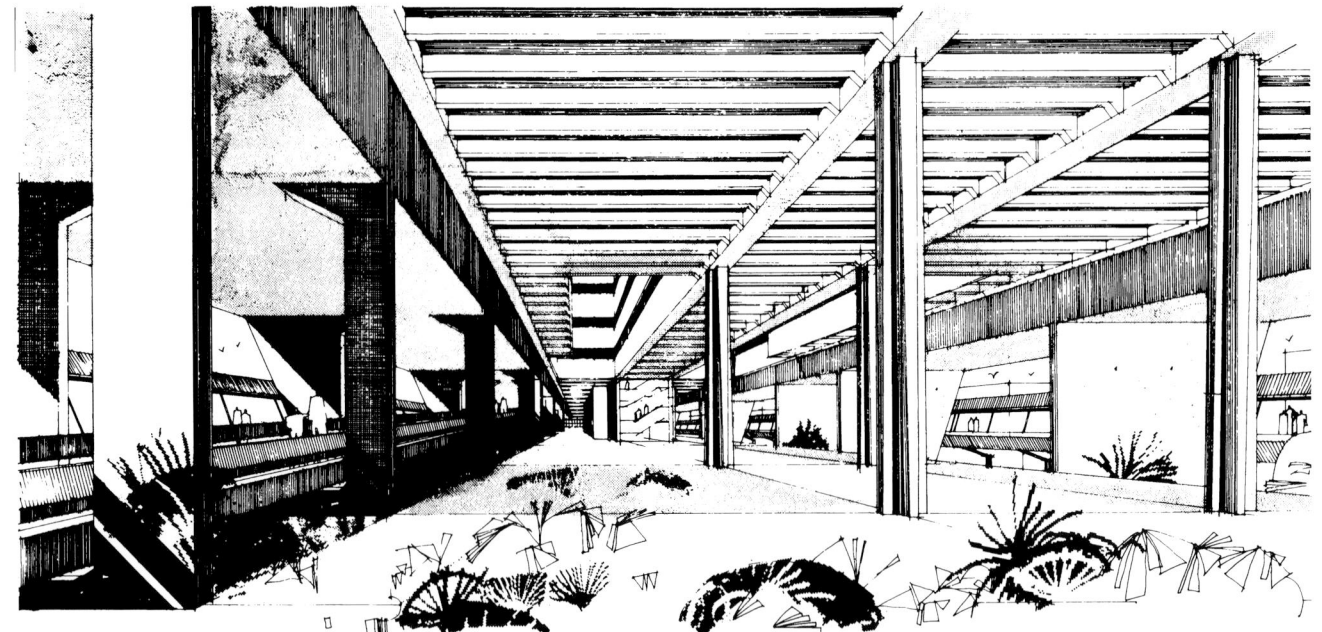

Entrance garden under the main building

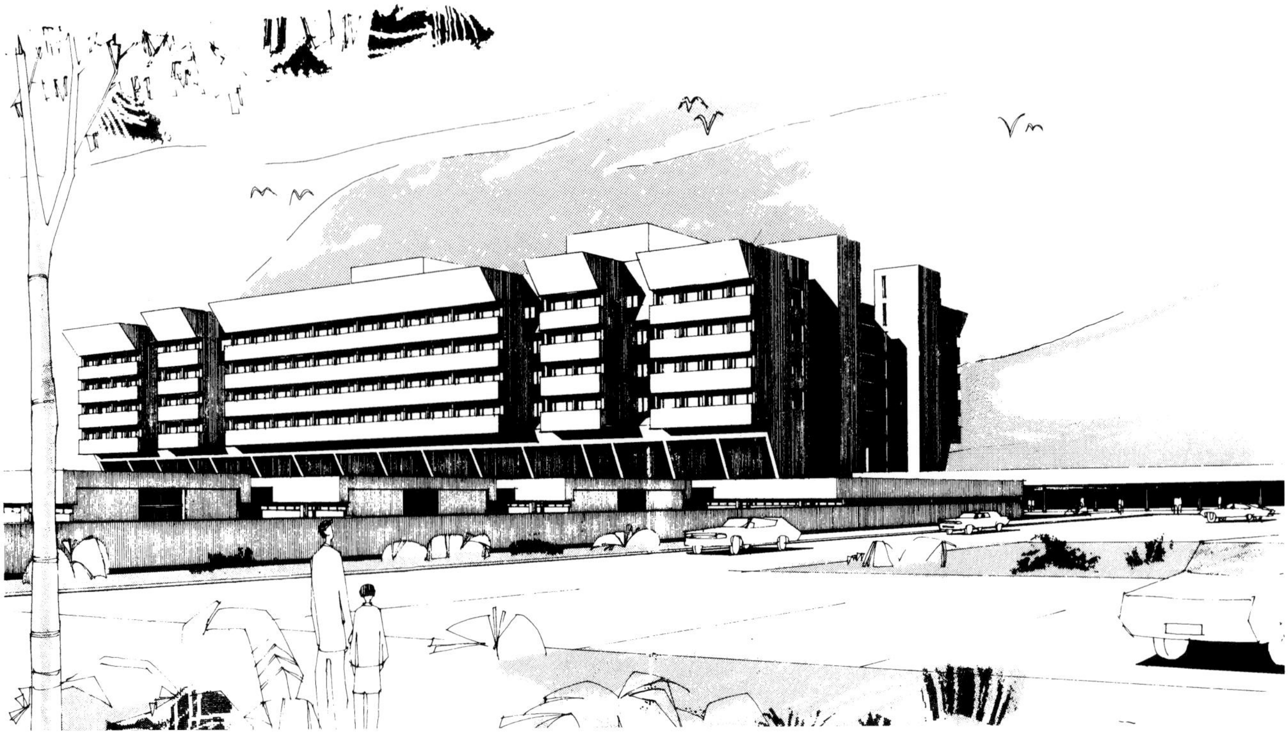

Division of Diagnostic Imaging

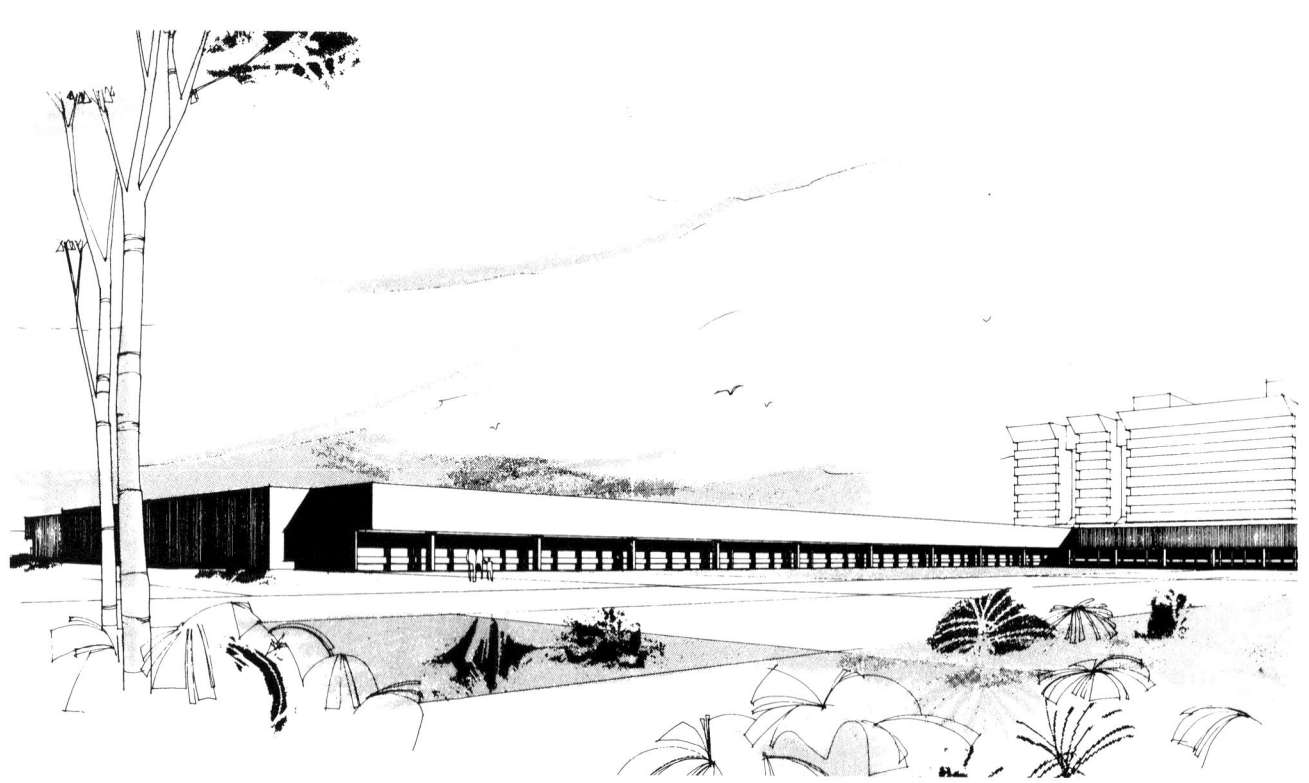

A. Conventional X-ray

1. Entrance
2. Waiting room
3. Reception
4. Nurses' office
5. Medical files and film archives
6. Cloak room
7. Demonstration / conference room
8. X-ray radiography
9. Standard radio diagnostic rooms
10. Dark room
11. General, abdominal, neurological and peripheral angiography
12. Future n.M.R. Activities
13. Seminars room
14. Staff lounge
15. Radiologists' and X-ray technicians' rooms, including radiography school
16. Immediate viewing and sorting room
17. Film processing room

B. C.T. scan and ultrasound

1. Entrance
2. Waiting area
3. C.T. Scanner
4. Operators' room
5. Medical files and film archives
6. Ultrasound room
7. Conference room
8. Preparation room
9. U.S. Physicians' rooms
10. C.T. Physicians' rooms
11. U.S. Physicians' rooms
12. Development room

C. Nuclear medicine

1. Entrance
2. Waiting room
3. Admission
4. Examination room
5. Radiopharmacy room
6. Preparation and injection room
7. Gamma camera
8. Computer room
9. Development room
10. Laboratory room
11. Seminars room
12. Physicians' rooms
13. Head of dept.
14. Secretary
15. Deputy to head of dept.
16. Physicist
17. Cloak room
18. Kitchen
19. Storeroom

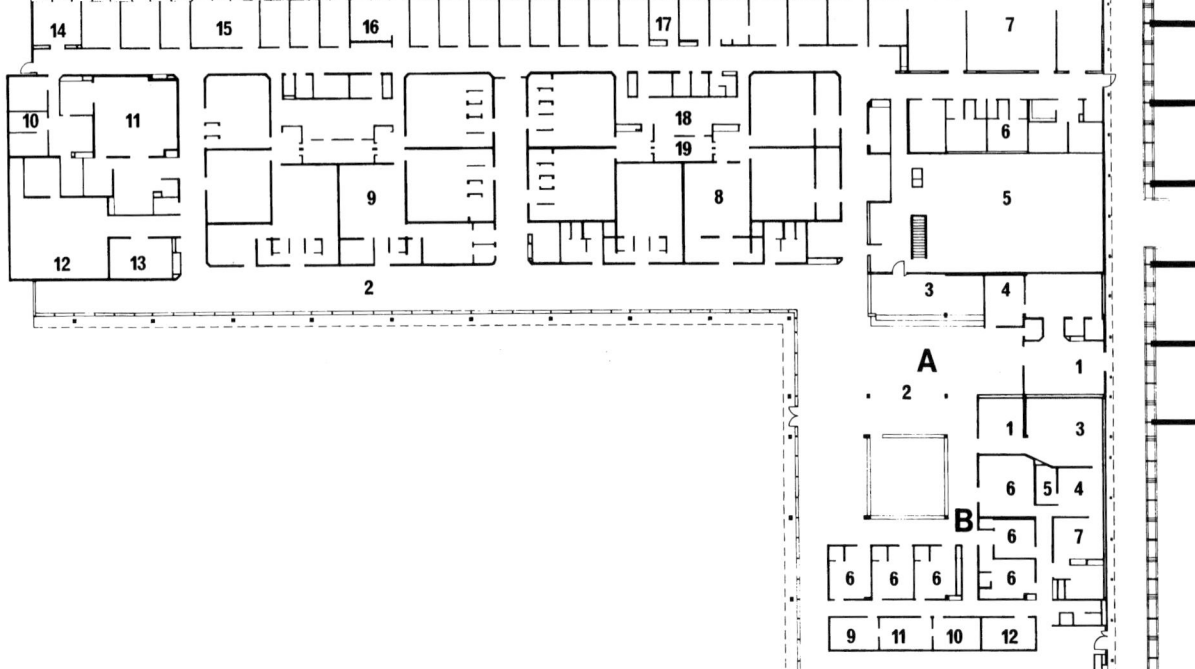

Outpatients Department and Institutes

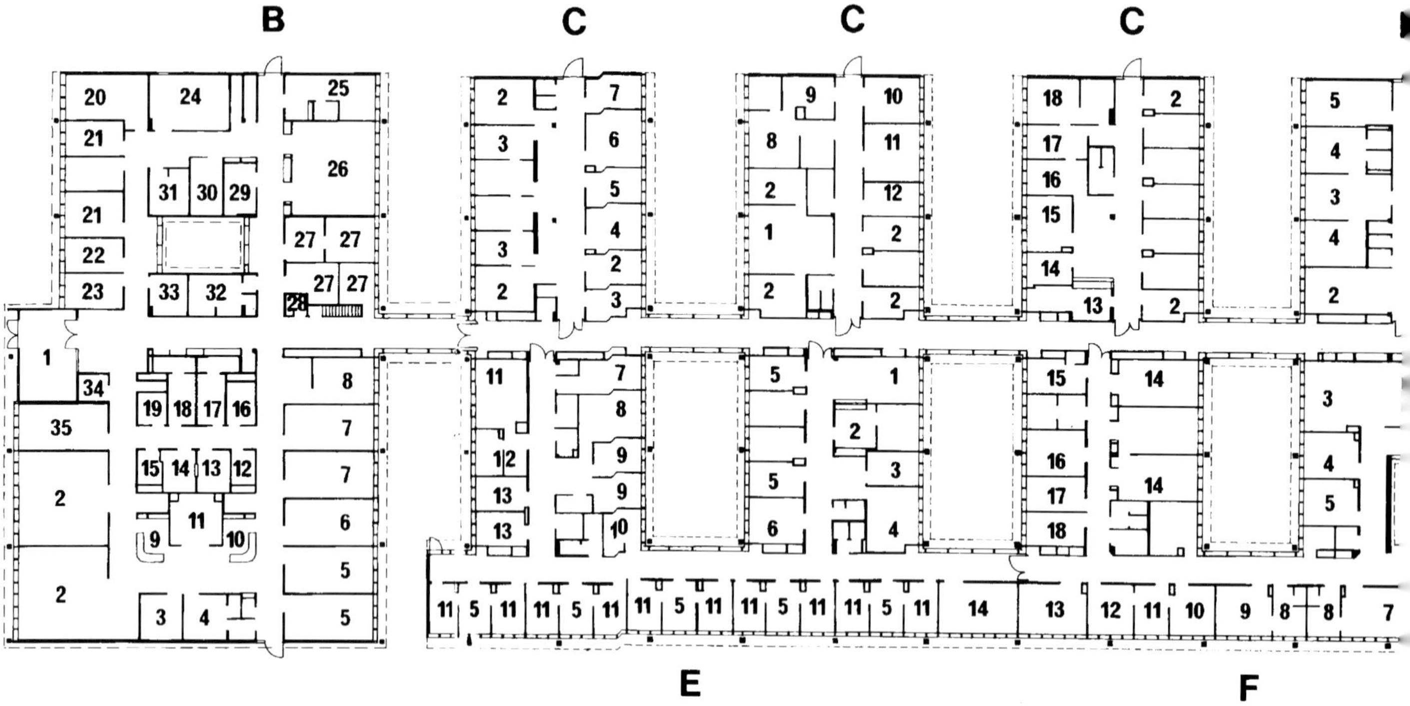

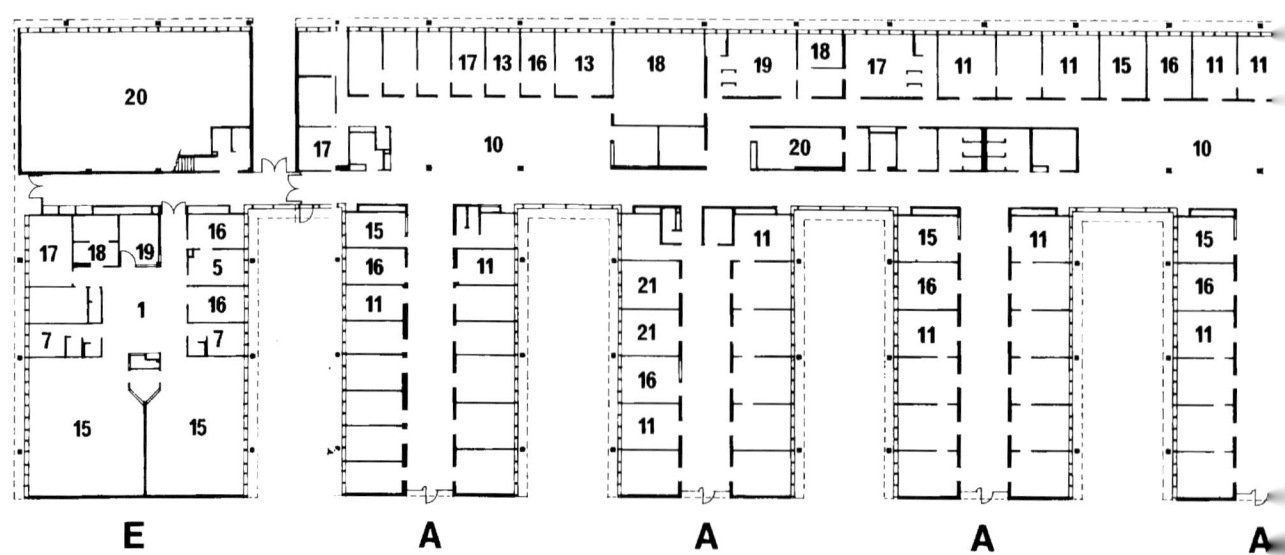

5. The Hospitals and Health Facilities of Zarhy Architects

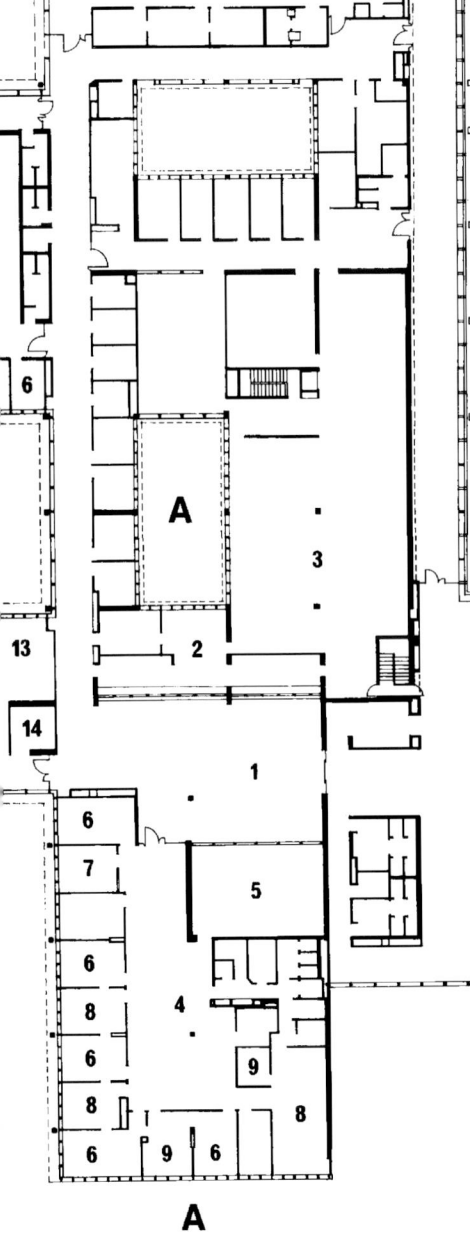

A.
Outpatients' department

General
1. Entrance hall
2. Reception
3. Patients' medical records

Orthopedics
4. Waiting area
5. Patio
6. Examination rooms
7. Secretary
8. Treatment room
9. Plaster storeroom

Outpatient – general purpose
10. Waiting room
11. Consulting and examination room
12. Pharmacy
13. Seminars room
14. Stretcher and wheelchair nook
15. Secretary
16. Nurse
17. Treatment room
18. Preparation room
19. Cystoscopy
20. Recovery
21. Laboratory

C.
Pulmonary function
1. Waiting room
2. Doctor's room
3. Examination room
4. Head of dept.
5. Computer
6. Library
7. Kitchenette
8. Treatment room
9. Preparation room
10. Laboratory
11. Physiotherapy
12. Inhalation room
13. Reception
14. Children treatment room
15. Treatment room
16. Head nurse
17. Secretary
18. Head of dept.

F.
Gastroenterology
1. Waiting room
2. Reception
3. Recovery
4. Endoscopy
5. Treatment room
6. Doctors' room
7. Colonoscopy
8. Preparation room
9. Rectoscopy
10. Deputy to head of dept.
11. Head of dept.
12. Seminars room
13. Laboratories
14. Cloakroom
15. Stool examination lab.
16. Microscopy
17. Kitchenette

D.
Neurology
1. Reception
2. Waiting room
3. Preparation for electroencephalography
4. Electro-encephalography
5. Examination room
6. Doctors' room
7. Kitchenette

E.
Cardiac rehabilitation
1. Waiting room
2. Reception
3. Secretary
4. Head of dept.
5. Doctors' room
6. Nurses' room
7. Cloakroom
8. Library
9. Halter
10. Kitchenette
11. Examination room
12. Blood-test room
13. Echocardiography
14. Seminars room
15. Gymnastic room
16. Ergometry
17. Treatment room
18. Storeroom
19. Office
20. Future expansion

B.
Nephrology
1. Main lobby and waiting room
2. Chronic hemodialysis
3. Hemodialysis for acute
4. Hemodialysis for isolated patients with hepatitis
5. Training for peritoneal self-treatment
6. Treatment of peritonitis
7. Ambulatory care and special investigations
8. Procedures' room
9. Nurse's station for hemodialysis
10. Nurse's station for dialysis and ambulatory care
11. Nurses
12. Laundry storage
13. Patients' dining room
14. Kitchenette
15. Sanitary equipment cleaning
16. Solutions' storage
17. Cloakroom
18. Cloakroom
19. Linen storage
20. Head of dept.
21. Doctors' room
22. Head nurse
23. Secretary
24. Seminars room
25. Small animals experimental laboratory
26. Laboratory
27. Medical equipment maintenance
28. Janitor
29. Laboratory office
30. Laboratory storage
31. Staff room
32. Nurses' cloakroom
33. Dietitian and social care
34. Garbage
35. General storage

Main Entrance Hall and Public Services

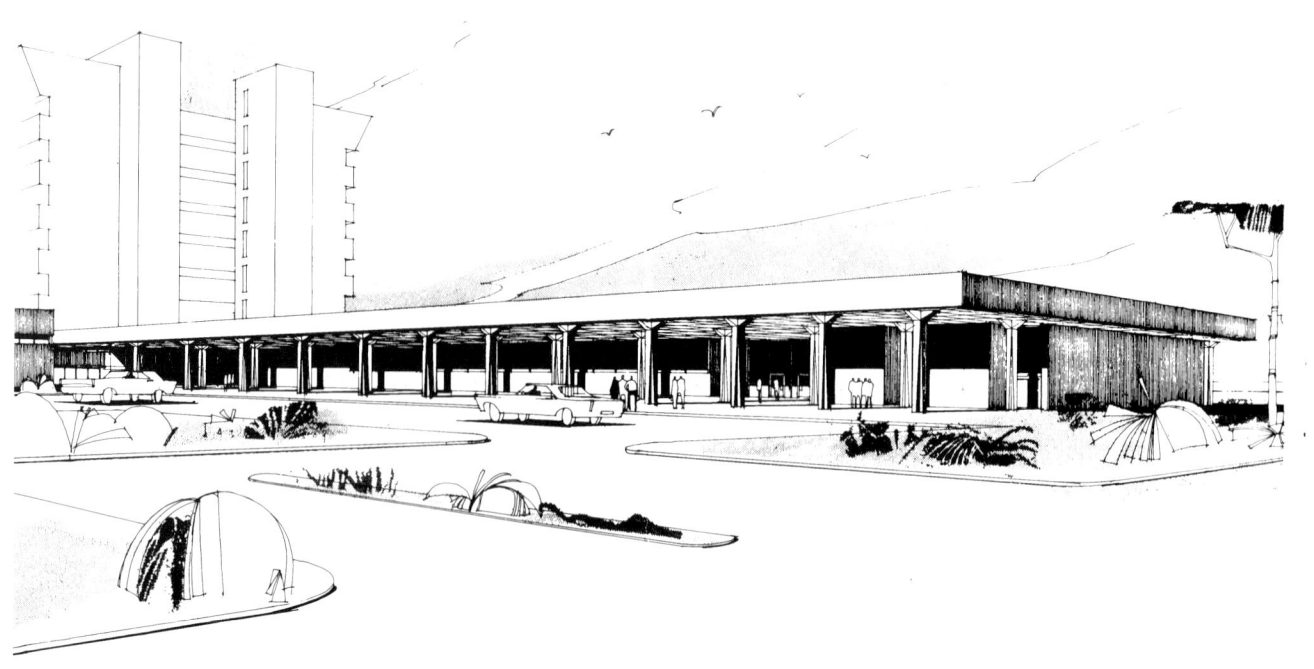

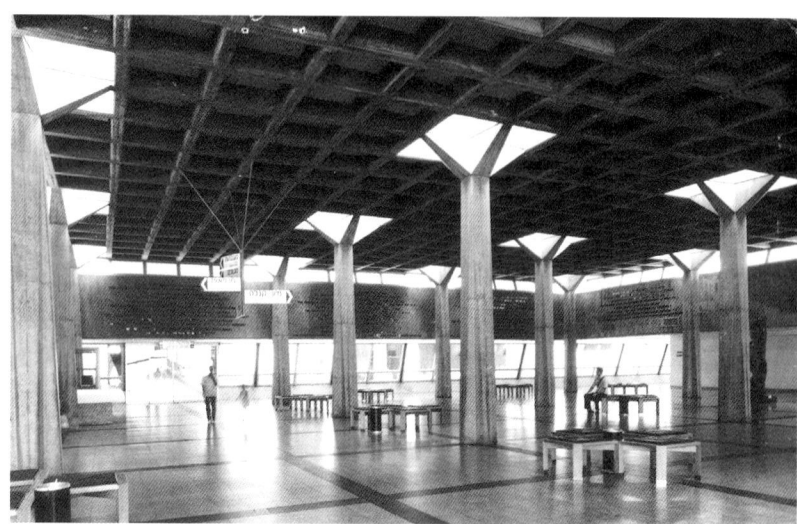

5. The Hospitals and Health Facilities of Zarhy Architects

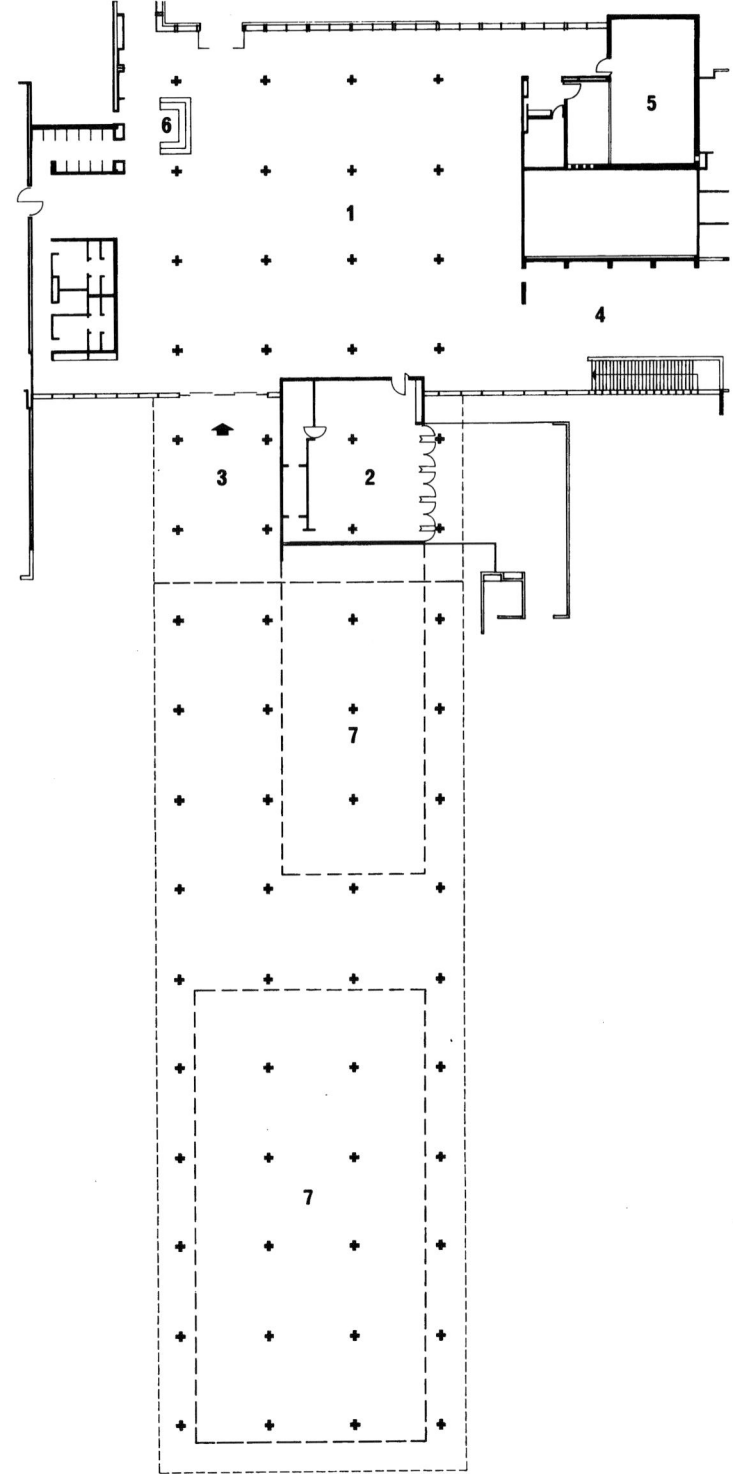

1. Entrance hall
2. Cafeteria
3. Main entrance to the hospital
4. Waiting room
5. Synagogue
6. Information
7. Future expansion

Casualty Department

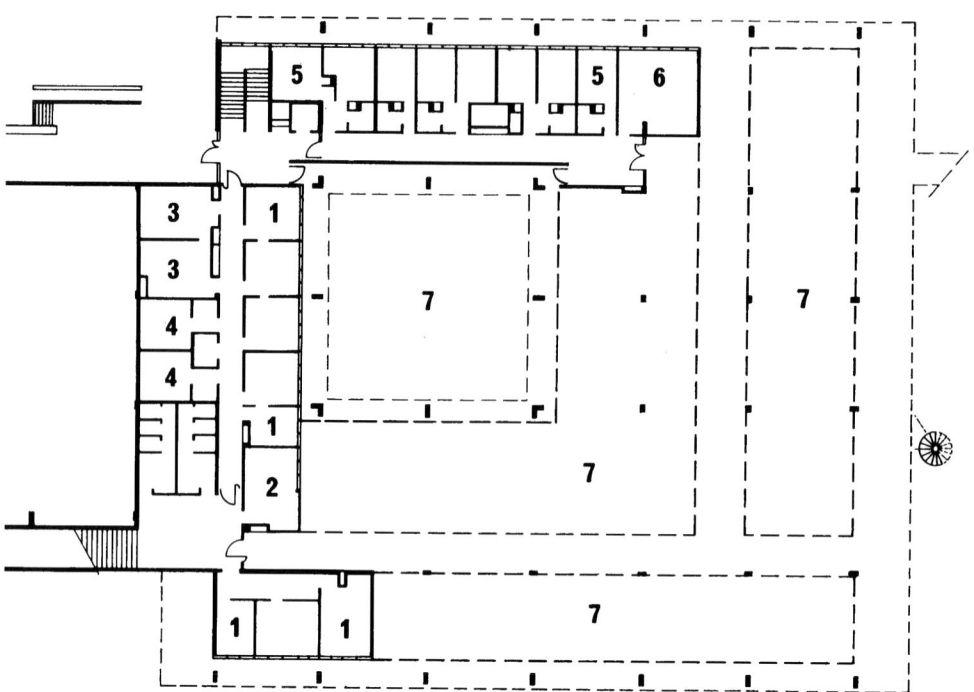

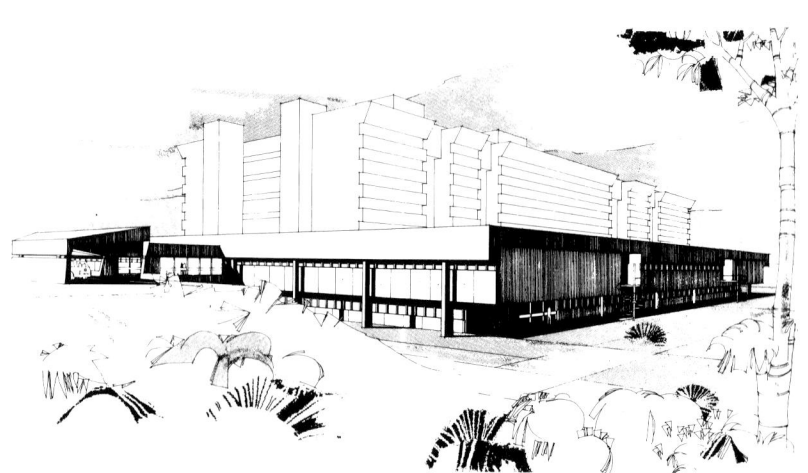

Ground floor

1. Office
2. Tea room
3. Archives
4. Cloakroom
5. On duty physician's room
6. Doctors' room
7. Future expansion

5. The Hospitals and Health Facilities of Zarhy Architects

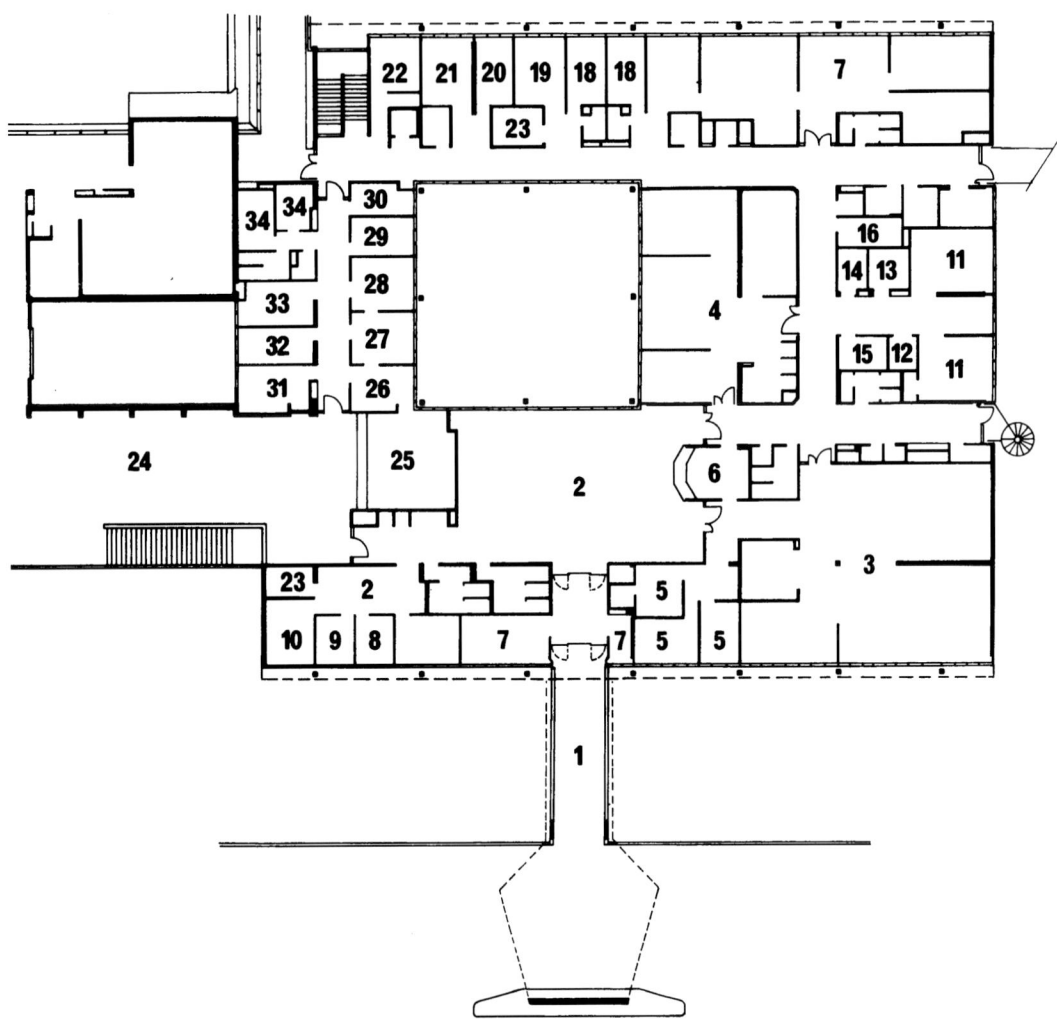

First floor

Casualty department

1. Covered entrance
2. Entrance and waiting hall
3. Stretchers ward – general
4. Stretchers ward – traumatology
5. Examination room
6. Information desk
7. Stretchers and wheelchairs
8. Nurses' room
9. Police
10. Family waiting room
11. Treatment room
12. X-ray nook
13. Laboratory
14. Clean linen room
15. Sluice room
16. Kitchenette
17. Observation rooms
18. On duty physician's rooms
19. Tea room
20. Head nurse
21. Head of dept.
22. Room for D.O.A (dead on arrival)
23. General storeroom

Admission

24. Waiting hall
25. Patients' admission and release office
26. Deputy to head of dept.
27. Secretary
28. Doctor in charge of patients' admission
29. Social worker
30. Nurse's room
31. Cashier
32. Soldiers' admission and release office
33. Office
34. Storeroom

Heart Institute:
Intensive Care Unit

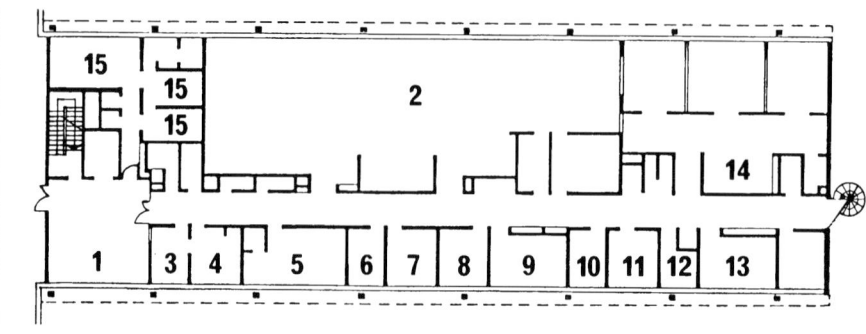

Intensive care unit
1. Entrance hall
2. 11-bed bay
3. Secretary
4. Head of dept.
5. Doctors' room
6. Head nurse
7. Nurses' room
8. Sluice room
9. General storeroom
10. Technician's room

11. Kitchenette
12. Laboratory
13. Bed cleaning room
14. 3-bed bay
15. Blood-gas analysis unit

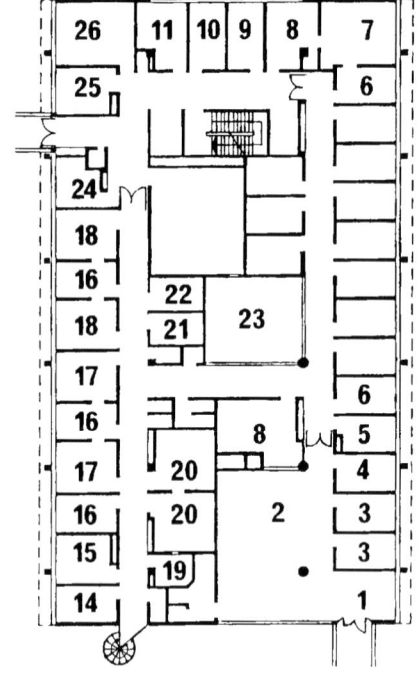

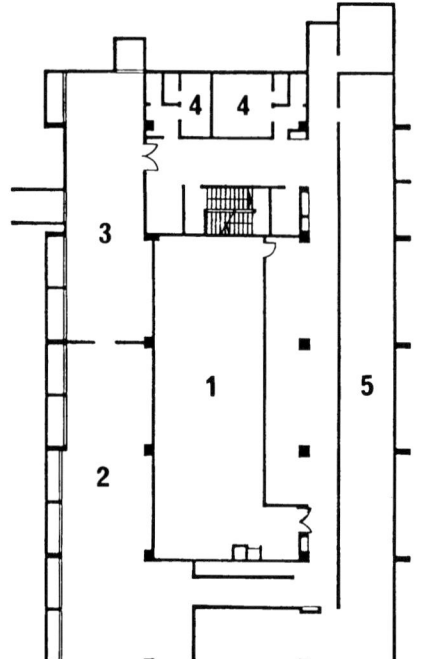

Basement floor
1. Medical records room
2. Machine room
3. Machine room
4. Cloakroom
5. Future expansion

First floor
1. Entrance to O.P.D.
2. Waiting room
3. E.C.G. room
4. Children's waiting room
5. Nurses' room
6. Examination room
7. Head of dept.
8. Secretary
9. Administrator
10. Head nurse
11. Deputy to head of dept.
12. Dietician's room
13. Pacemaker examination room

14. Physicist's room
15. Technicians' room
16. Doctors' room
17. Ergometry room
18. Echocardiography room
19. Radioactive material room
20. Camera room
21. Halter diagnostic room
22. Halter connecting room
23. Lectures hall
24. Computer room
25. Library

5. The Hospitals and Health Facilities of Zarhy Architects

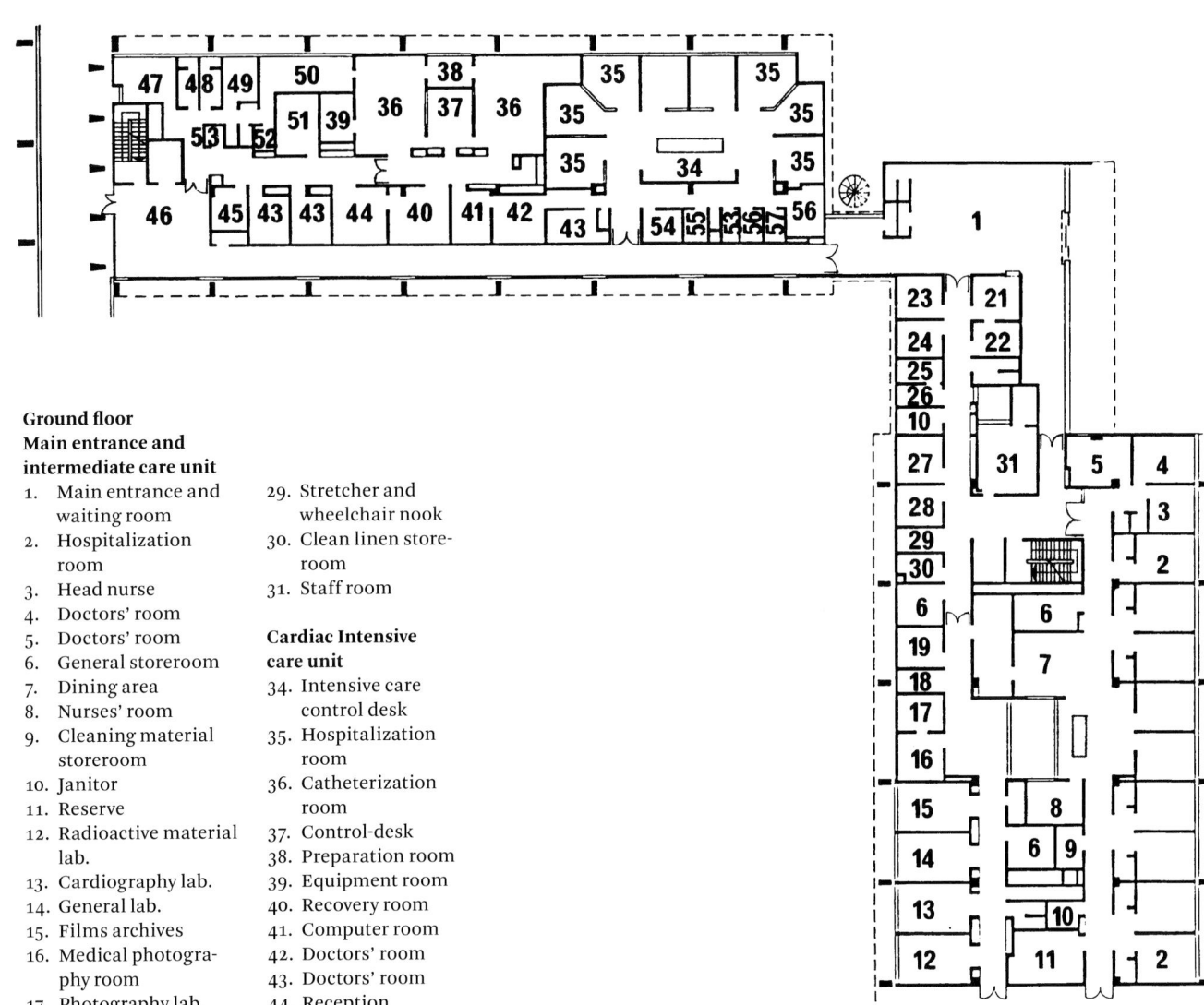

Ground floor
Main entrance and intermediate care unit

1. Main entrance and waiting room
2. Hospitalization room
3. Head nurse
4. Doctors' room
5. Doctors' room
6. General storeroom
7. Dining area
8. Nurses' room
9. Cleaning material storeroom
10. Janitor
11. Reserve
12. Radioactive material lab.
13. Cardiography lab.
14. General lab.
15. Films archives
16. Medical photography room
17. Photography lab.
18. Mobile X-ray unit
19. Solutions storeroom
20. Kitchen
21. Secretary and information
22. Computer section
23. Social worker's office
24. Psychologist's office
25. Soiled linen storeroom
26. Garbage
27. Cleaning material storeroom
28. Housekeeper's room
29. Stretcher and wheelchair nook
30. Clean linen storeroom
31. Staff room

Cardiac Intensive care unit

34. Intensive care control desk
35. Hospitalization room
36. Catheterization room
37. Control-desk
38. Preparation room
39. Equipment room
40. Recovery room
41. Computer room
42. Doctors' room
43. Doctors' room
44. Reception
45. Secretary
46. Waiting room
47. Staff room
48. Cloak room
49. Materials storeroom
50. Laboratory
51. Development room
52. Cleaning equipment storeroom
53. Soiled linen storeroom
54. Head nurse
55. Cleaning material storeroom
56. General storeroom
57. Kitchenette

Operating Theatres

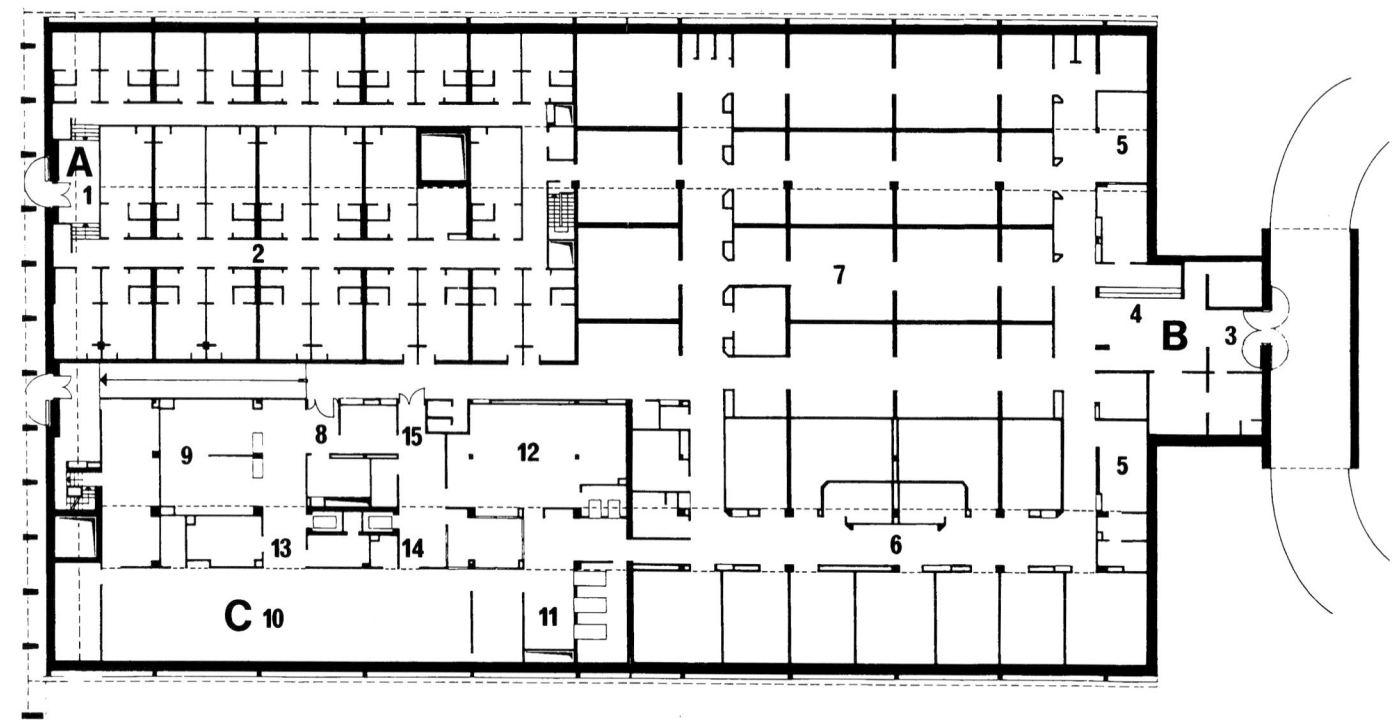

Supply services level

A. Central cloakrooms

1. Entrance
2. Cloakrooms and toilets

B. Emergency casualty unit

3. Entrance
4. Receptionist
5. Nurse and treatment
6. Operating theatres
7. Casualty admission rooms

C. Central sterile supply dept.

8. Entrance
9. Cleaning and stores
10. Working space for inspection and assembly
11. Sterilization
12. Clean store
13. Clean equipment elevator
14. Supply elevator

5. The Hospitals and Health Facilities of Zarhy Architects

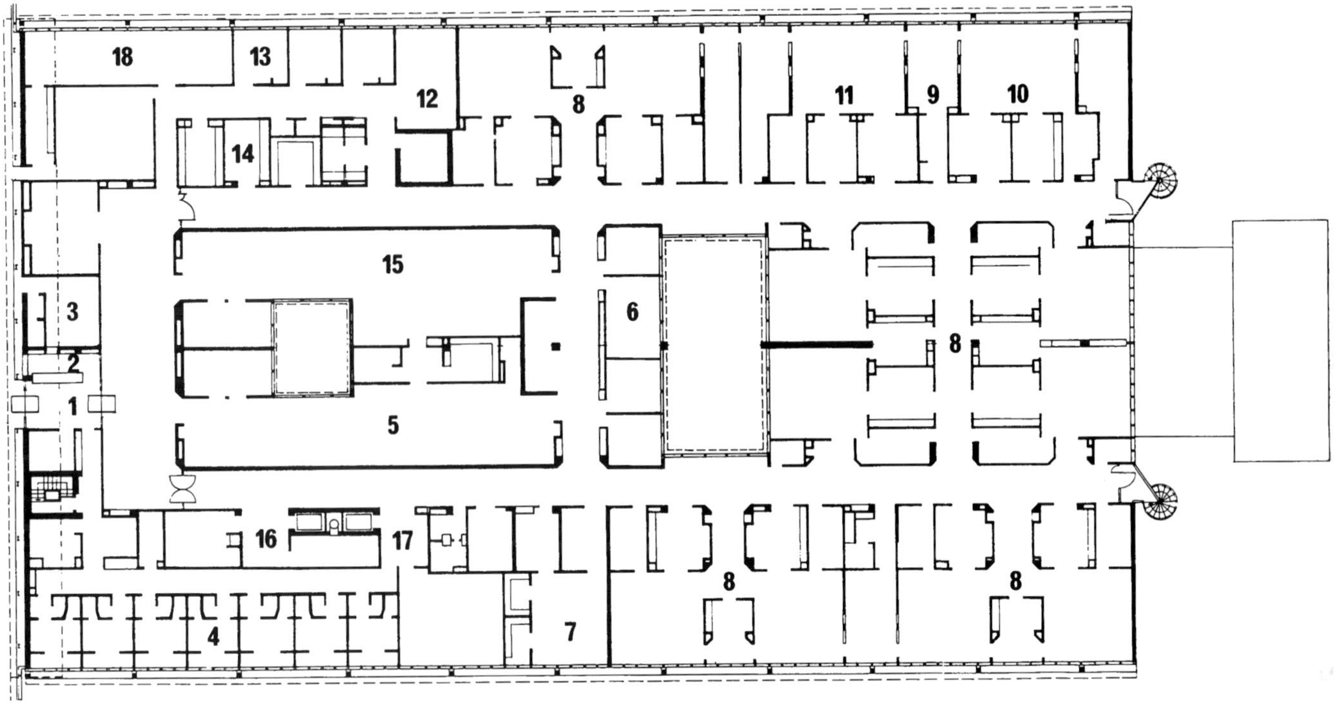

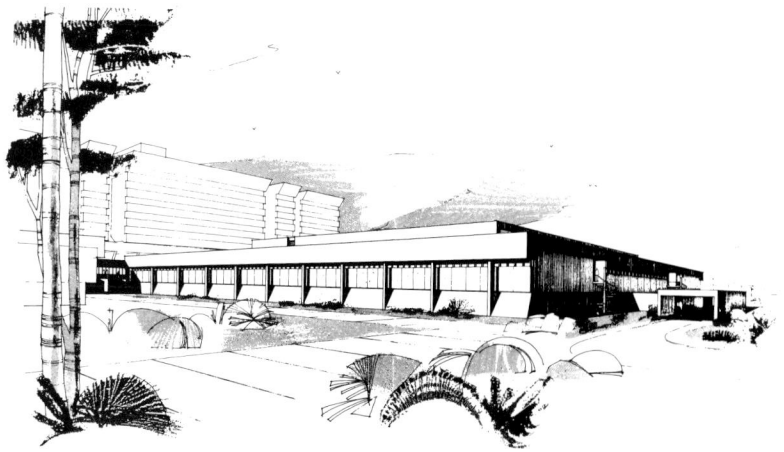

Entrance and medical services level

1. Entrance
2. Receptionist and information
3. Family waiting room
4. Staff cloakroom
5. Patient admission and preparation
6. Nurses' utility room
7. Plaster room
8. Standard theatre suite
9. Control room
10. Cardiac surgery
11. Neurosurgery
12. Seminars room
13. Surgeons' offices
14. Laboratories
15. Recovery room
16. Unclean equipment elevator
17. Clean supply elevator
18. Staff tea room

Medical Supply Store and Pharmacy:
Rehabilitation Wards

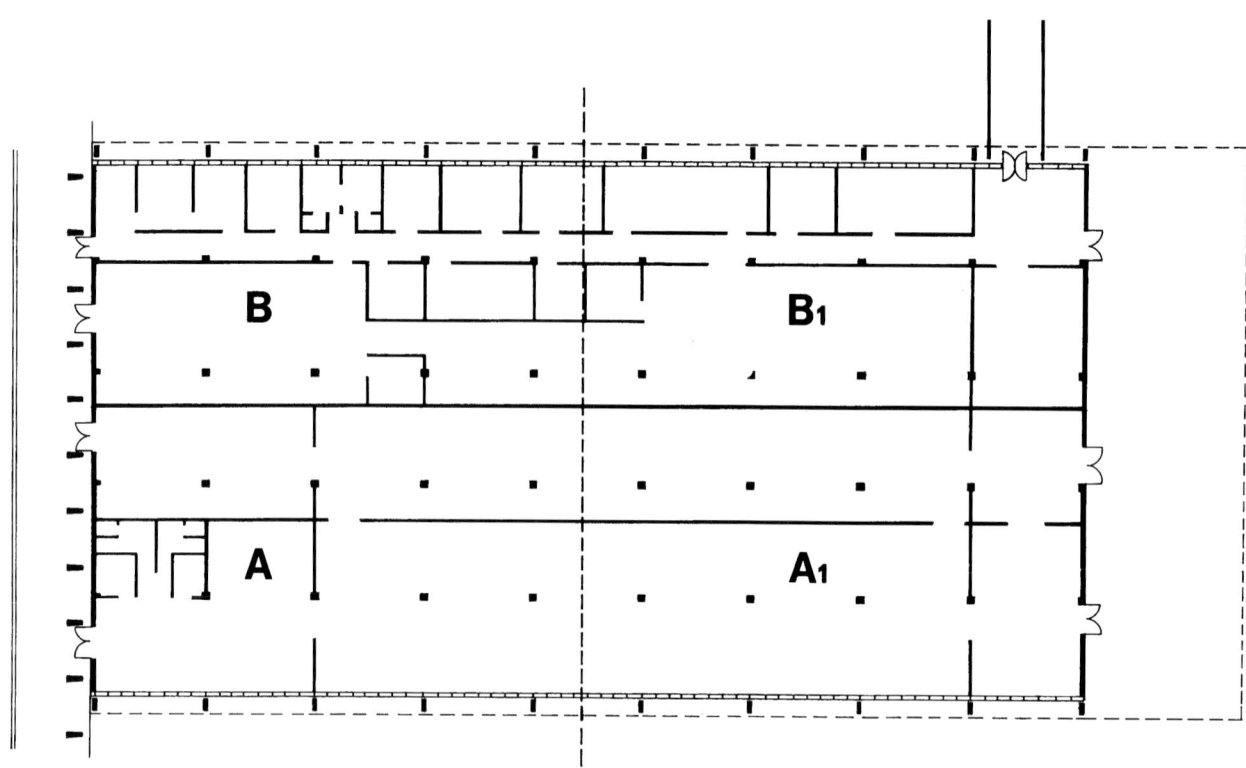

Ground floor
A.   Medical supply store
A1. Future expansion to A
B.   Future pharmacy
B1. Future expansion to B

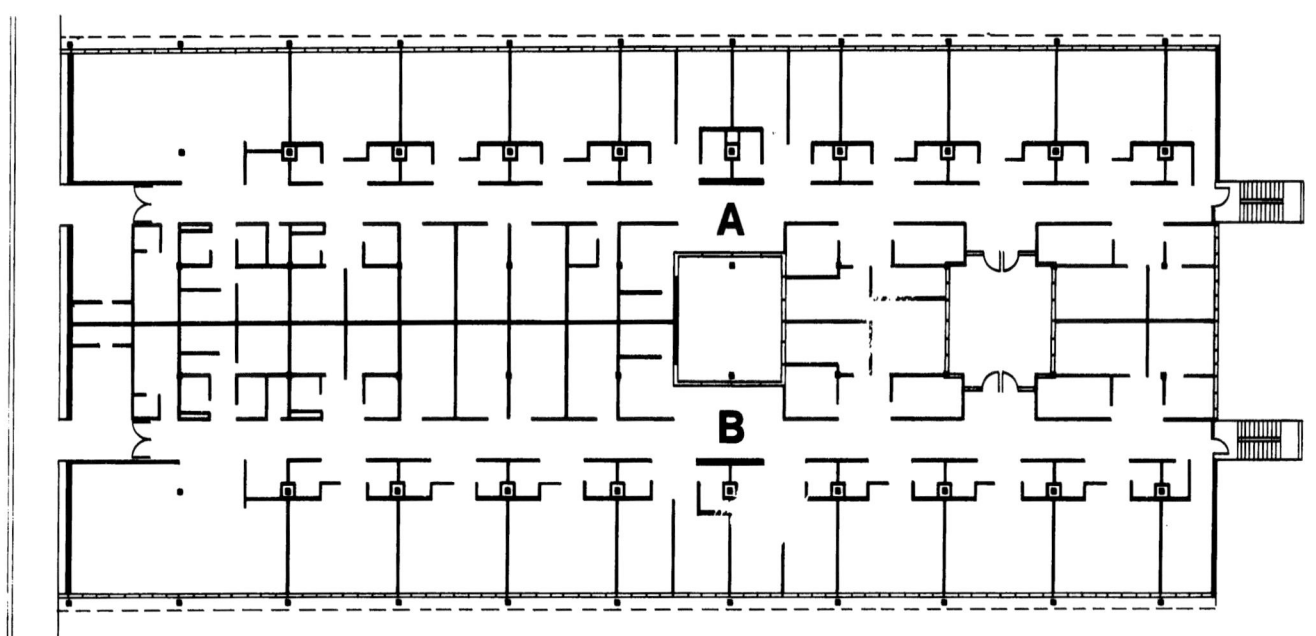

First floor

A. Future rehabilitation ward I
B. Future rehabilitation ward II

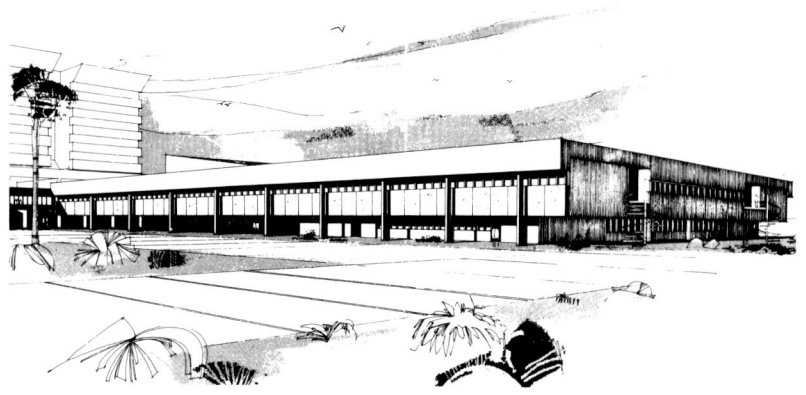

Service and Power Centre

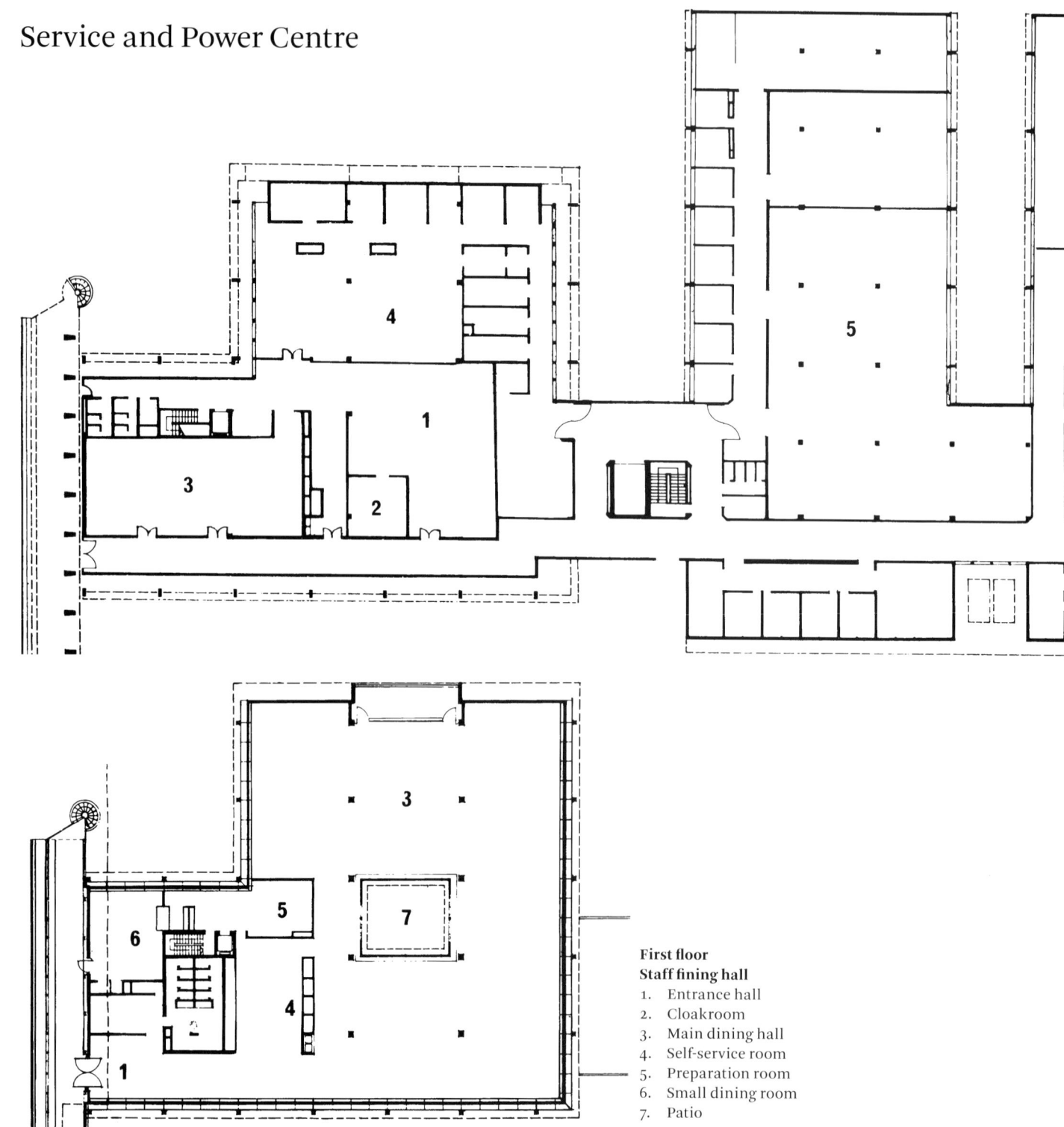

First floor
Staff fining hall
1. Entrance hall
2. Cloakroom
3. Main dining hall
4. Self-service room
5. Preparation room
6. Small dining room
7. Patio

5. The Hospitals and Health Facilities of Zarhy Architects

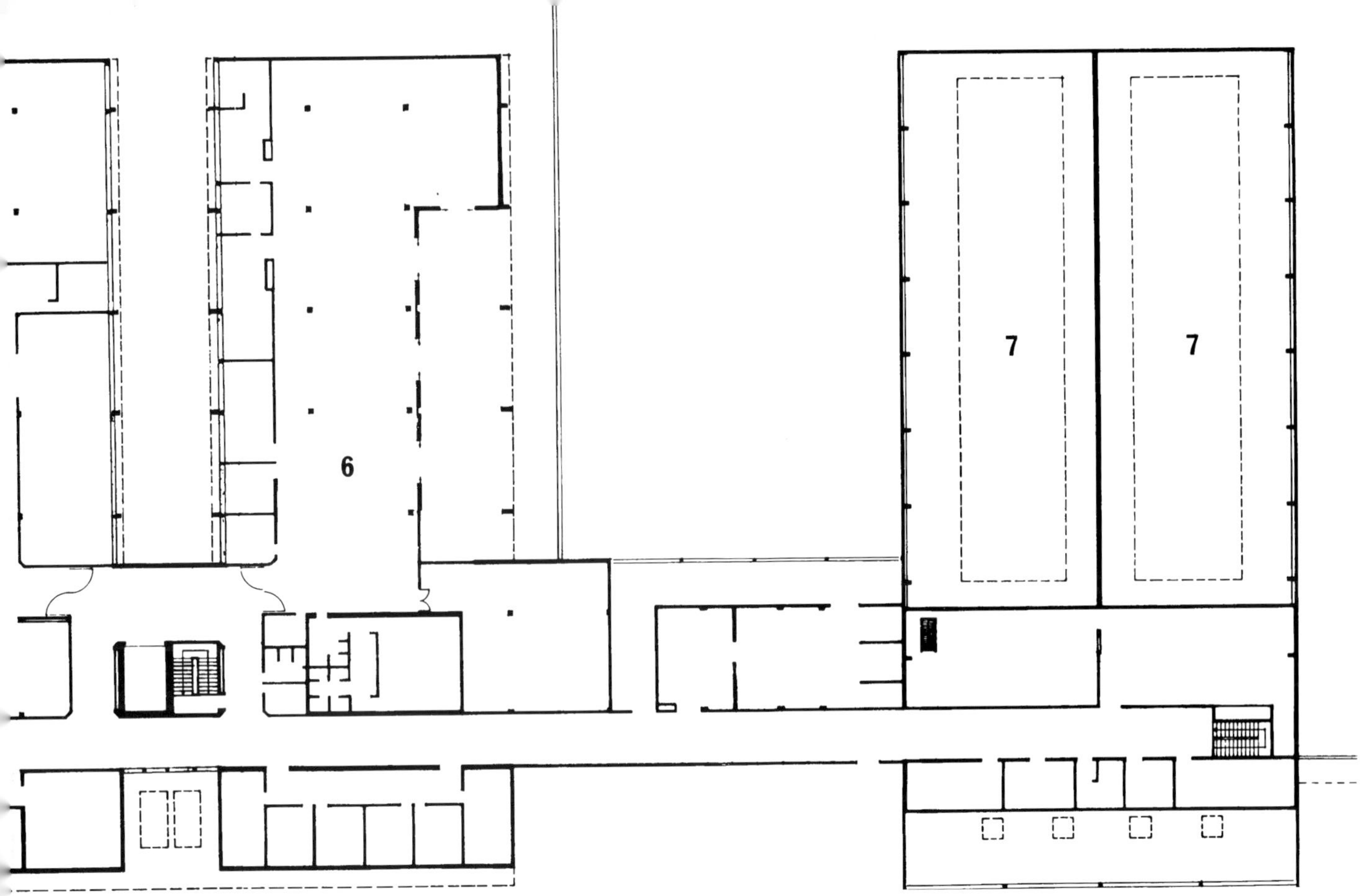

Ground floor

1. Food trolleys room
2. Refrigerated storeroom
3. Dish-washing room
4. Main kitchen (future expansion)
5. Central store (future expansion)
6. Workshops (future expansion)
7. Machine rooms

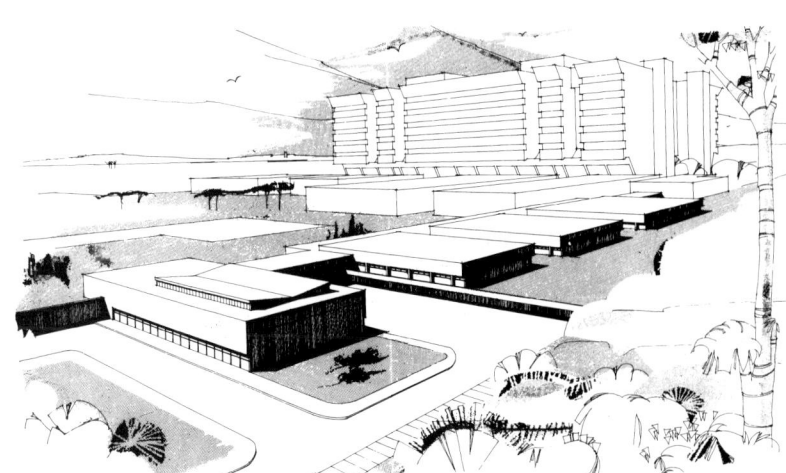

Clinical and Research Laboratories

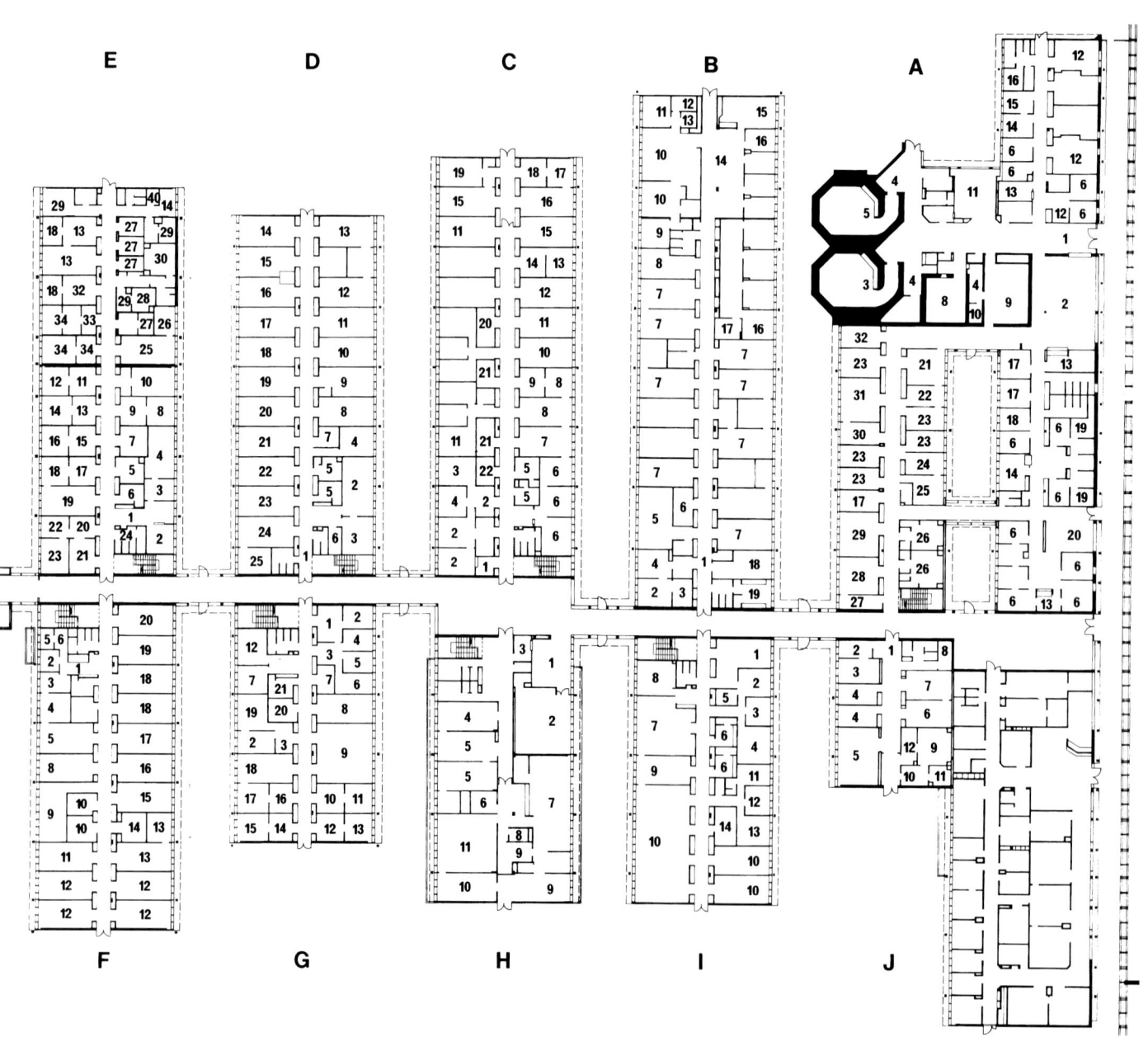

A. Oncology

1. Entrance
2. Main waiting area
3. Linear accelerator room
4. Control desk
5. Cobalt room
6. Doctor's room
7. Dressing room
8. Conventional therapy
9. Simulator room
10. Darkroom
11. Waiting room
12. Patients' ward (chemotherapy)
13. Secretary and information
14. Nurse's room
15. Injection room
16. Sluice room
17. Secretary
18. Head of dept.
19. Examination room
20. Waiting room
21. Treatment planning
22. Office
23. Laboratory
24. Physicist's office
25. Storeroom
26. Cloakroom
27. Kitchenette
28. Seminars room
29. Library
30. Scrub-up room
31. Treatment
32. Shielded radioactive storage

B. Haemtalogy

1. Entrance
2. Head of dept.
3. Examination cubicle
4. Secretary
5. Seminars and library
6. Cold room
7. Laboratory
8. On duty physician's room
9. Treatment room
10. Day-care roam
11. Nurse's room
12. Storeroom
13. Sterile storeroom
14. Waiting room
15. Reception and medical records
16. Doctors' room
17. Social worker
18. General storeroom
19. Cloakroom

C. Histology

1. Entrance
2. Secretary
3. Head of dept.
4. Deputy to the head of dept.
5. Cloakroom
6. Specimen reception and preparations
7. Laboratory (staining)
8. Histochemistry and staining
9. Ultra-microtomes
10. Cytology
11. Doctor's room
12. Seminars room
13. Tea room
14. Kitchenette
15. Laboratory
16. Photography
17. Head of medical photography sect.
18. Office
19. Development
20. Instruments room
21. Storeroom
22. Glassware washing

D. Biochemistry

1. Entrance
2. Head of dept.
3. Secretary
4. Deputy to head of dept.
5. Cloakroom
6. Janitor
7. Cold room
8. Research laboratory
9. Glassware washing
10. Automatic testing II
11. S.M.A.
12. Automatic testing I
13. Office
14. Storeroom
15. Urine laboratory
16. Specimen allocation
17. Laboratory (flame photom. electrophone)
18. Instruments
19. Glassware washing
20. Atomic absorption
21. Laboratory – enzymes I
22. Laboratory – enzymes II
23. Research laboratory
24. P.K.U.
25. Sterilization room

E. Virology and cross-infections

1. Entrance and waiting
2. Reception
3. Secretary
4. Head of dept.
5. Storeroom
6. Cloakroom
7. Preparation for serology
8. Radioactive room
9. Instruments
10. Tissue culture room
11. Preparation
12. Research laboratory
13. Radioactive room I
14. Radioactive room II
I5. Laboratory
16. Serology
17. Laboratory
18. Office
19. Antibiotics – level determination
20. Waiting room
21. Doctors' room
22. Secretary
23. Head of section1
24. Janitor and toilets
25. Clinical virology lab.
26. Head of section II
27. Cold room
28. Photography
29. Dark room
30. Isolation room
31. State smallpox centre
32. Skin rash laboratory
33. Tissue culture laboratory
34. Laboratory

F. Bacteriology

1. Entrance
2. Specimen recreation
3. Secretary
4. Head of dept.
5. Laboratory – head of dept.
6. Preparation
7. Stool examination laboratory
8. Instruments
9. Storeroom
10. Cold room
11. Sterilizers
12. Standard laboratory
13. Culture preparation
14. Sterile room
15. Blood culture
16. Urine culture
17. Laboratory – deputy to head dept.
18. Laboratory (general bacteriology)
19. Serology
20. T.B. laboratory

G. Toxicology

1. Reception and registration
2. Secretary
3. Waiting area
4. Head of toxicology section
5. Head of pharmacology section
6. Head of laboratory section
7. Chemicals storeroom
8. Laboratory
9. Laboratory (gas chromatography)
10. Laboratory (liquid chromatography)
11. Spectrometer
12. Optical instruments
13. Atomic reabsorption
14. Radioactive room
15. Centrifuges
16. Laboratory
17. Fractionation
18. Autoanalyzer
19. Head of dept.
20. Cold room
21. Cloakroom
22. Glassware washing-room

H. Shored laboratory services

1. Lecture hall lobby
2. Lecture hall
3. Kitchenette
4. Workshop
5. Maintenance workshop
6. Central glassware washing office
7. Central glassware washing room
8. Trolleys cleaning
9. Sterilizers
10. Pocking
11. Glassware storeroom

I. Blood bank

1. Entrance and waiting area
2. Secretary
3. Administrator
4. Head of dept.
5. Archives
6. Cloakroom
7. Blood donors' room
8. Kitchenette tea room
9. Psychophysics lab.
10. Laboratory

J. Hypertension research section

1. Entrance
2. Secretary
3. Head of dept.
4. Doctor's room
5. Treatment room
6. Laboratory I
7. Laboratory II
8. Kitchenette
9. Experimental surgery
10. Preparation room
11. Animas room
12. Scrub-up room

Funeral Parlour

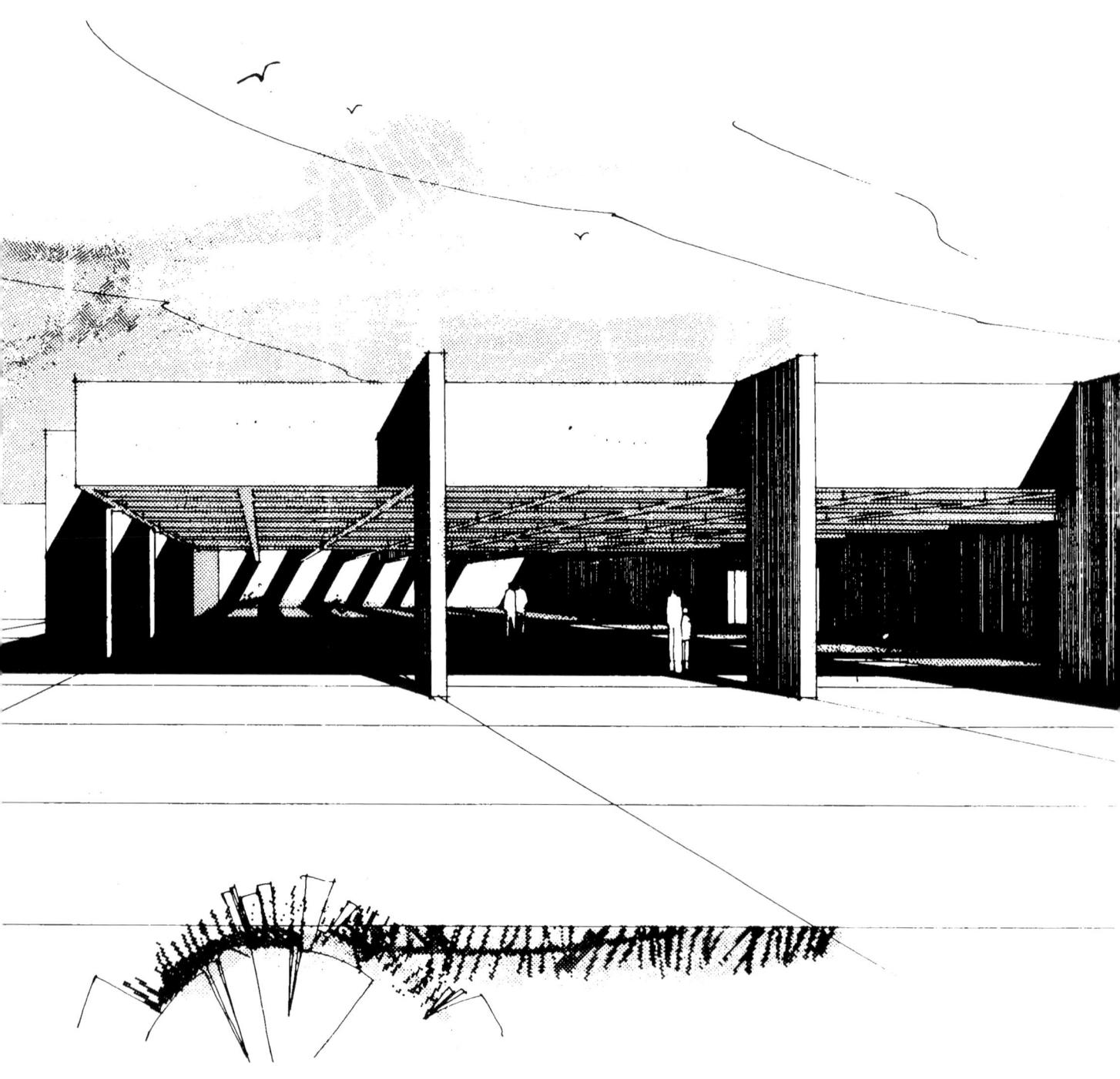

5. The Hospitals and Health Facilities of Zarhy Architects

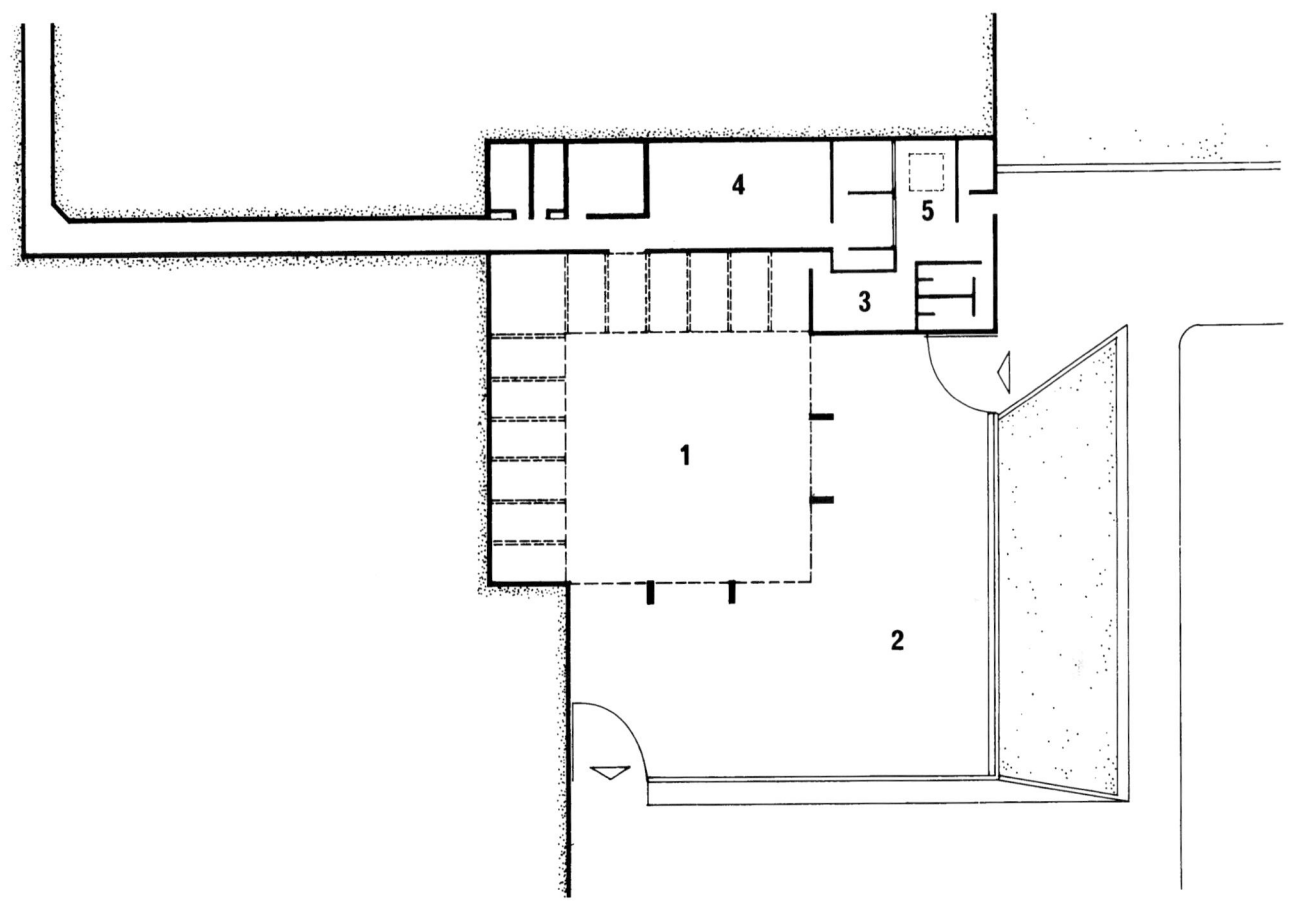

1. Mourners hall
2. Mourners court
3. Room for the family of the deceased
4. "Tahara" room
5. "Hevra kadisha"

Eye Institute

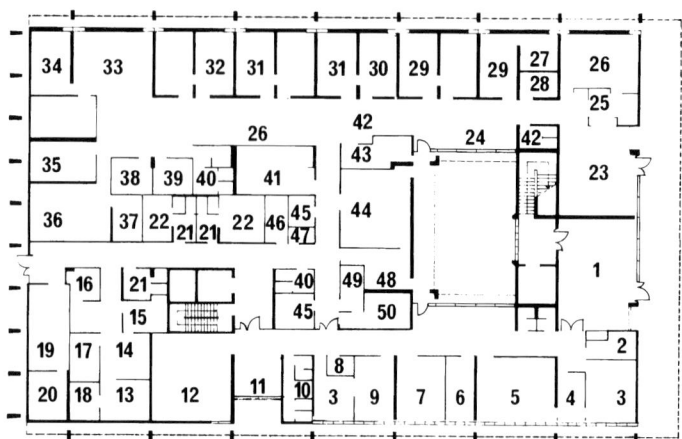

Ground floor

Administration
1. Entrance and waiting area
2. Information and telephone
3. Office switchboard
4. Secretary
5. Library
6. Social nurse
7. Rehabilitation room
8. Cleaning utensils
9. Administrator's room
10. Toilets
11. Waiting room
12. Conference room
44. Head of Institute

Electron microscope
13. Electron microscope
14. Reserve room for election
I5. Office microscope
16. Engine room
17. Ultra tome room
18. Dark room
19. Laser room
20. Laser room

Shared Area
21. Dressing room
22. Cloakroom

Outpatient department
23. Entrance and waiting area
24. Waiting area
25. Office
26. Out-patient medical files
27. Minor surgery examination
28. Head nurse

29. General examination room
30. Outer-eye disease's examination
31. Retina patient's examination
32. Glaucoma patient's examination
33. Waiting area for children
34. Strabismus room
35. Contact lenses and low vision
36. Photolaboratory
37. Dark room

38. Tonography dynamometry
39. Perimetry
40. Toilets
41. Laser and xenon photocoagulator
42. Nurses' stations
43. Nurses' room
44. Head of institute
45. Storeroom
46. Soiled linen
47. Cleaning utensils
48. Secretary
49. Kitchenette
50. Tea room

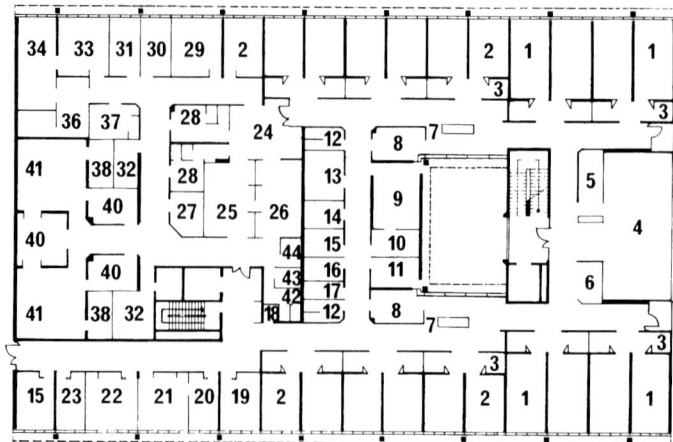

5. The Hospitals and Health Facilities of Zarhy Architects

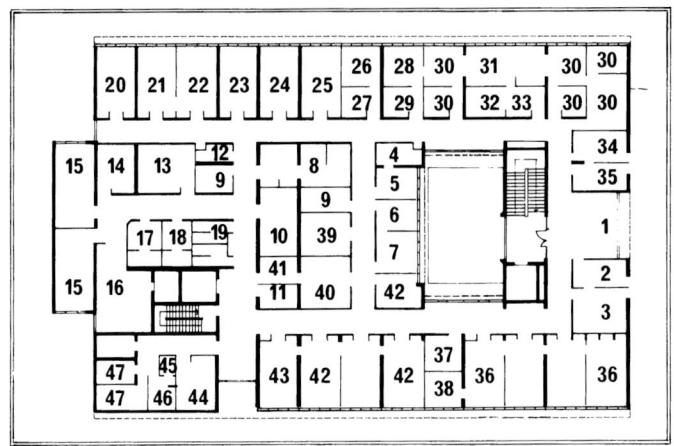

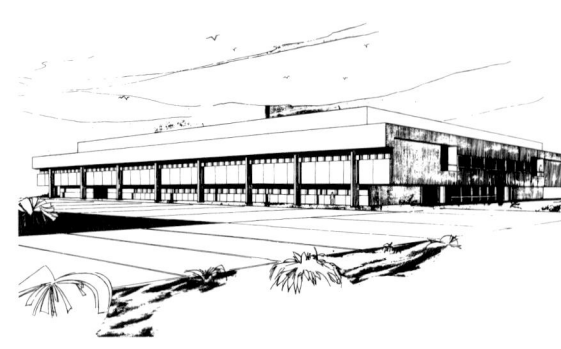

Second floor
Research department general

1. Waiting area
2. Secretary
3. Head of dept.
4. Eye bank
5. Xerox room
6. Kitchenette
7. tea room
8. Laboratory kitchen
9. General storeroom
10. Heavy equipment
11. Scintillator
12. Cleaning utensils
13. Special apparatus
14. Office

15. Laboratory
16. Machine room
17. Cold roam
18. Constant temp. room
19. Toilets
20. Workshop

Pathology

21. Reagents
22. Processing
23. Light microscopy and photogr.
24. General storeroom
25. Tissue cultures

Electrophysiology of vision

26. Data processing
27. Dark room
28. Electronics workshop
29. Dark adaptation room
30. Laboratory
31. Computer
32. Patients' room
33. E.R.G.
34. Office
35. Secretary

Biochemistry and pharmacology

36. Laboratory
37. Instruments
38. Office

Microbiology of the eye

39. Immunology
40. Culture preparation
41. General storeroom
42. Laboratory

Animal quarters

43. Laboratory
44. Drying room
45. Washing room
46. Food preparation
47. Animal room

First floor
In-patient department

1. 3-bed room
2. 2-bed room
3. Patients' W.C.
4. Patients' day / dining room
5. Kitchenette
6. Stretcher and wheelchair nook
7. Nurses' station
8. Nurses' workroom
9. Examination roam
10. Treatment room

11. Head nurse
12. Staff toilets
13. Sluice room
14. Clean storage
15. General storage
16. Soiled linen
17. Cleaning utensils
18. Garbage
19. Staff tea room
20. Secretary
21. Head of dept.
22. Doctors' room
23. Superintendent's room

Operating theatres suite

24. Entrance
25. Reception room
26. Recovery roam
27. Anesthetist's storeroom
28. Cloakrooms and toilets
29. Head nurse
30. Doctors' room
31. Clean storeroom
32. General storeroom
33. Nurses' workroom
34. Sterile storeroom

35. Sterilization roam
36. Washing room
37. Sluice room
38. Instruments roam
39. Scrub-up and gowning rooms
40. Preparation and induction room
41. Operating theatres
42. Patients toilets
43. Cleaning utensils
44. Soiled linen

Women Hospital

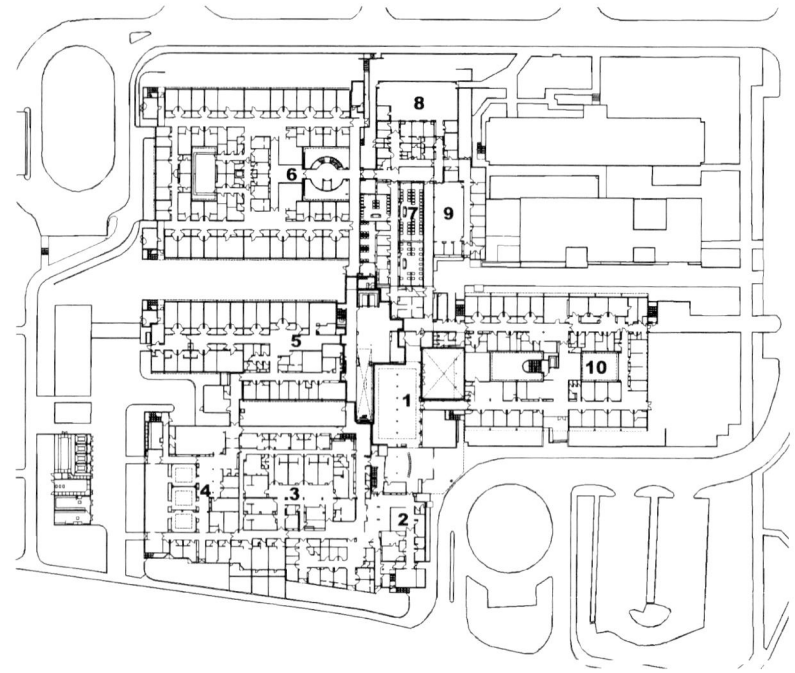

Ground floor plan
1. Main entrance hall
2. Admittance and examination rooms
3. Delivery rooms
4. Intervention and operating theatres
5. Obstetrics and gynecology Department
6. Hospitalization wards
7. New born ward
8. Premature babies' ward
9. Intensvive care unit
10. Out patients' department

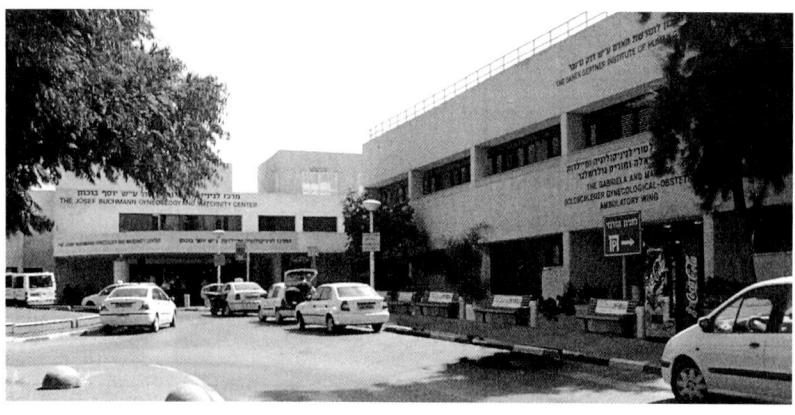

View to the main entrance

5. The Hospitals and Health Facilities of Zarhy Architects

First floor plan

11. Medical hotel
12. High risk pregnancy unit
13. Research laboratories
14. Genetic research laboratories

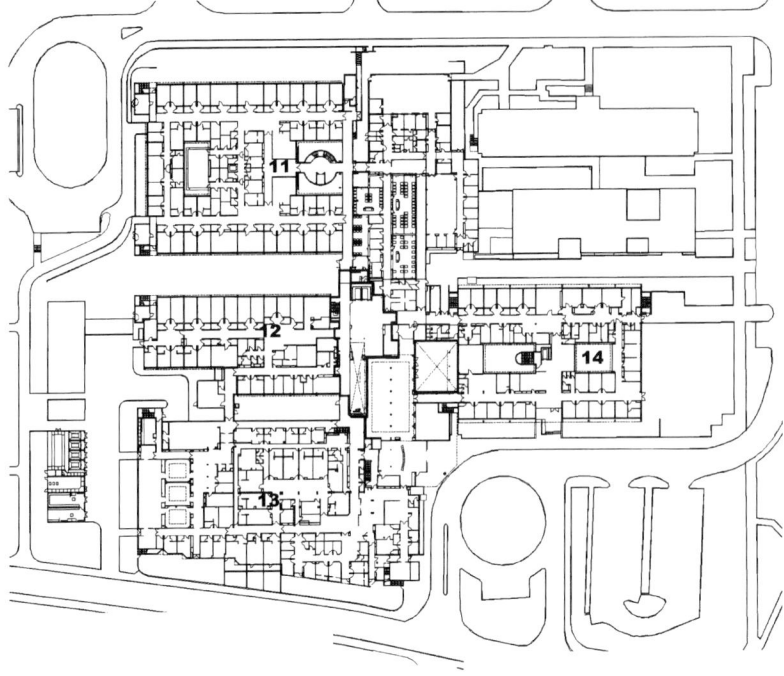

West elevation

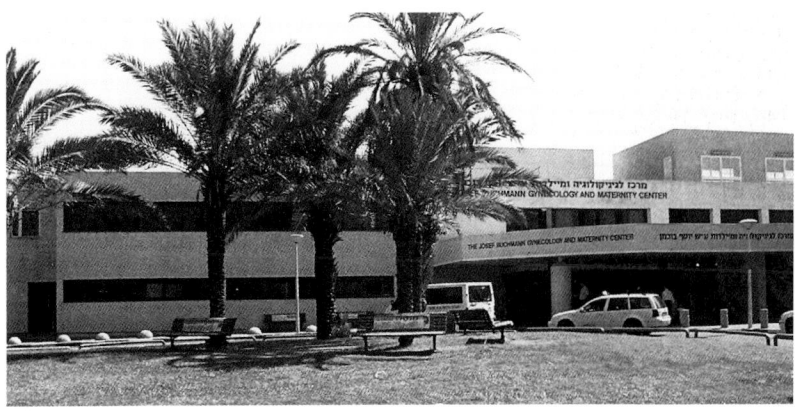

Rehabilitation Hospital

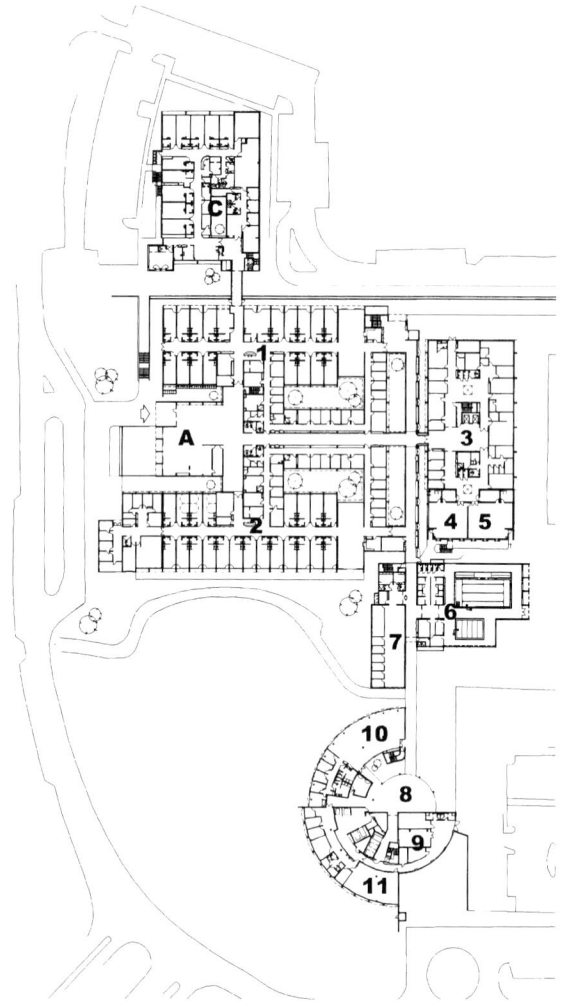

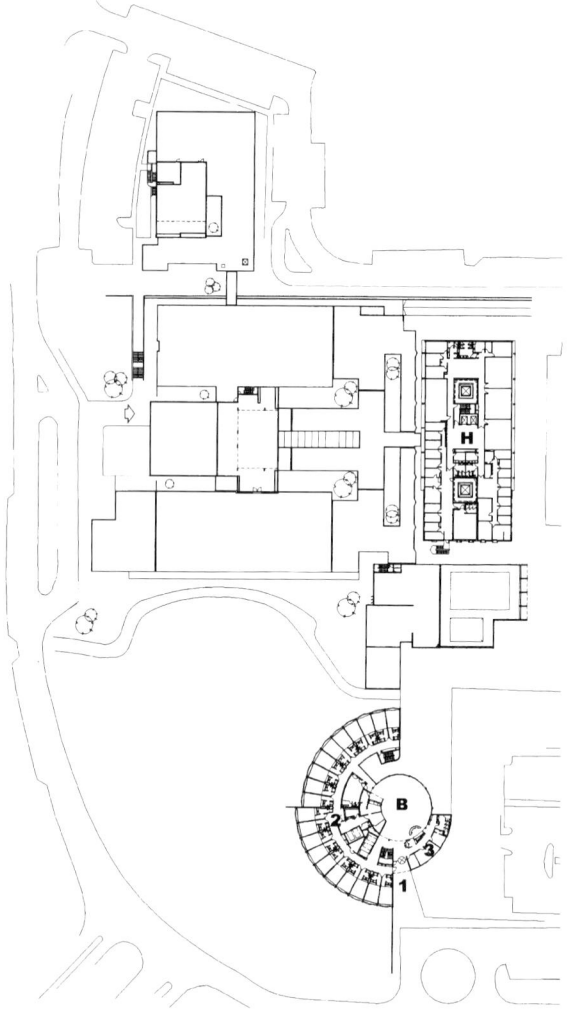

Ground floor plan

A Main entrance hall
1. Neurological department
2. Orthopaedical department
3. Treatment department
4. Physiotherapy
5. Occupational therapy
6. Therapeutical swimming pools

7. Fitness department
8. Lower ground floor entrance
9. Machine room
10. Fitness hall and spa
11. Motion lab.

C Respiratory rehabilitation center

Lower floor plan

D Multiple sclerosis department
E Out patients' department
F Entrance hall to O.P.D
G Machine room

5. The Hospitals and Health Facilities of Zarhy Architects

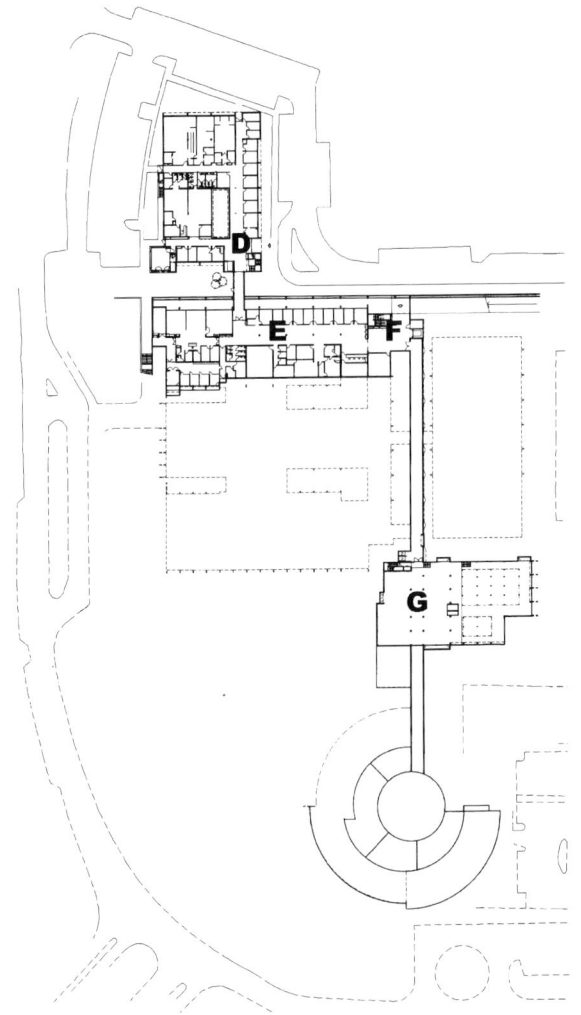

Upper floor plan
B   Medical hotel lounge
1. Main entrance to the medical hotel
2. Patients' rooms
3. Examination rooms
H. Physiotherapy school

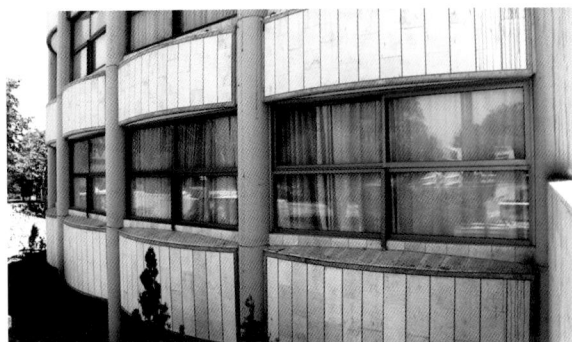

Detail of the facade
Photo: Pawlik 2013

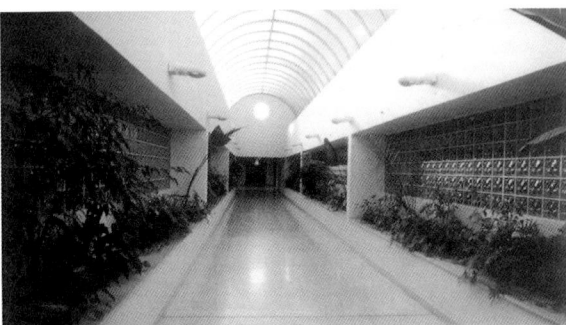

The hospital street

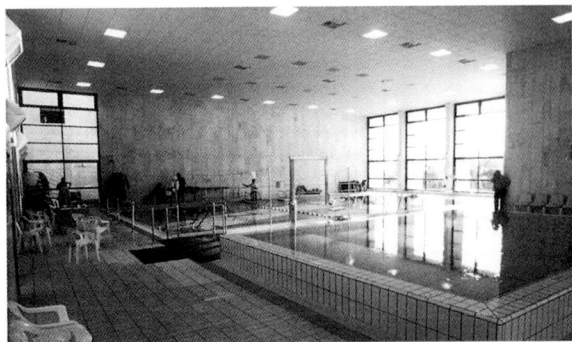

The therapeutical swimming pool

Psychiatric Hospital

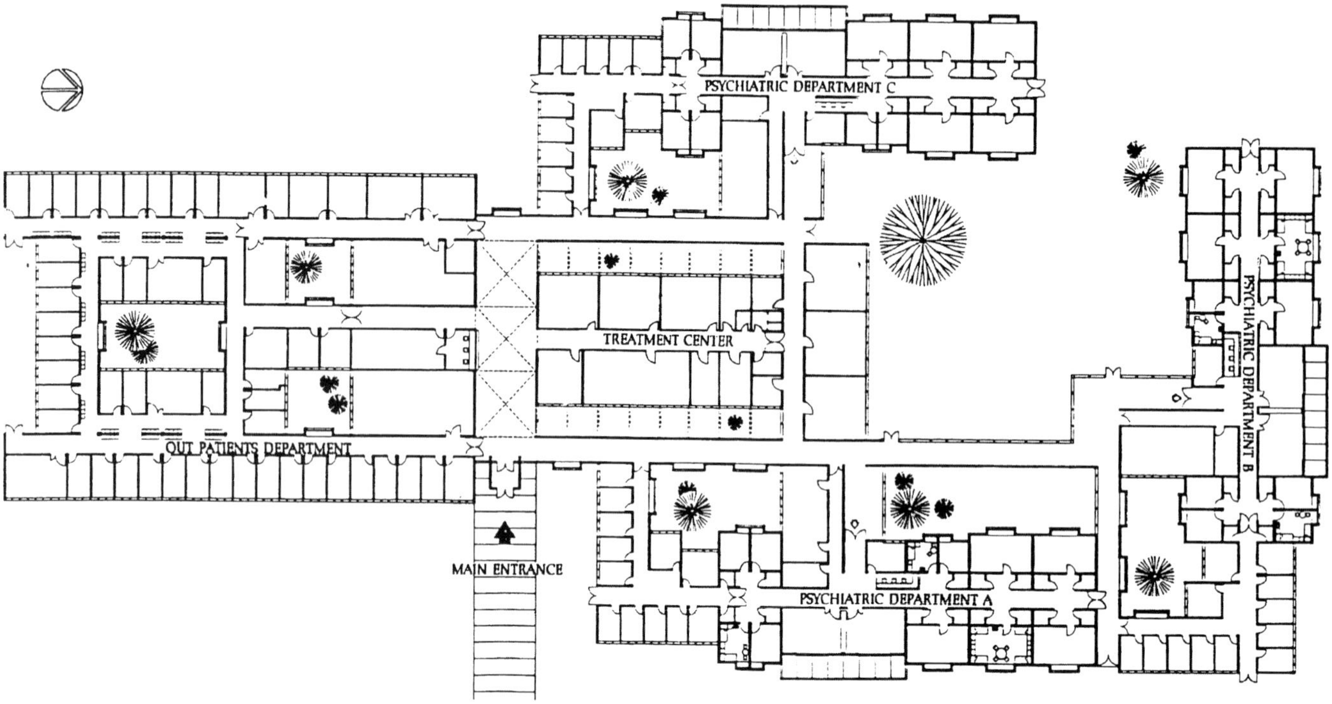

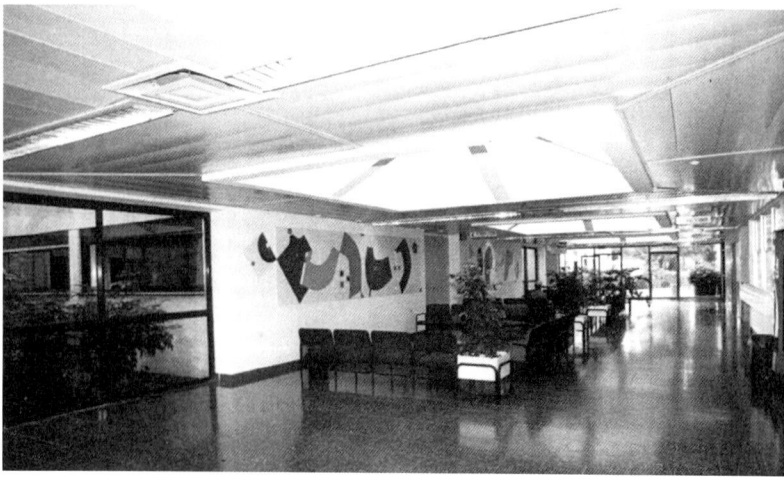

PSYCHIATRIC DEPARTMENT C

TREATMENT CENTER

PSYCHIATRIC DEPARTMENT B

OUT PATIENTS DEPARTMENT

MAIN ENTRANCE

PSYCHIATRIC DEPARTMENT A

Ground floor

The main entrance hall

5. The Hospitals and Health Facilities of Zarhy Architects

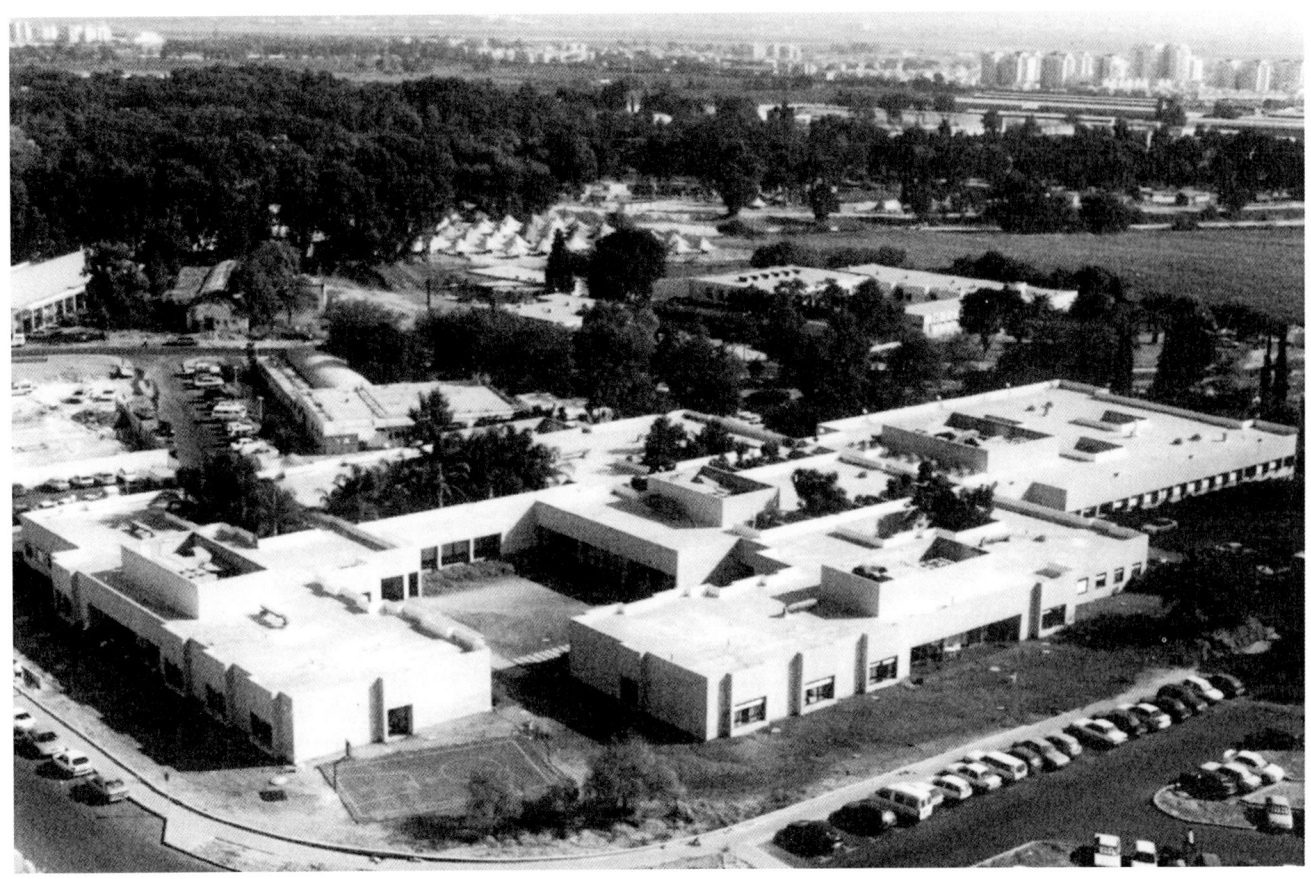

Birds view of the psychiatric hospital

The psychiatric hospital consists of 3 inpatients departments of 30 beds each, a large outpatient clinic and a day care facility. It offers the following services and facilities:

· Full or partial inward treatment,
· Comprehensive outpatient treatment, including a specialized mood disorder clinic,
· A rehabilitation day care service,
· The liaison and consultation service,
· An advisory facility for medical clinics in our catchment area,
· Psychology and Social Work services,
· Occupational therapy,
· Training programs,
· Research.

Medical Training and Teaching Institute

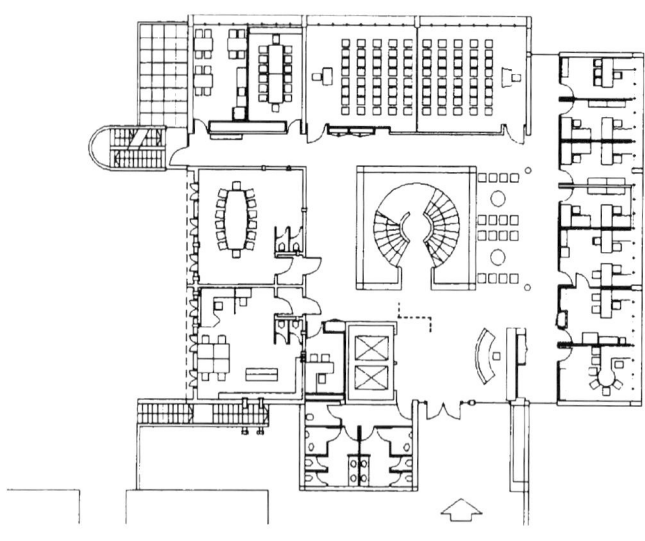

Entrance floor plan

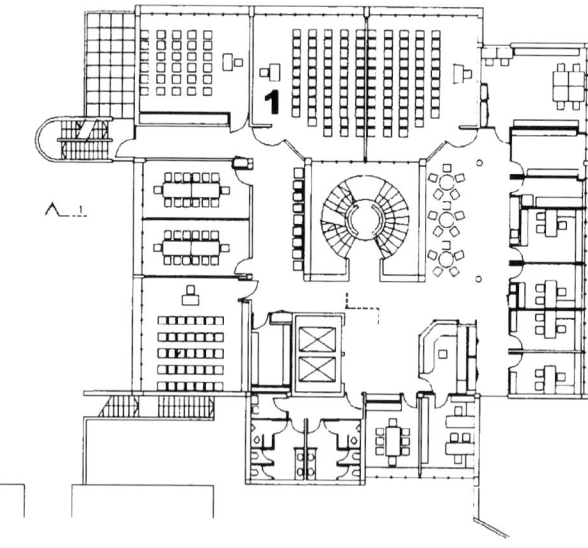

First floor plan

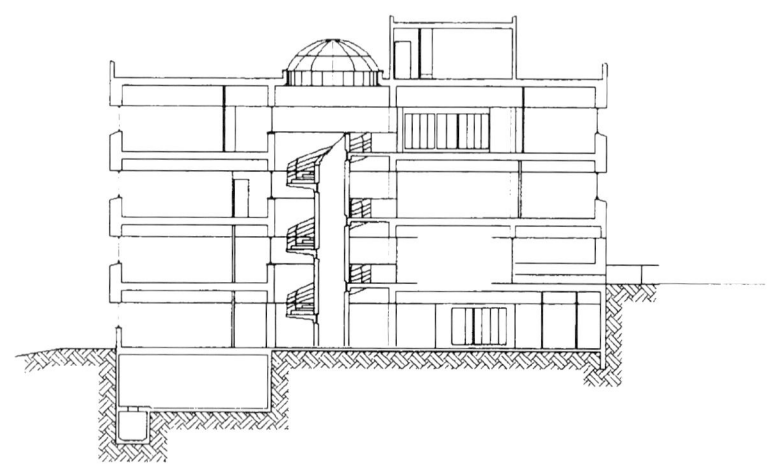

Cross Section

1. Lecture room
2. Class room
3. Physicians' examination section
4. Simulated operating theatres

5. The Hospitals and Health Facilities of Zarhy Architects

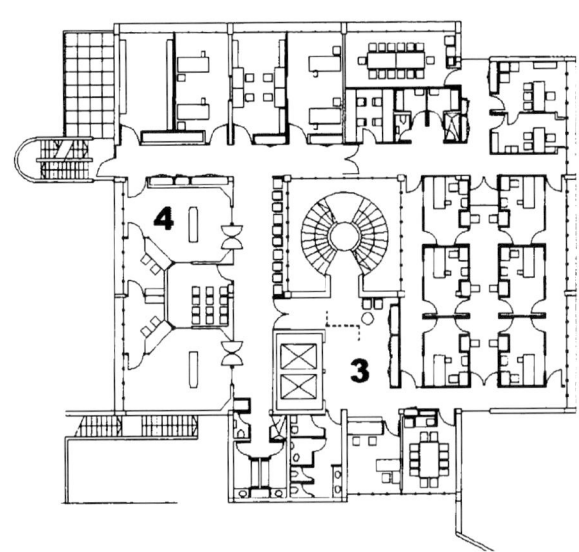

Second floor plan

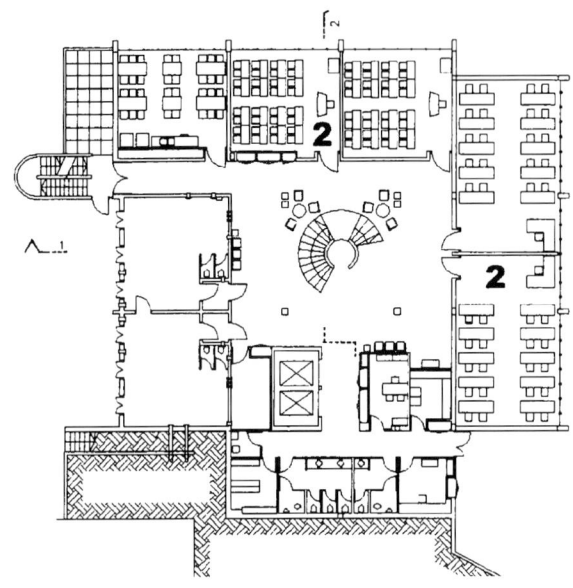

Lower floor plan

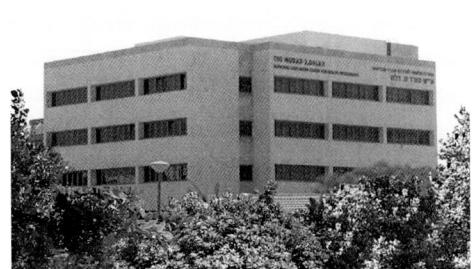

Main view from south-west

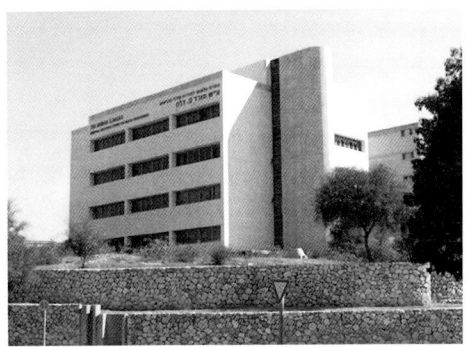

Main view from north-east

Oral and Maxillofacial Institute

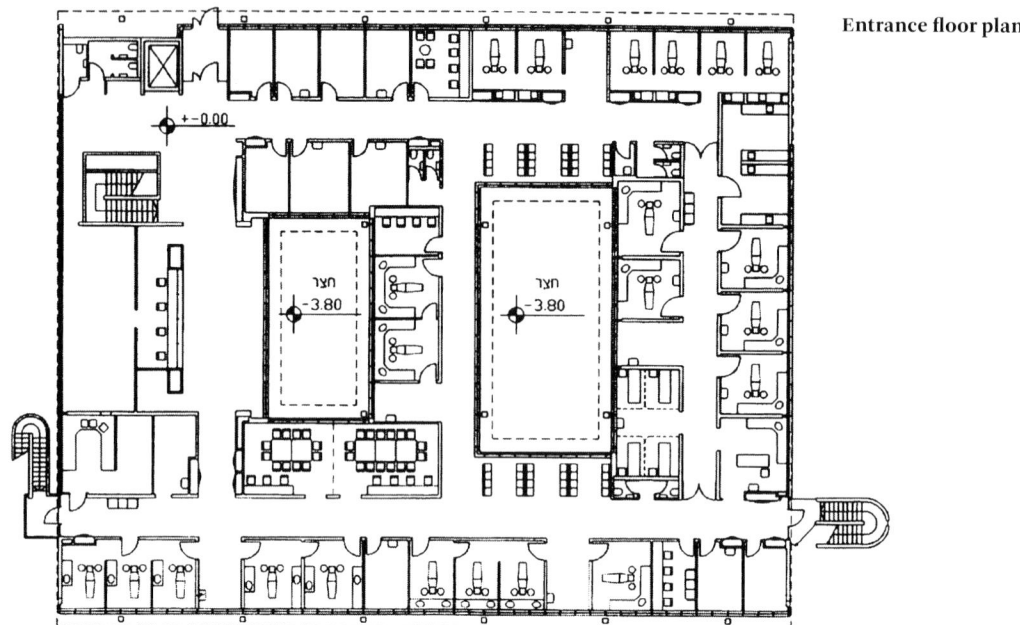

The Oral and Maxillofacial Institute is a two stories building. The admittance is at the entrance floor which is the ground floor. The institute has about forty five modular treatment rooms and all the ancillary rooms. The total floor area is 2,900 sqm.

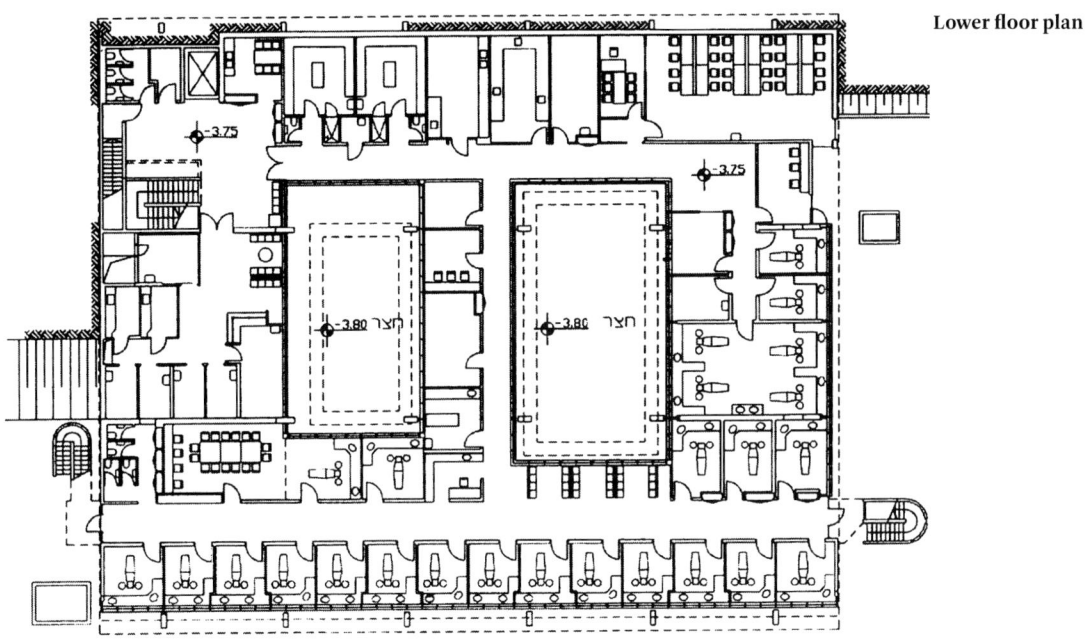

Lower floor plan

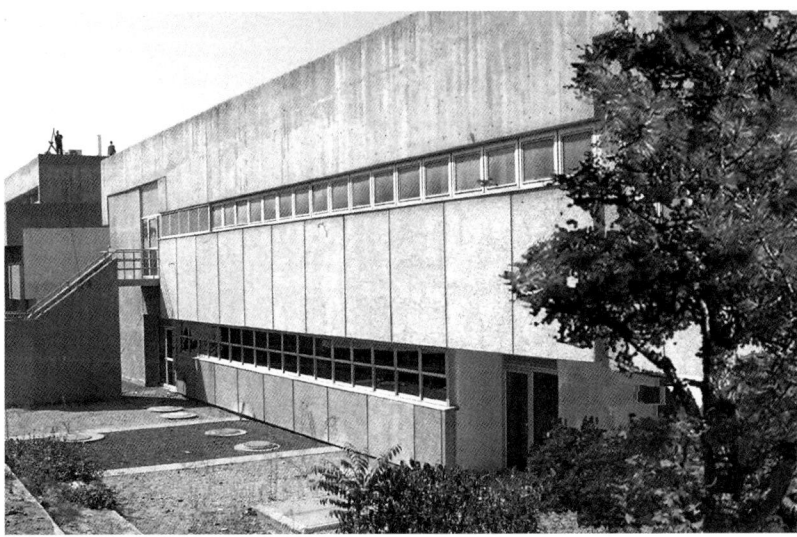

View to the entrance

Administration and Management Building

The administration and management building is located centrally in Sheba Medical Center. It is a one story building comprised of wings of offices and meeting rooms surrounding a courtyard.

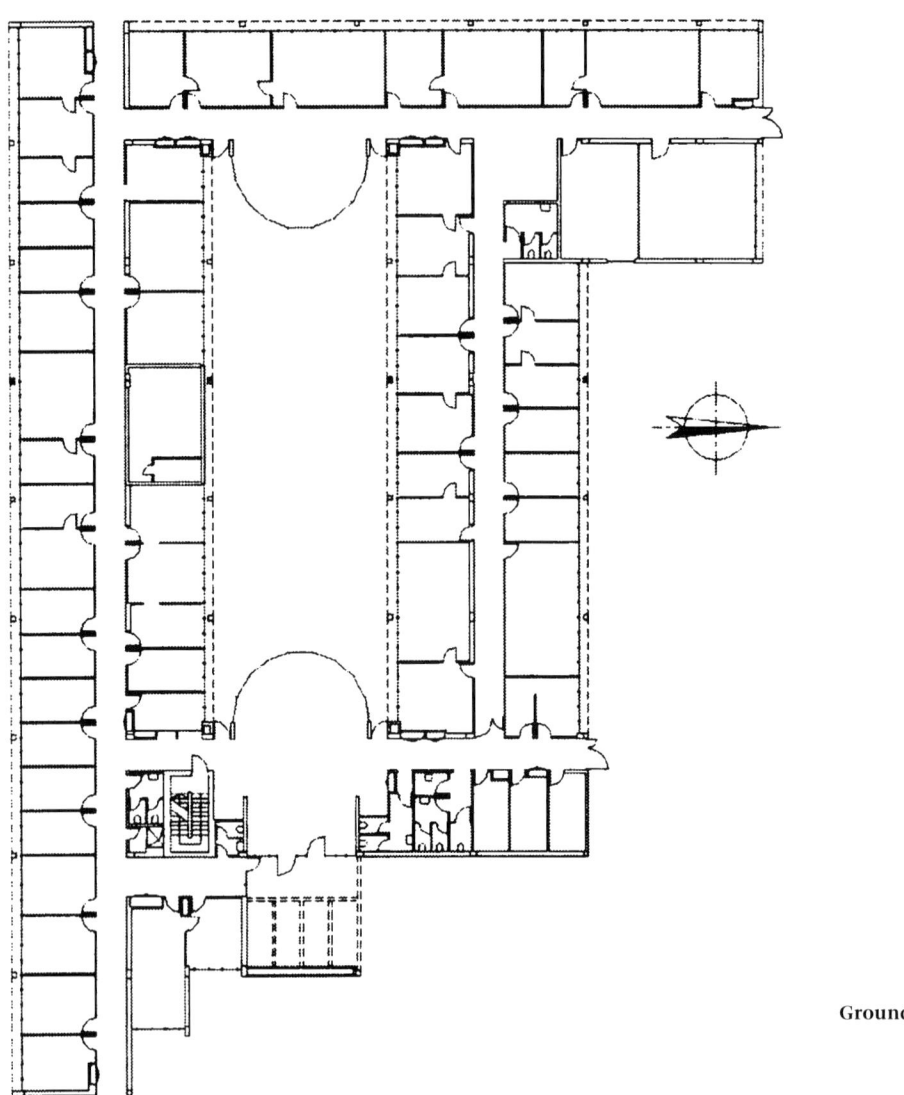

Ground floor plan

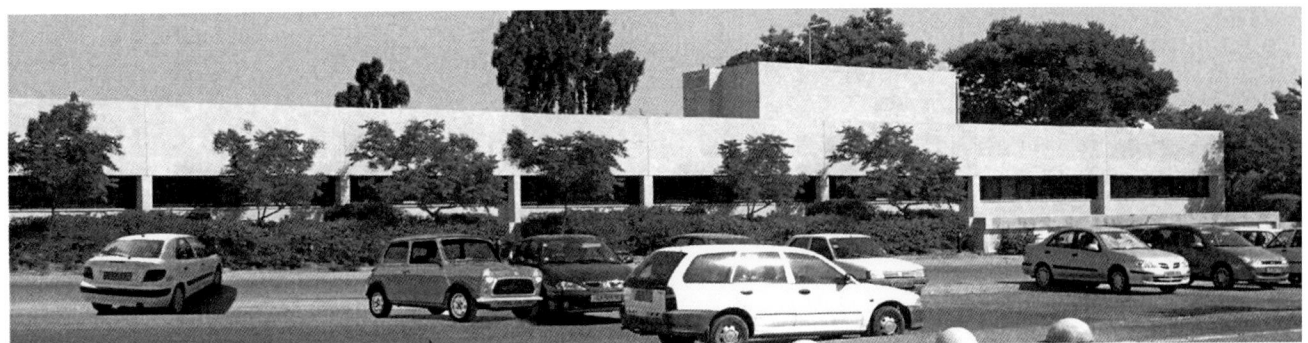

Main view

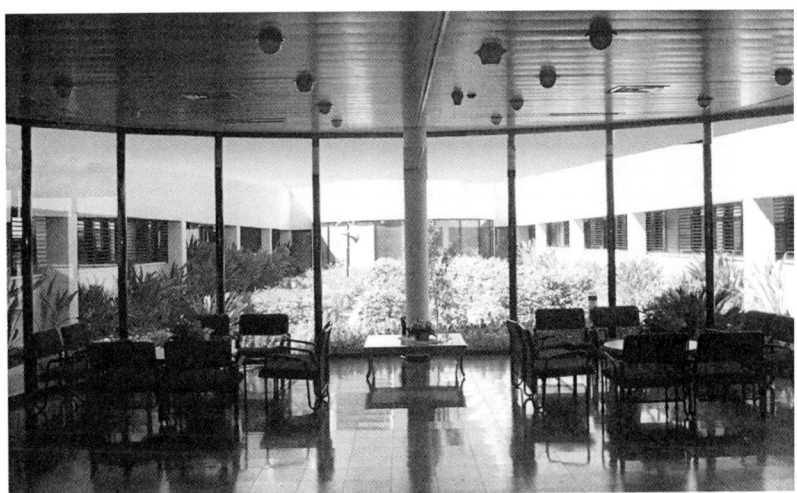

View into the inner courtyard

Public Health Research Institute

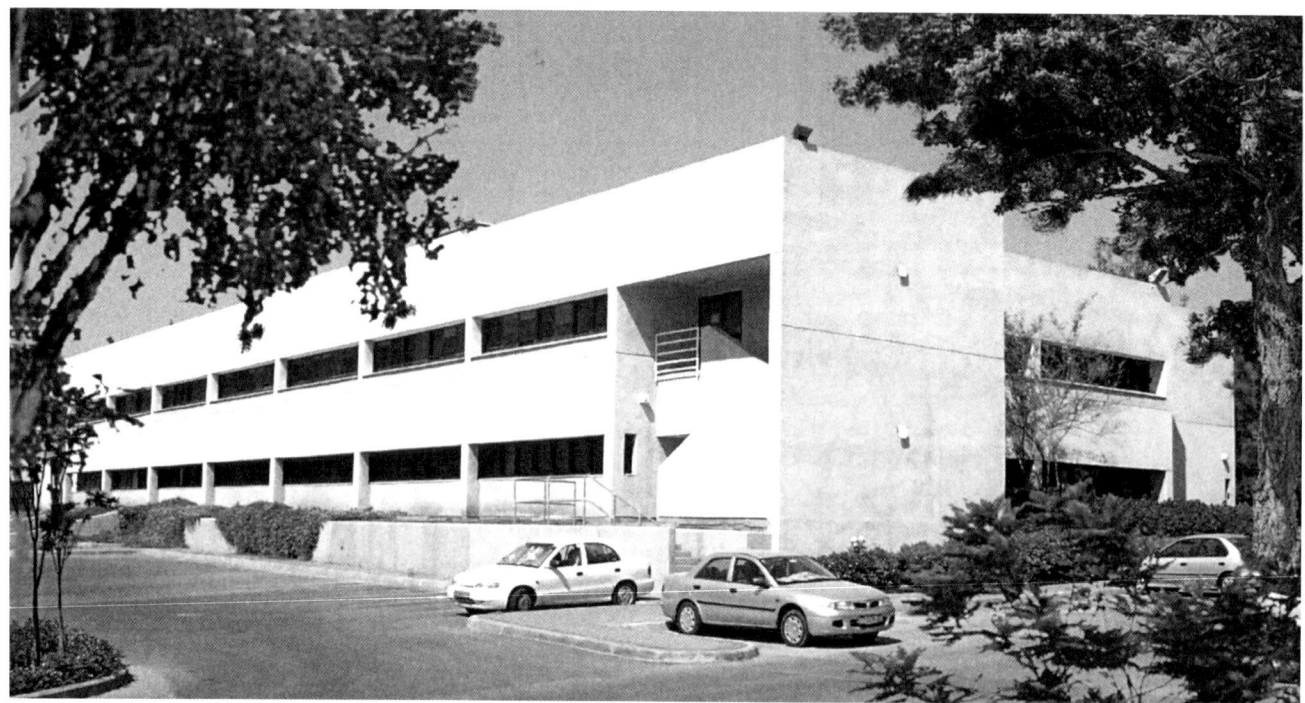

Main view

First floor plan

1. Director
2. Deputy director
3. Secretary
4. Researcher
5. Associate researcher
6. Unit director
7. Office
8. Statistician
9. Conference room
10. Computers room
11. Library
12. Office services
13. Kitchenette
14. Storage
15. Shelter
16. Archives

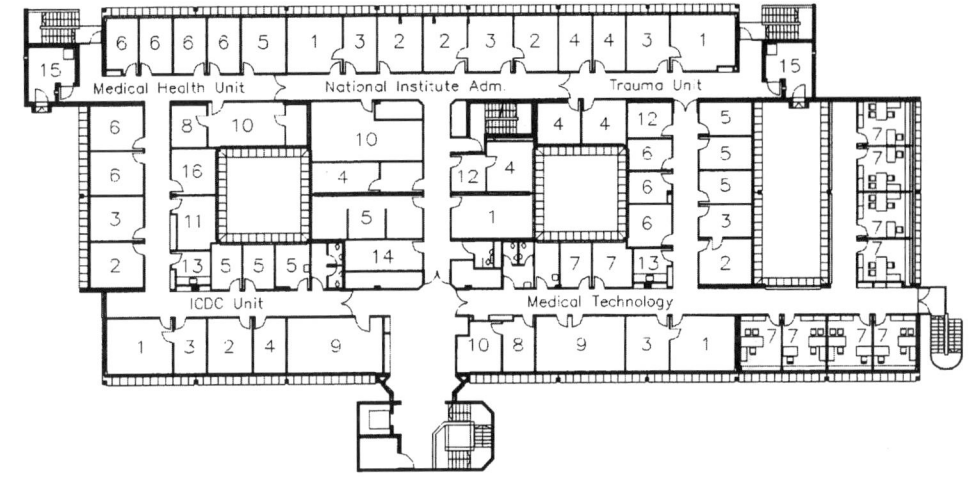

Ground floor plan

1. Director
2. Deputy director
3. Secretary
4. Researcher
5. Associate researcher
6. Typing room
7. Office
8. Statistician
9. Conference room
10. Computers room
11. Library
12. Office services
13. Kitchenette
14. Storage
15. Shelter
16. Archives
17. Medical advisors
18. Programmer

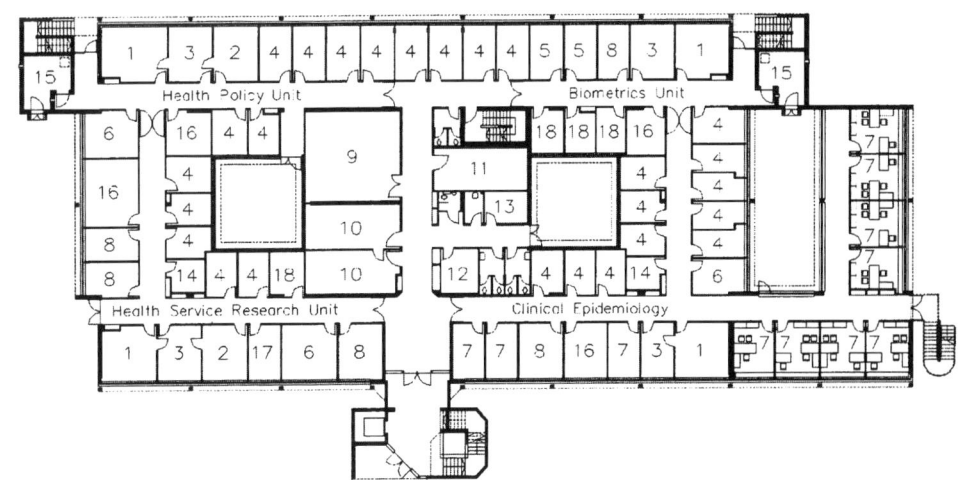

E.N.T. and Audiology Institute

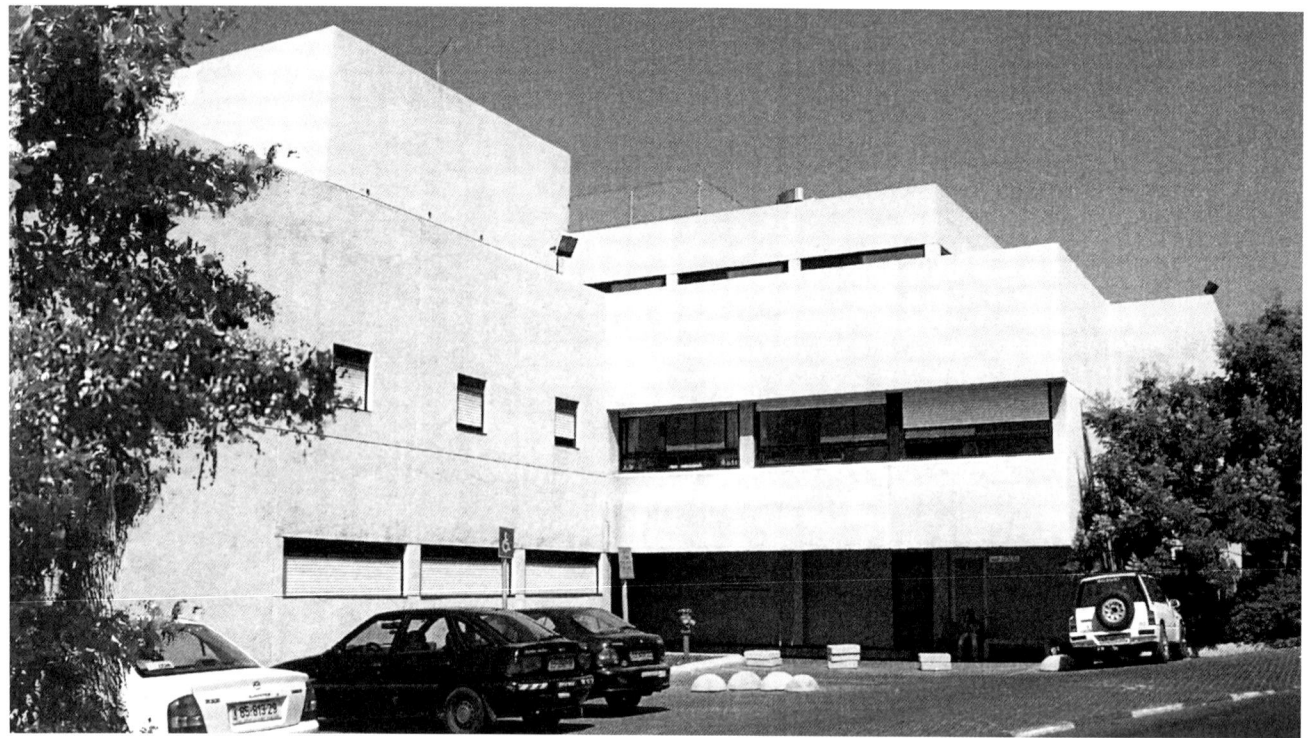

View to the main entrance

First floor plan
4. Ward
5. Operating theatres

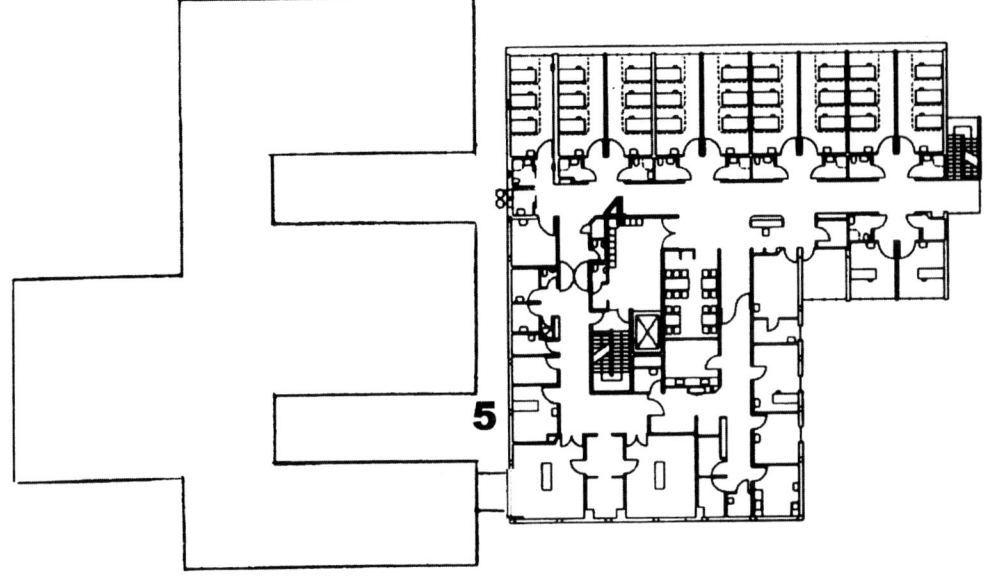

Ground floor plan
1. Out patients' department
2. Administration
3. Audiology department

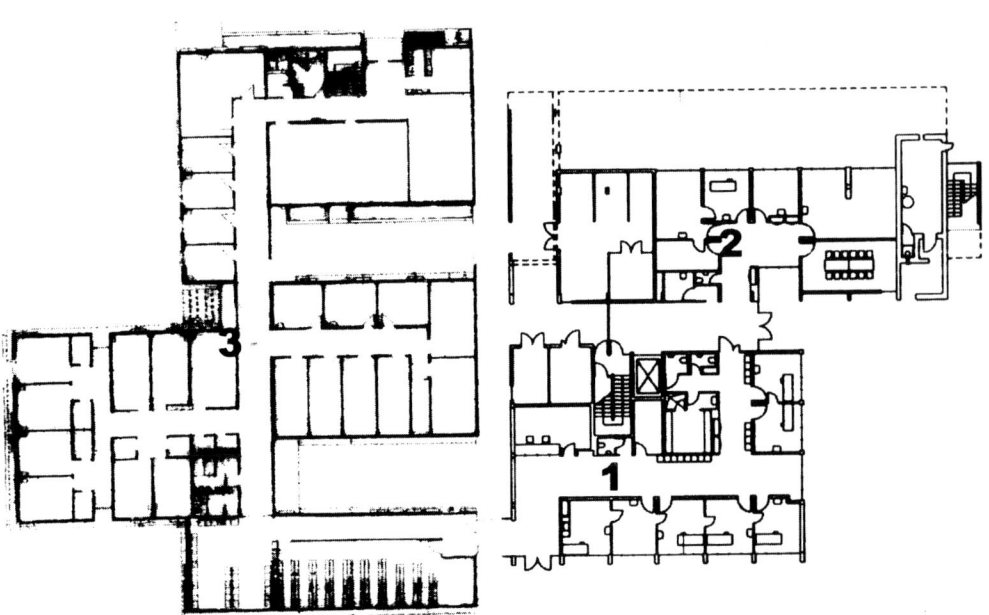

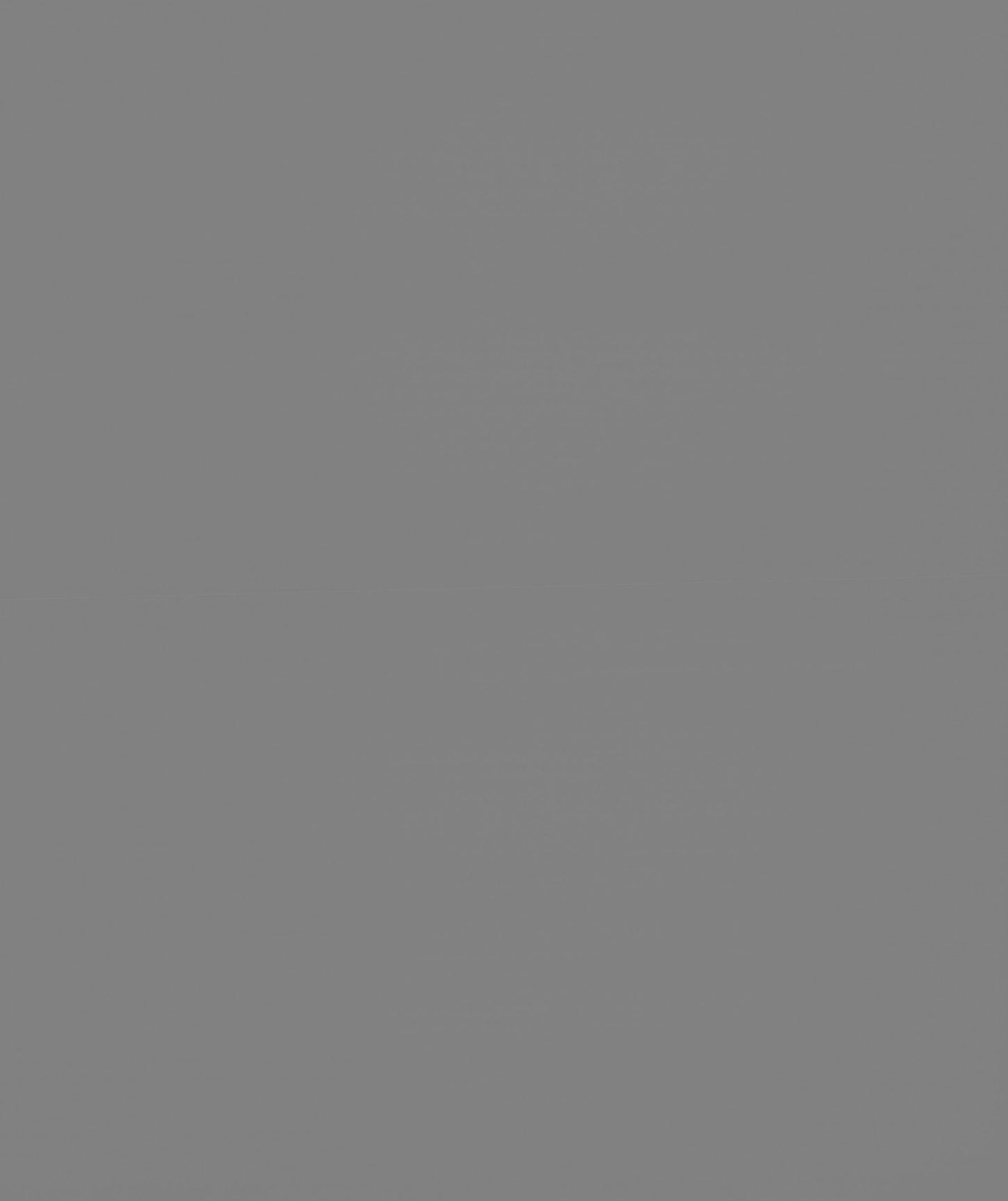

2. Meir Medical Center

Sapir Medical Center
Kfar Saba, 620 Beds, 65,000 sqm, 1952–2010

Meir Hospital is located in Kfar Saba and serves the population of the Sharon Valley. It was financed and is operated by the Health Organization of the Labour Union (Kupat-Holim).

The design of the hospital is based on plans submitted to an architectural competition in 1947, which won first prize. The hospital was planned as a T.B. hospital based on an explicit programme for a specialized hospital for lung diseases. It was intended to treat the new immigrants of the early fifties. Later, as a consequence of changing conditions of hospitalization requirements, it was transformed into a general hospital. New wings to house medical services were added and it developed into a medical centre, consisting of the various facilities to provide comprehensive medical care.

The building consists of three main blocks. The ward block, the largest one, contains 10 typical medical wards, 40 beds each, in five typical floors.

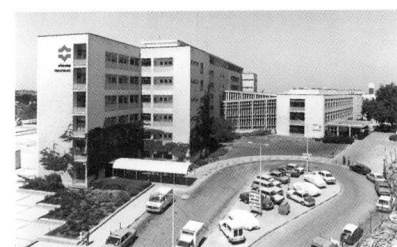 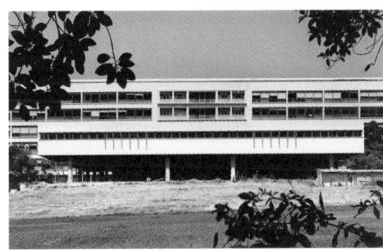

Left: main view
Right: garden view

Sapir Medical Center

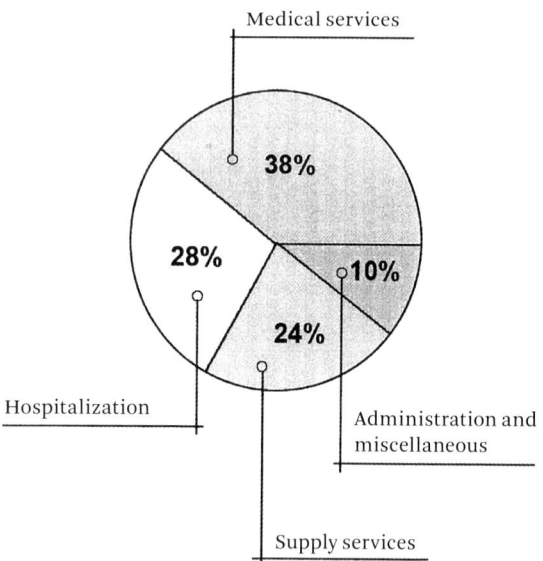

Medical services

38%

28%

10%

24%

Hospitalization

Administration and
miscellaneous

Supply services

Total area
102,427 sqm
Medical services
39,460 sqm
Hospitalization
28,245 sqm
Supply services
24,222 sqm
Administration and miscellaneous
10,500 sqm

The disposition of the main ward block and the basic composition of the whole edifice were based on the requirement to have southern orientation for all patients' rooms. Cross-ventilation was made possible by leaving spaces along the corridor, facing the northern wall of the building.

Operating theatres and outpatient departments are located on the southern part of the hospital. The operating theatres suite is located on the same level as the first ward floor and forms a "cul-de-sac" as far as circulation is concerned.

The outpatient department is spread over three floors and has its own separate public entrance. This main entrance and the waiting hall are located at the intermediate floor, in order to save on patients' circulation. This is made possible by the terrain that slopes gently to the south.

The inter-relationship of the main functIonal divisions of the hospital

1. Hospitalization services
2. Medical services
3. Administrative services and miscellaneous
4. Supply services
5. Outpatient department
A. Main entrance
B. Entrance to casualty department
C. Service entrance

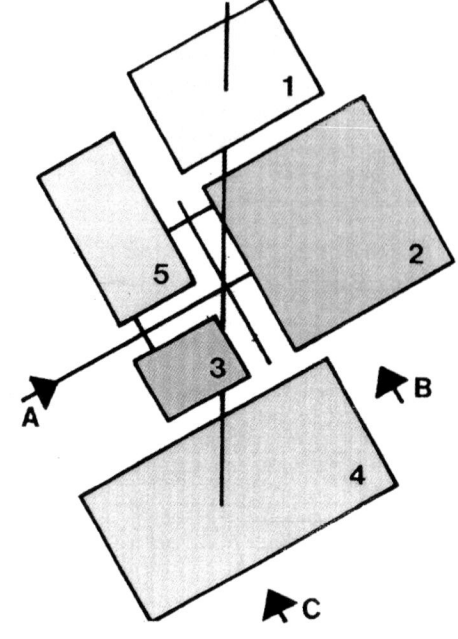

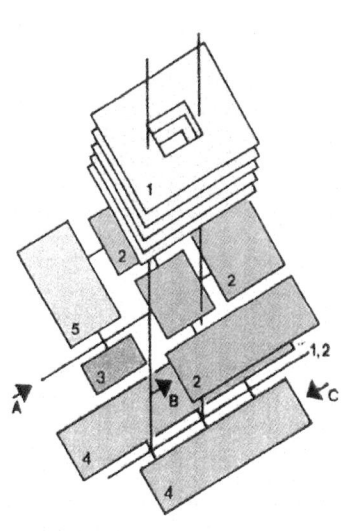

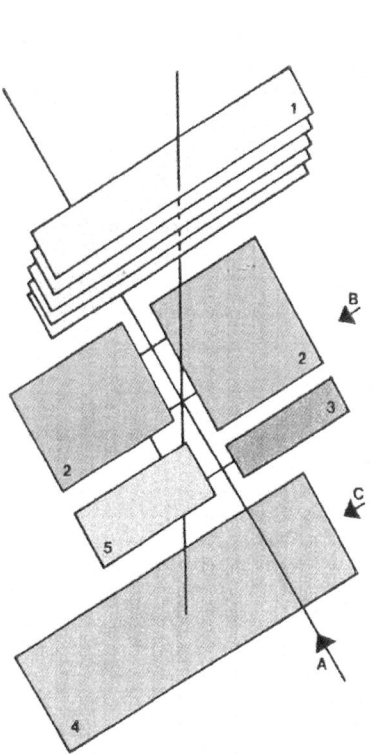

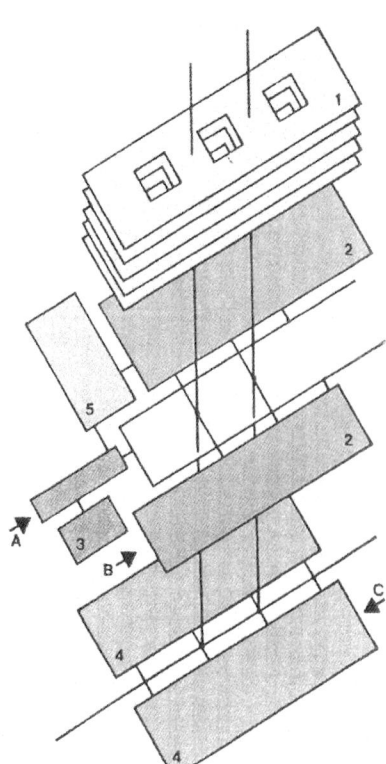

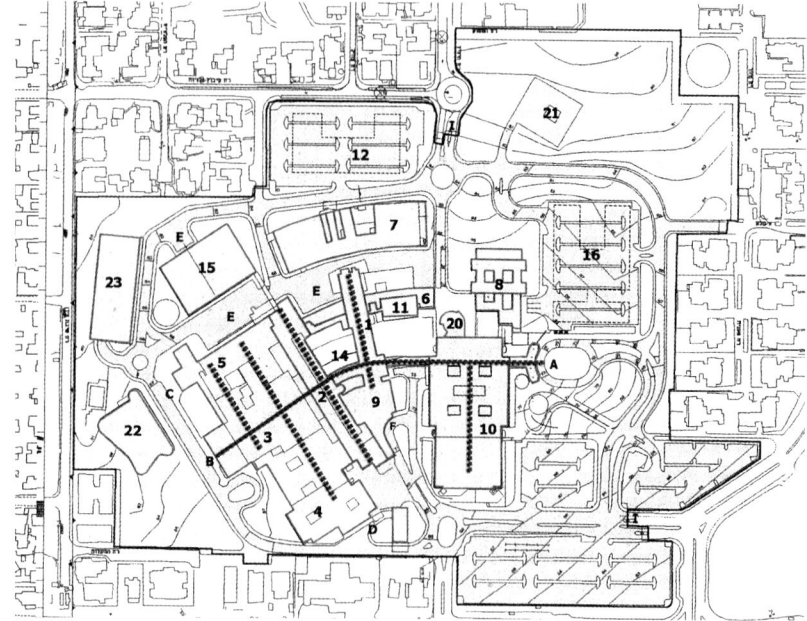

Future expansion is planned on the southwest corner of the main block. This wing will contain the Central Supply Service Department and a pharmacy on the lower ground floor and a children's hospital at the entrance level which will be facing the main garden of the hospital. The origin master plan made it possible, that the hospital could still develop into a modern facility. The final master plan from Zarhy Architects is from the year 2010.

5. The Hospitals and Health Facilities of Zarhy Architects

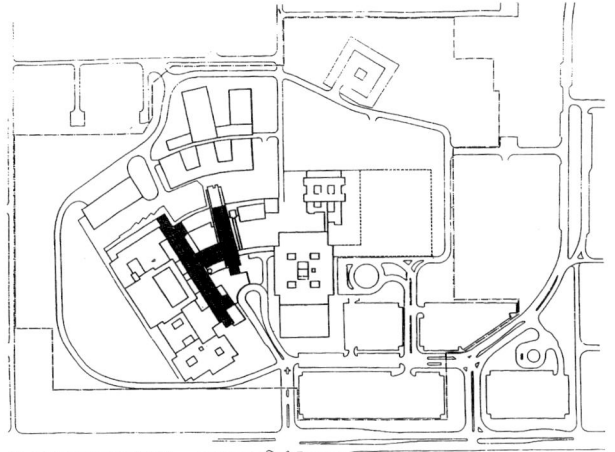

Master plan 1956

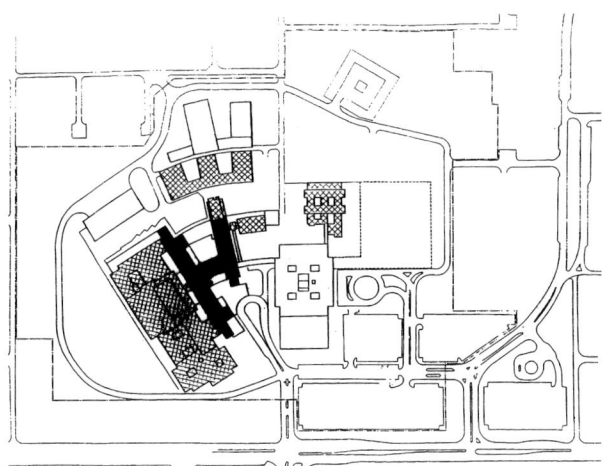

Master plan 1976

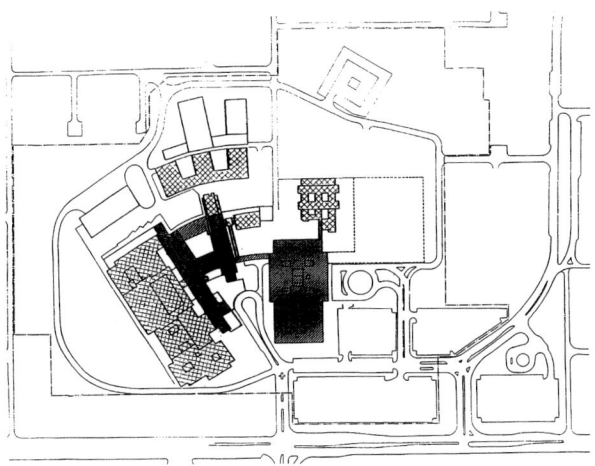

Master plan 1996

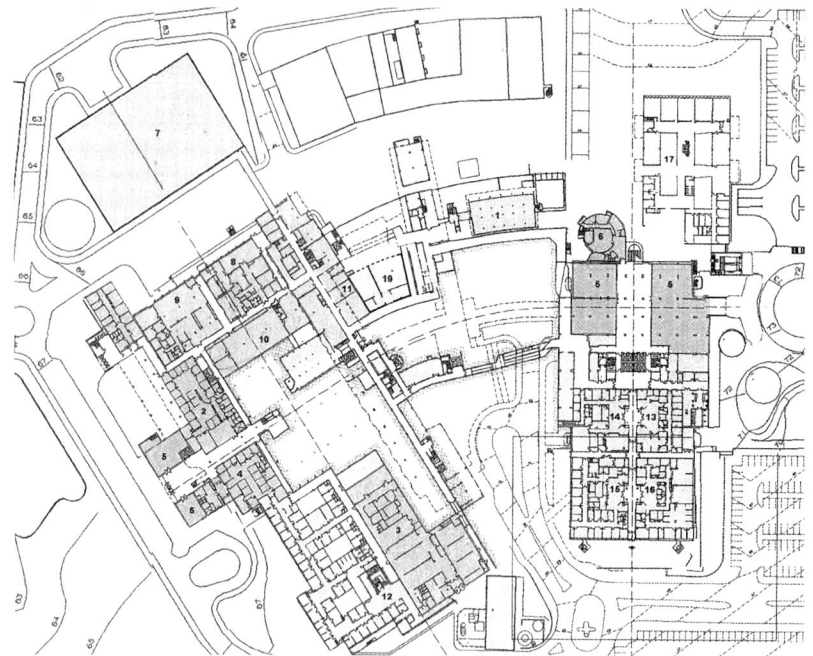

The campus level 2
+67.80 and +69.95

Medical services
1. Research laboratories
2. Schildren day ward unit
3. Sheltered emergency hospital
4. Children casualty department

Administrative services and miscellaneous
5. Recreation services
6. Synagogue

Supply services
7. Logistics center
8. Sterile supply department
9. Pharmacy
10. Clean laundry services
11. Stores

Outpatient department
12. Out patients' department
13. Haemotology
14. Cardiology rehabilitation
15. Mamography
16. Physiotherapy
17. School for nurses

Services corridor
18. Service corridors

Technical room
19. Technical room

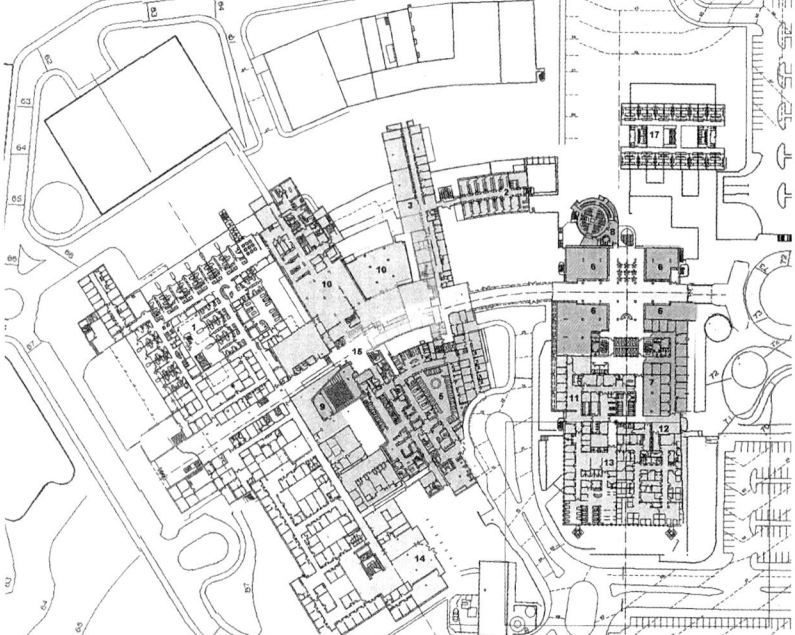

The campus level 3
+71.75 and +73.55

Hospitalization services
1. Childrens' hospital

Medical services
2. Research laboratories
3. Radiology
4. Day hospital
5. Casualty department

Administrative services and miscellaneous
6. Recreation services
7. Administration
8. Synagogue
9. Lecture hall

Supply services
10. Kitchen and dining halls

Outpatient department
11. Gastro-antrology
12. Nephrology
13. Oncology
14. Out patients' department

Service corridor
15. Hospital street and service corridor

Technical room
16. Technical room
17. School for nurses

5. The Hospitals and Health Facilities of Zarhy Architects

The campus level 4
+75.35 and +77.15

Hospitalization services
1. Ward units

Hospitalization services
2. Radiology
3. Intensive care unit
4. Research laboratories
5. Operatlng theatres
6. Day hospital
7. IVF and medical photography

Administrative services and miseallaneous
8. Administratlon

Outpatient department
9. Out patients' department

Service corridor
10. Hospital street and service corridor

Technical room
11. Technical room
12. School for nurses

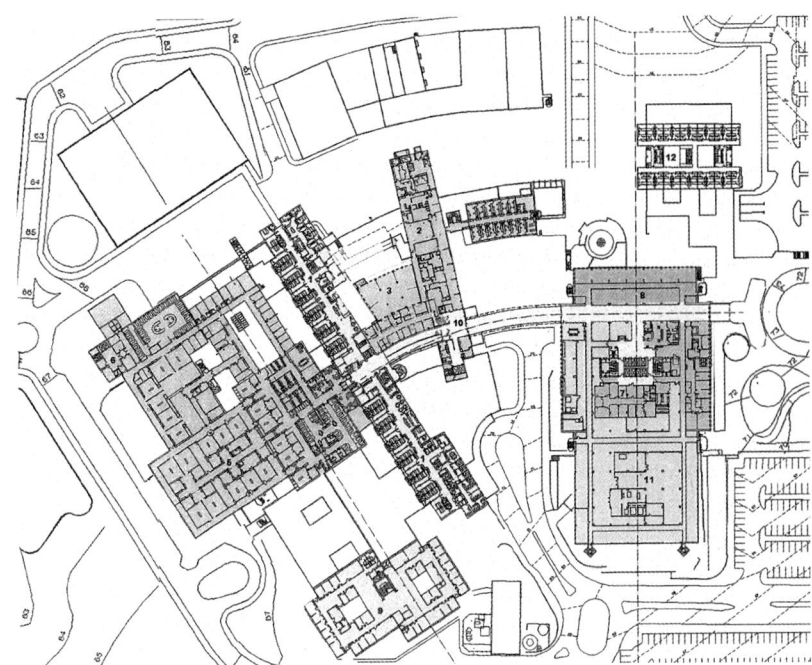

The campus level 5
+78.95 and +80.75

Hospitalization services
1. Ward units

Medical services
2. Research laboratories
3. Operating theaters
4. Cllnical laboratories
5. Babies department
6. Delivery rooms

Outpatient department
7. Out patients' department

Service corridor
8. Elevator lobby

Technical room
9. Technical room
10. School for nurses

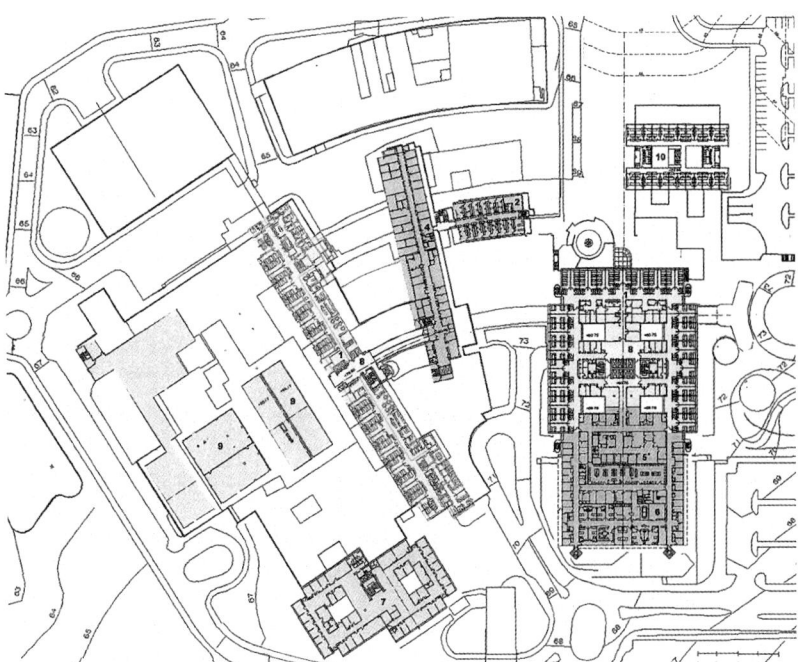

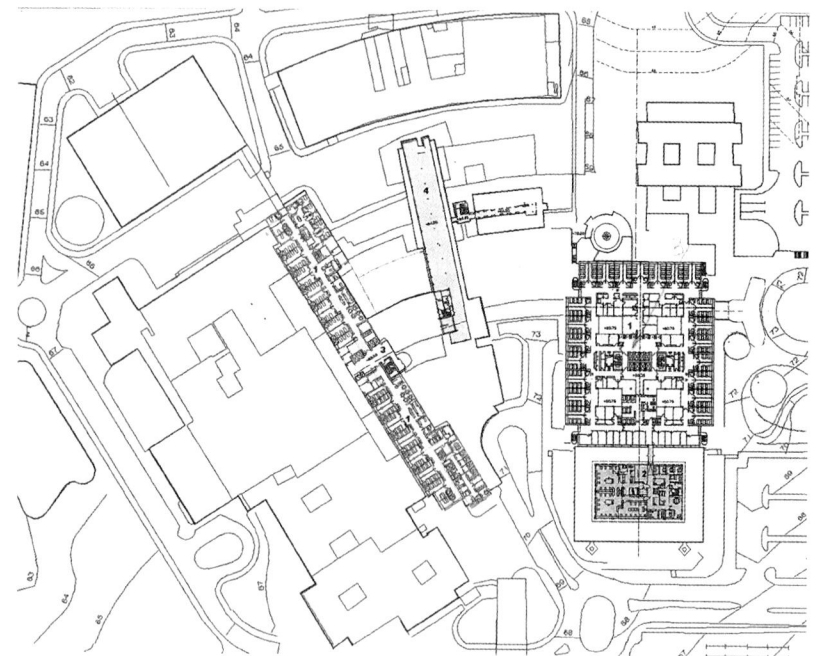

The campus level 6
+82.55 and +84.35

Hospitalization services
1. Ward units

Medical services
2. Premature babies'
   department

Service corridor
3. Elevators' lobby

Technical room
4. Technical room

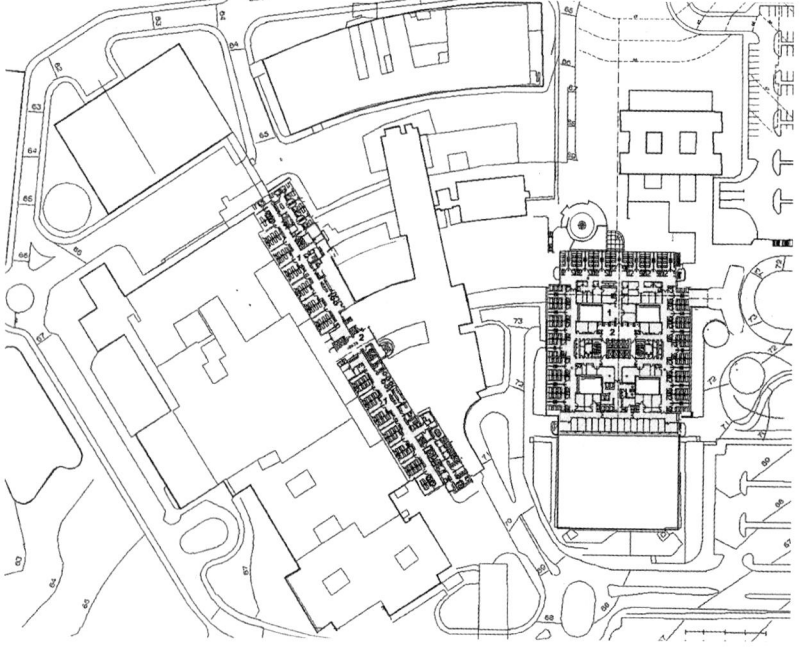

The campus level 8
+89.75 and +91.55

Hospitalization services
1. Ward units

Service corridor
2. Elevators' lobby

5. The Hospitals and Health Facilities of Zarhy Architects

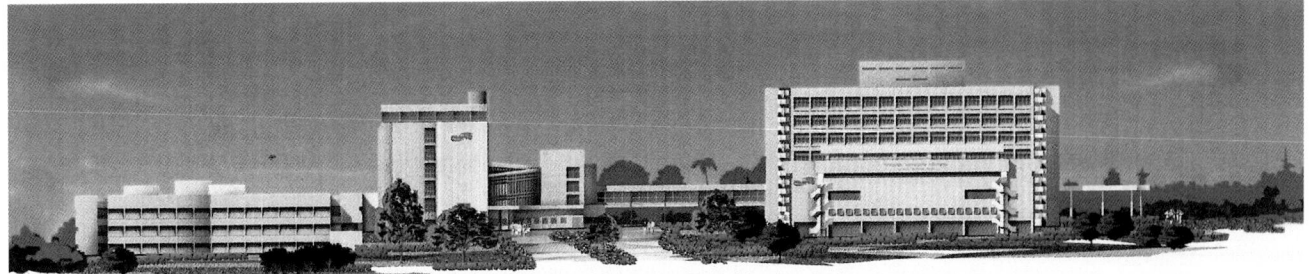

East elevation

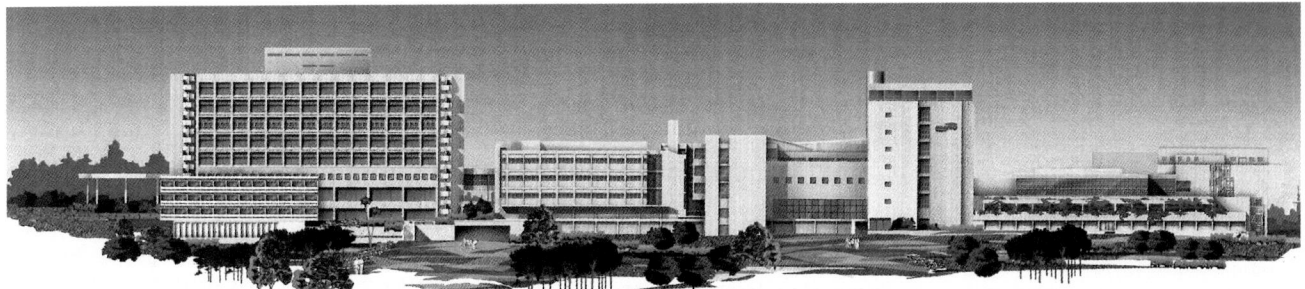

West elevation

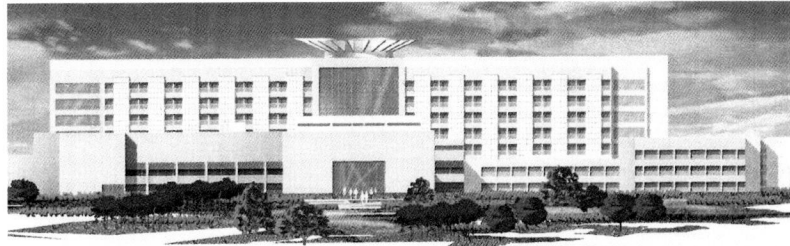

North elevation

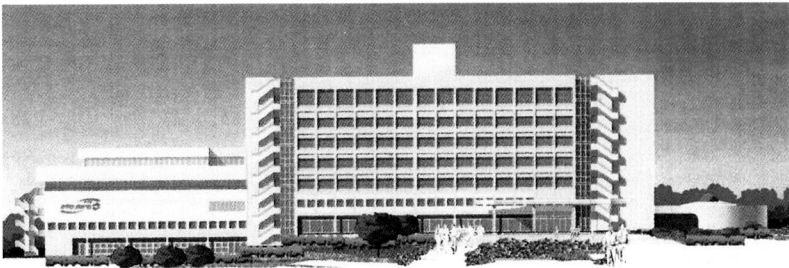

South elevation

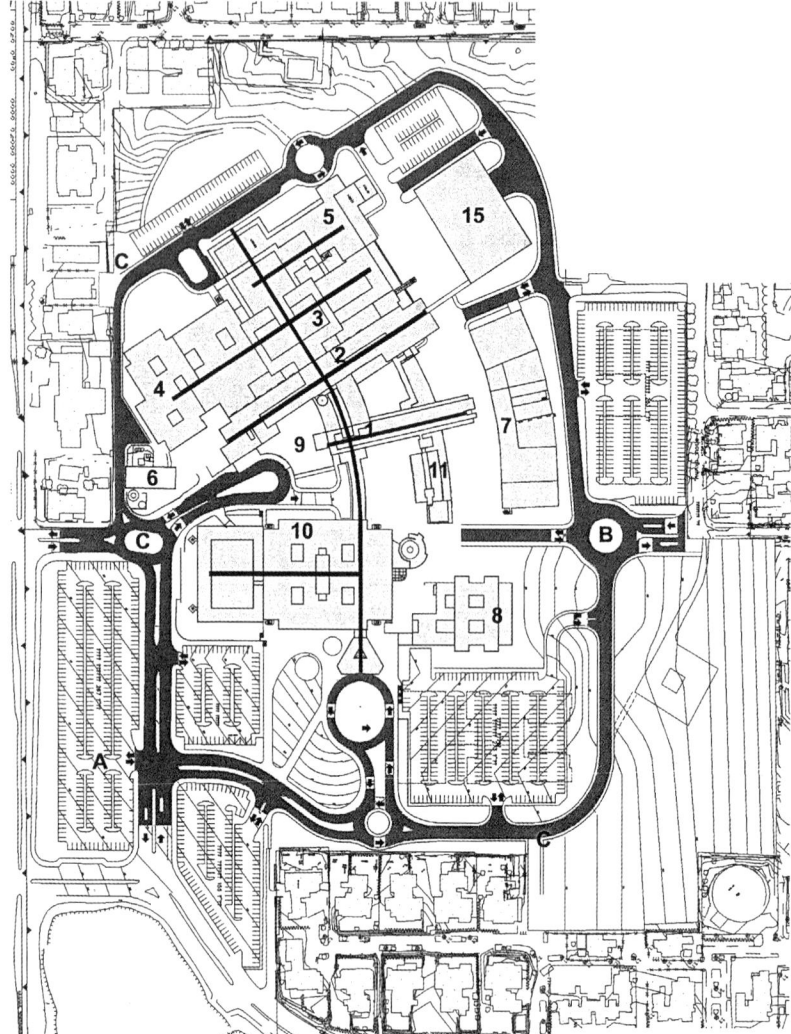

Circulation master plan

1. Laboratories, radiology,
   admittance and medical records
2. Surgical wards
3. Operating theatres
4. Out patient department
5. Children hospital
   Day hospital
6. Power plant
7. Supply services and power plant
8. School for nurses
9. Emergency department
10. Internal medicine wards,
    obstetrics and gynecological wards
11. Research laboratories
15. Logistics center

▬ Circumferential road
▭ Pedestrian hospital street

A. Main entrance
B. Service entrance
C. Emergency entrance

5. The Hospitals and Health Facilities of Zarhy Architects

Ramps in the entrance

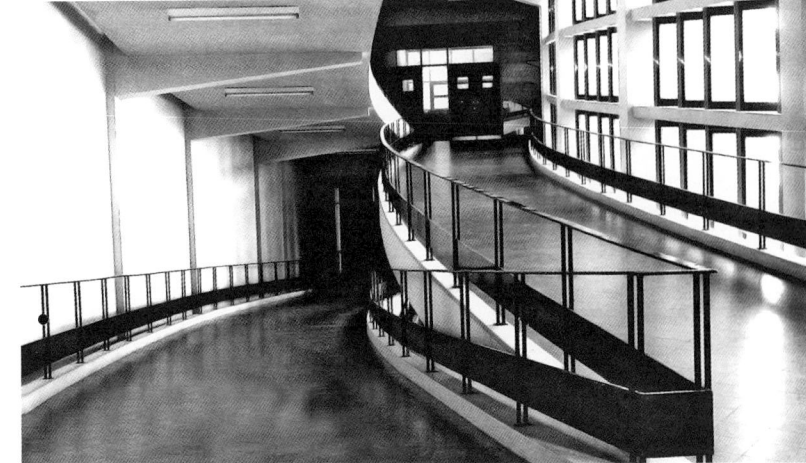

3 Bed room
Photo: Pawlik 2013

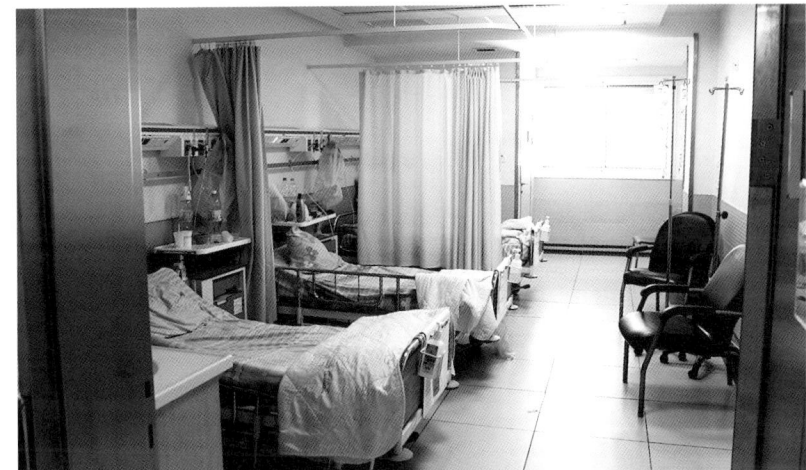

Inner courtyard
Photo: Pawlik 2013

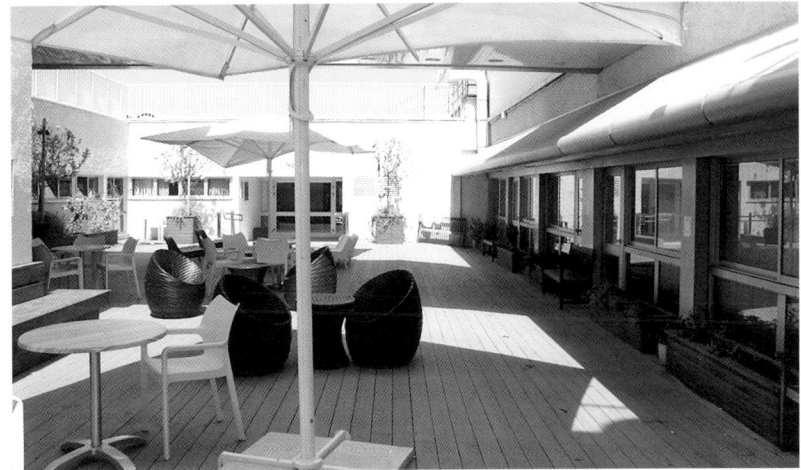

School for Nurses

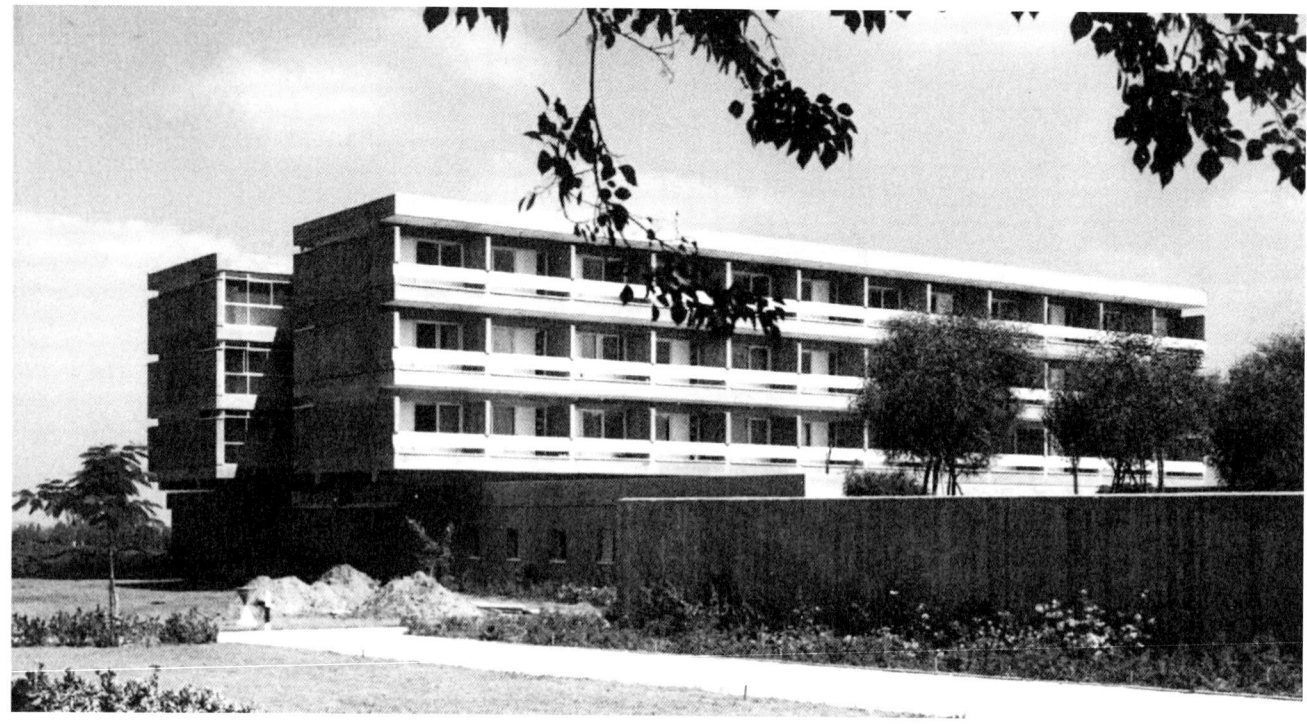

The Meir School of Nurses is composed of an upper block and a lower block. The upper block contains the students' living quarters, and the lower block house the school itself.

The upper block is composed of three floors, four groups of six rooms each, two students in each room (altogether 150 students). Every group of six rooms has its own convenience.

The lower block consists of classrooms, teaching facilities, recreation room and administration.

The intention was to base the concept of the building on an "open plan". It was intended to give the students a feeling of home, a place where they can live and study and have their recreation.

The school is integrated in Meir Hospital. It grants a registered nurse diploma, plus university credits for a B.A. in nursing. The Nursing School also runs special courses and programs, such as oncological nursing training program, retraining programs for new immigrants and others.

Main view nursing school

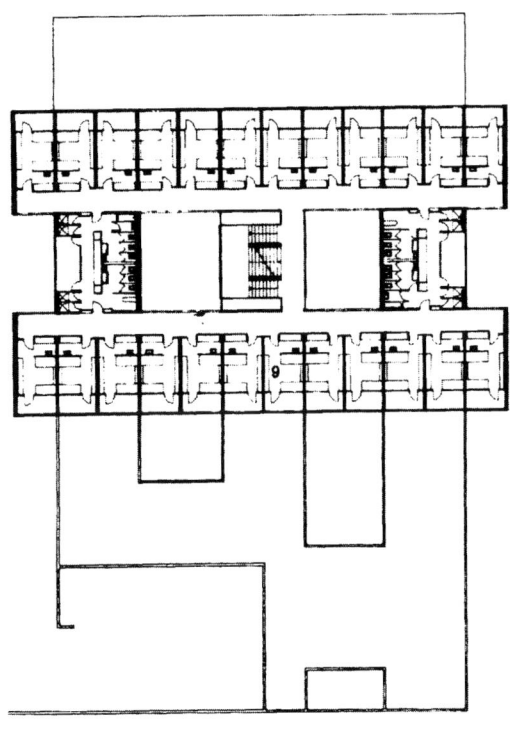

1. Entrance court
2. Entrance hall
3. Administration
4. Classrooms
5. Library
6. Recreation room
7. Teaching laboratory
8. House mother' living quarters
9. Students' living quarters

Ground floor

Typical floor

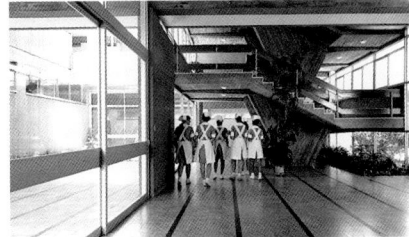

Nursing students in the main hall

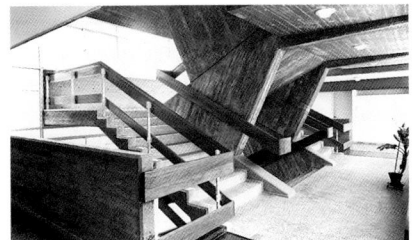

Main staircase

The Synagogue

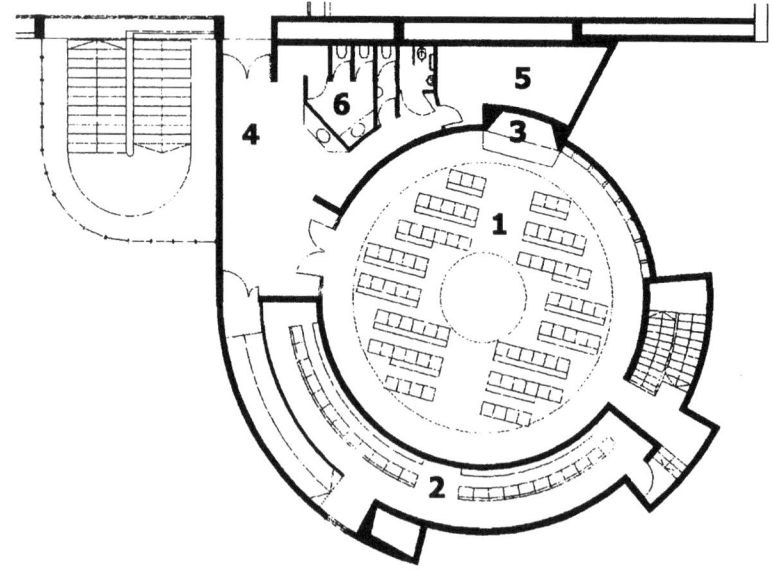

1. Synagogue hall
2. Women's gallery
3. Aron kodesh
4. Mevuah
5. Storage
6. Toilets

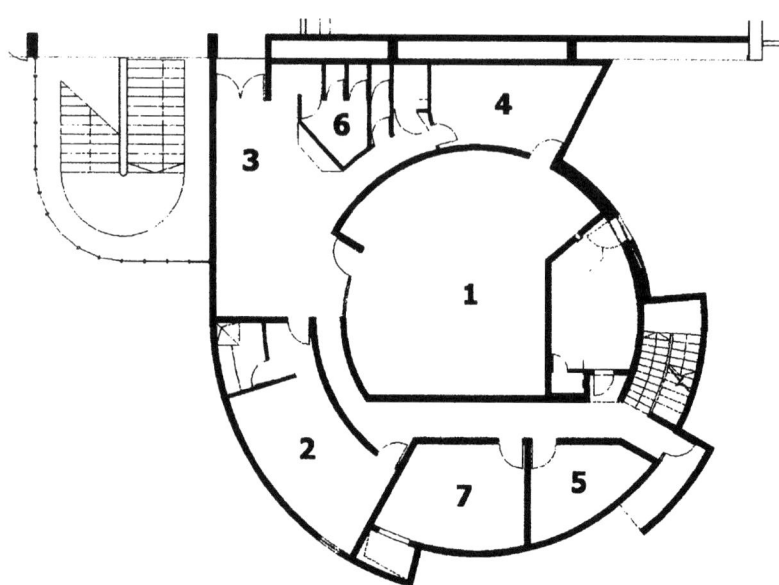

1. Function hall
2. Office of the rabbi
3. Entrance
4. Storage
5. Shelter
6. Toilets
7. Technical room

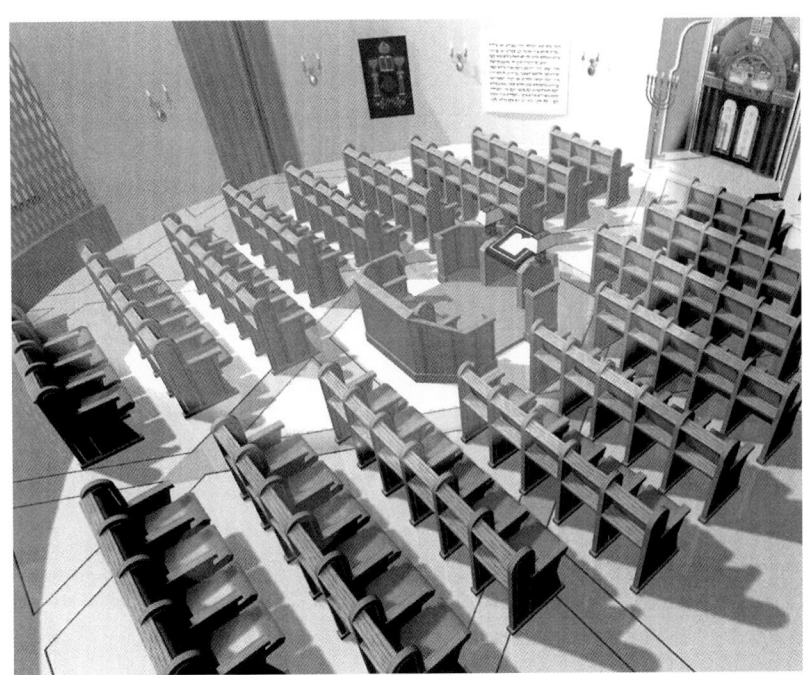

Interior view

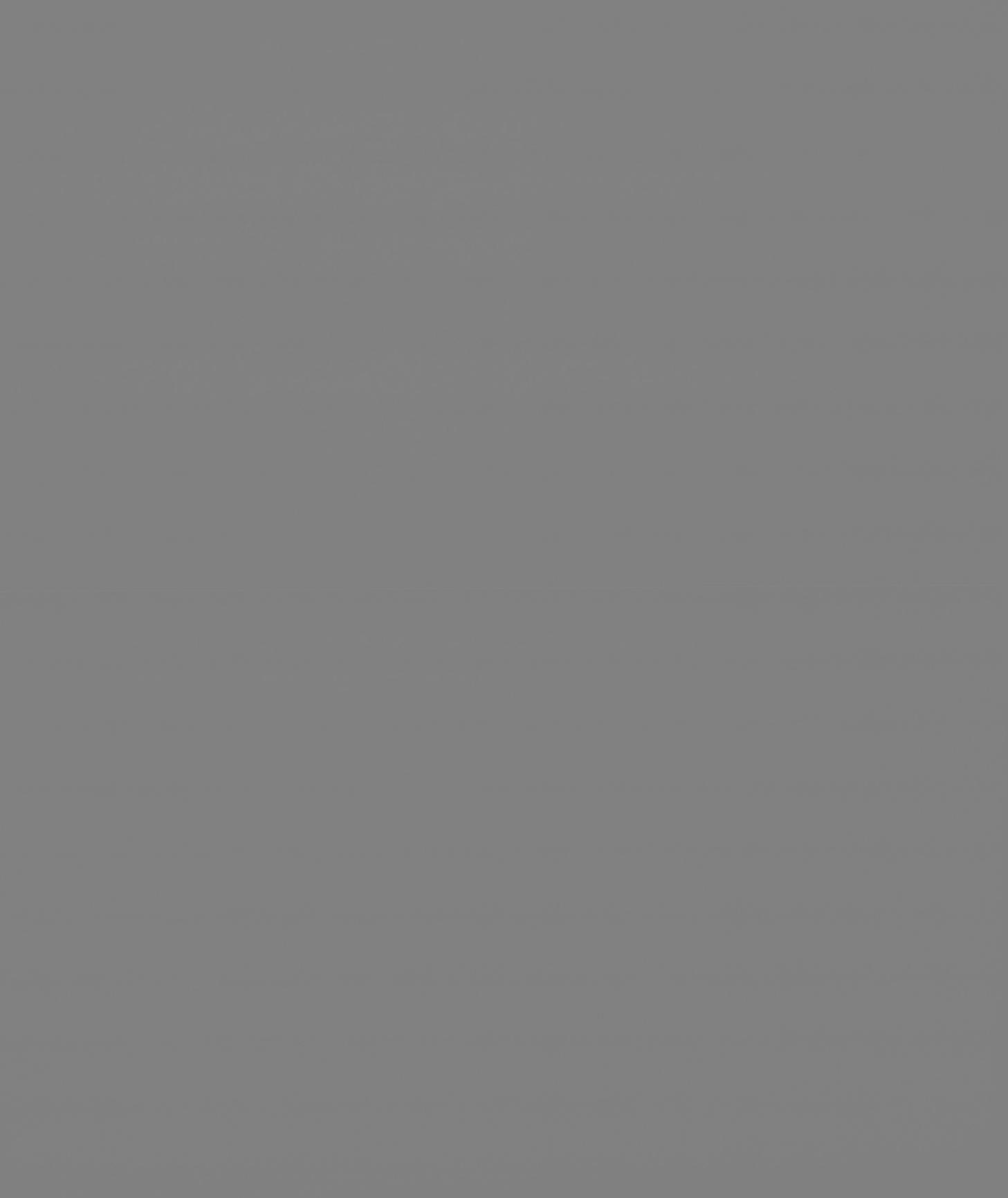

3. The Safed Government Hospital

The Rebecca Sieff Government Hospital

Safed, Upper Galilee, 300 Beds, 30,000 sqm, 1962–1973

From the dedication ceremony address by the Architect Moshe Zarhy

Mrs. Prime Minister, Lord Sieff, Minister of Finance, Minister of Health, Ladies and Gentlemen.

Our colleague Rabbi Yossi Habanai, the Cabalist builder, flourished in this town some 400 years ago. There is a story related to Yossi the builder. He was once asked: How was the Earth first created?" and he answered: "The Holy One, blessed be He, took dust from beneath the Throne of Glory and cast it into the water and it became land, and the pebbles became hills and mountains"; I am sure that only one who was living in Safed could express himself with such imagination and sense of scale.

Having been assigned the task of building on one of Rabbi Yossi's pebbles we tried to harmonize the building with its surroundings and also to create a frame through which the beautiful view is seen, while the building itself is kept humble, satisfied in doing its job.

The program called for a large regional hospital serving the entire community of the Upper Galilee. The crucial architectural problem was how to relate so large a building to the intimate scale of the town of Safed. Rather than dwarf the town, we adopted the concept of scaling down the general appearance of the building by following the contours of the hillside, and keeping the building as low as possible. The building consists of an upper block and lower blocks, which blend with landscape, flanking the main structure. The upper blocks contain all the hospital wards – close to 250 beds –including maternity ward and delivery rooms. The lower block, at the entrance level, houses the medical services, such as: Admittance and casualty department, operating theatres, X-Rays, Laboratories, outpatient department and so on. The lower two levels consist of the various supply services and 50-bed underground hospital hewn into the hillside for times of emergency. The cover-all plan makes full allowance for future extension up to a total of 500 beds. Careful consideration was given to the optimal centralization of the different medical services in order to save in equipment and personnel.

The Safed Hospital is a product of teamwork, the team consists of the hospital Planning Unit of the Ministry of Health, the Public Works Department, the various consultants, the construction supervisors, the contractors, who are building it and, of course, the architects and engineers who designed it.

There is something very exceptional about the process that brought this hospital into being and that is took an absolutely normal course. The site was chosen, the plans were submitted and approved, construction started and being continued until, very soon we hope, it will be completed as Rabbi Yossi, the cabalist, would have said it.

Thank you!

The History of Safed General Hospital

The history of Safed's present hospital may be said to have begun in the year 1912, when an institution with approximately 60 beds was founded by Baron Edmond de Rothschild. It served the Jewish and non-Jewish communities, as well as the Turkish Army during the 1914–1918 First World War, and in 1918 with British Occupation, was transferred to the Hadassah Medical Organization. In 1927 the first lung-department in the country was opened by Hadassah, with approximately 40 beds, and in 1937 beds for tuberculosis treatment was also opened at the Rothschild Hospital. The advent of antibiotic drugs towards the end of the nineteen-forties ended its period of importance as a lung hospital. During the 1936–1939 riots, as in the War of Independence, hundreds of wounded were treated there.

The immigration streams to the Upper Galilee of the early fifties necessitated re-founding of the general hospital. In 1954 the Ministry of Health started maternity section in the existing Rothschild building. In 1957 the Hadassah Medical Organization also transferred the lung disease hospital to the Government and departments for internal medicine and surgery were initiated in one of the buildings. A children's section was added to the maternity hospital. In the course of time various medical services were added, and recently an orthopedic department was opened.

It was clear that these buildings could not meet the hospitalization needs of Safed and the Galilee, expected to increase to 70,000 in a relatively short time. It was decided to build a new hospital to satisfy this need.

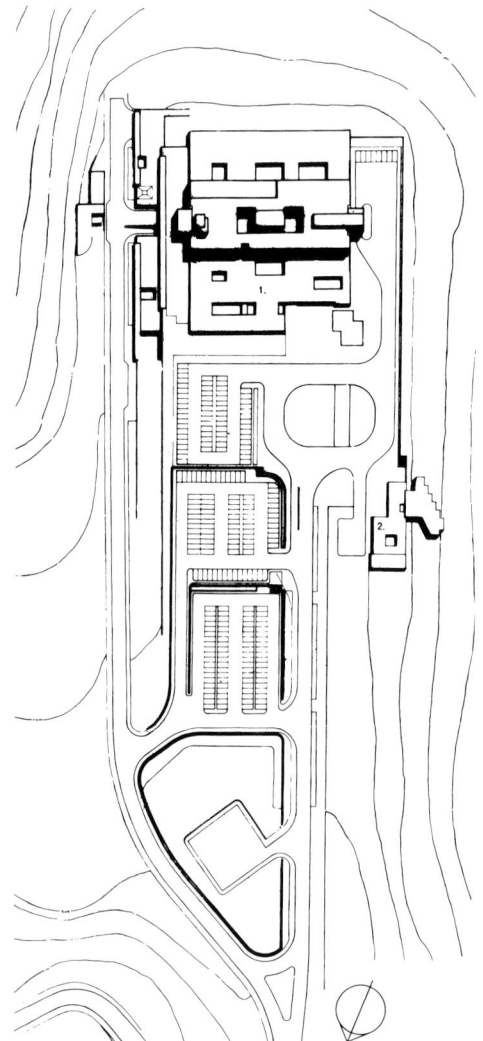

Site plan
First stage
1. Hospital
2. Nurses' training school

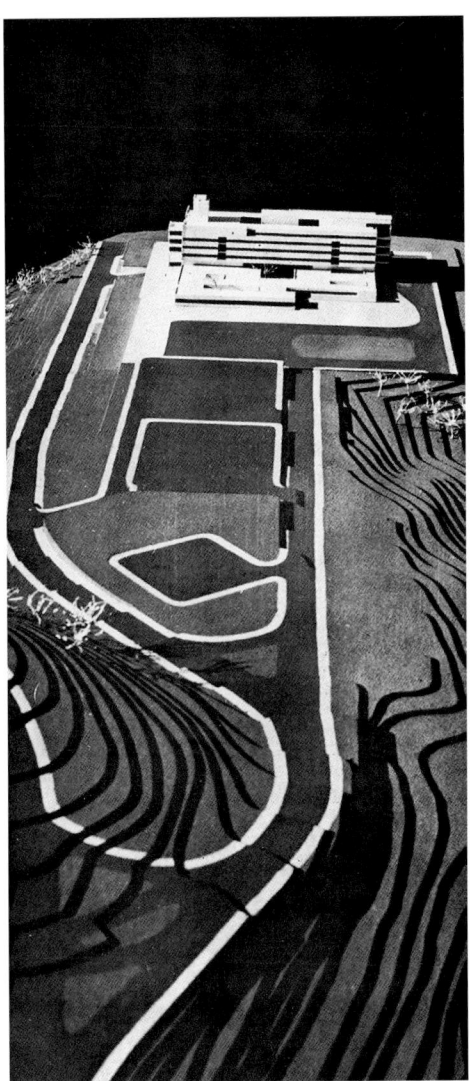

View from north, model

The Master Plan

The master plan enables a large general hospital to be built in stages. In the first stage there will be close to 250 general beds with the possibility of rationally increasing the size to 500 beds, including beds for chronic diseases and psychiatry. All the medical and technical services are planned so that they can be expanded considerably with minimum interference to the running of the hospital.

The new building is situated on a site of 112,000 sqm. on one of the ridges of the mountains of the town's outskirts. Although the steep slopes gave rise to problems in the hospital's design, the site was ideal from the point of view of location, climate and view. The crucial architectural problem was to relate the scale of this very large building with the more intimate one of the town of Safed. Advantage was taken of the site to suitably scale down the building by conceiving it as a superstructure, containing the wards, resting on a base of two floors, which blend into the site. Medical and technical service areas are located in the lower part of the building.

Future wards are planned on the sloping ground adjoining the medical and technical services.

The program called for a large regional hospital serving the entire community of the Upper Galilee.

The upper block contains all the wards, including maternity ward and delivery rooms. The lower block, at the entrance level contains the medical services such as: admittance and casualty department, operating theatres, X-rays, laboratories, outpatients' department and various supply services. It also contains a 50-bed underground hospital for time of emergency.

Careful consideration was given to the optimal centralization of the different medical services to save in equipment and personnel.

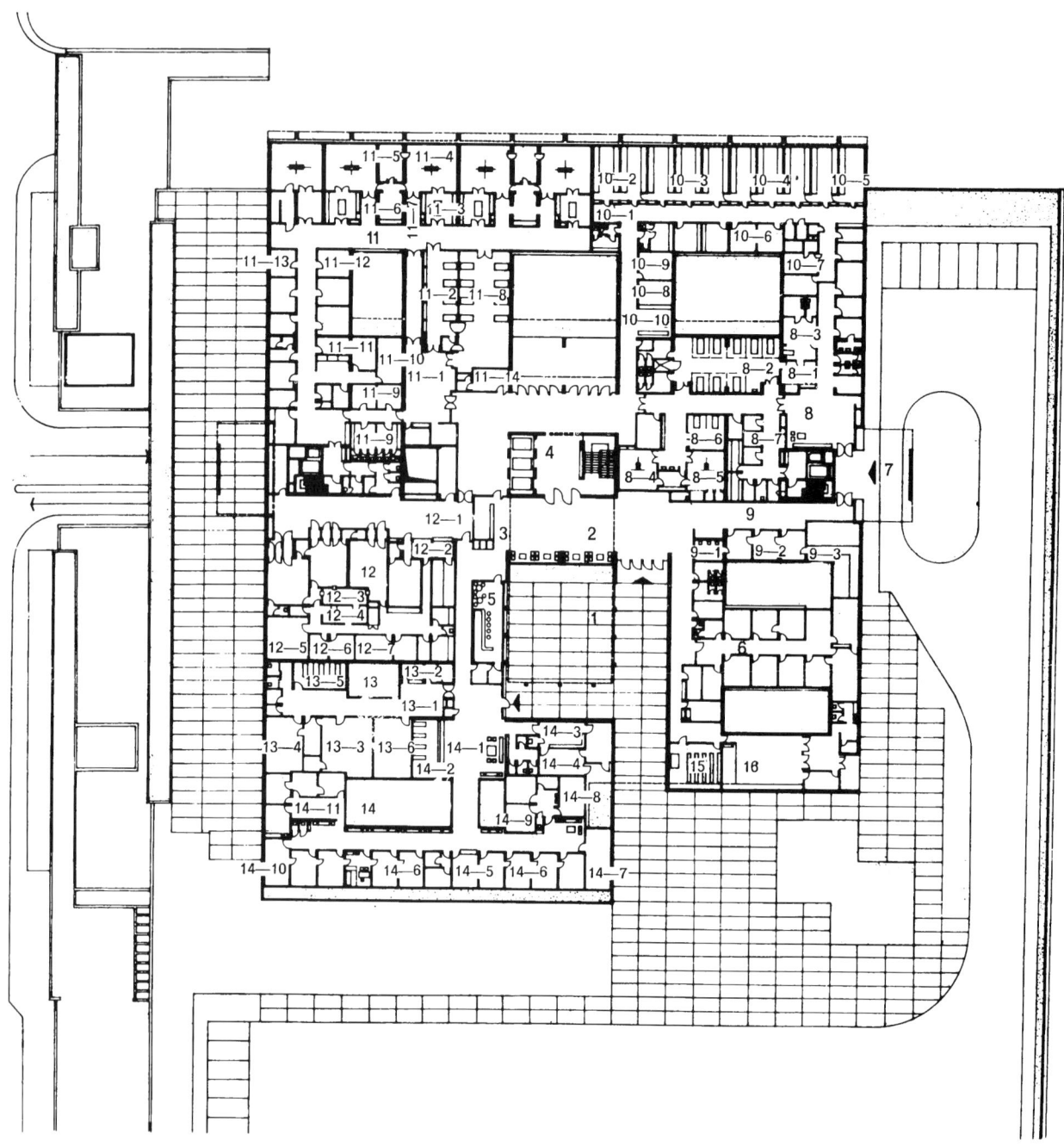

Entrance floor

1. Patio
2. Entrance hall
3. Information
4. Elevator's lobby
5. Cateteria
6. Administration

Casualty department

7. Covered entrance to casualty department
8. Casualty department's entrance hall
9. Nurses' utility room
10. Stretcher ward
11. Children's casualty ward
12. Plaster room
13. General treatment room
14. Preparation and post-operative room
15. Ancillary rooms

Admission department

16. Admission department – waiting
17. Patients' admission office
18. Clerical offices
19. Medical archives

Laboratories wing

20. Blood Bank
21. Haematology
22. Bacteriology
23. Virology
24. Cyto-genetics and cyto chemistry
25. Laboratories' offices
26. Laboratories' kitchen
27. Patient's and specimen reception
28. Specimen taking and examination room
29. Waiting

Operating theatres

30. Operating theatres' clean corridor
31. Entrance hall
32. Admission and reception
33. Anaesthetic room
34. Operating theatres
35. Lay-up room
36. Scrub-up room
37. Exit bay
38. Recovery room (short stay)
39. Staff changing room
40. Surgeons' lounge
41. Nurses' lounge
42. Chief nurse's office
43. Chief anaesthetist
44. Family waiting room

Radiology

45. General purpose radio diagnostic room
46. Radiology department waiting room
47. Reception
48. Processing room
49. Immediate viewing and sorting room
50. Demonstration / conference room
51. Technician's room
52. Chief of radiology department's room

Physiotherapy

53. Patio
54. Entrance hall and waiting
55. Reception desk
56. Gymnasium
57. Hydrotherapy
58. Examination and treatment
59. Occupational therapy room

Outpatients' department

60. Patio
61. General Waiting
62. Information and registration
63. Children's waiting room
64. Consultation and examination room
65. Nurses' room
66. Combined consultation and examination room
67. Plaster room
68. General treatment room
69. Cystoscopy
70. Gynaecology
71. Ophthalmology
72. Synagogue
73. Circumcision hall

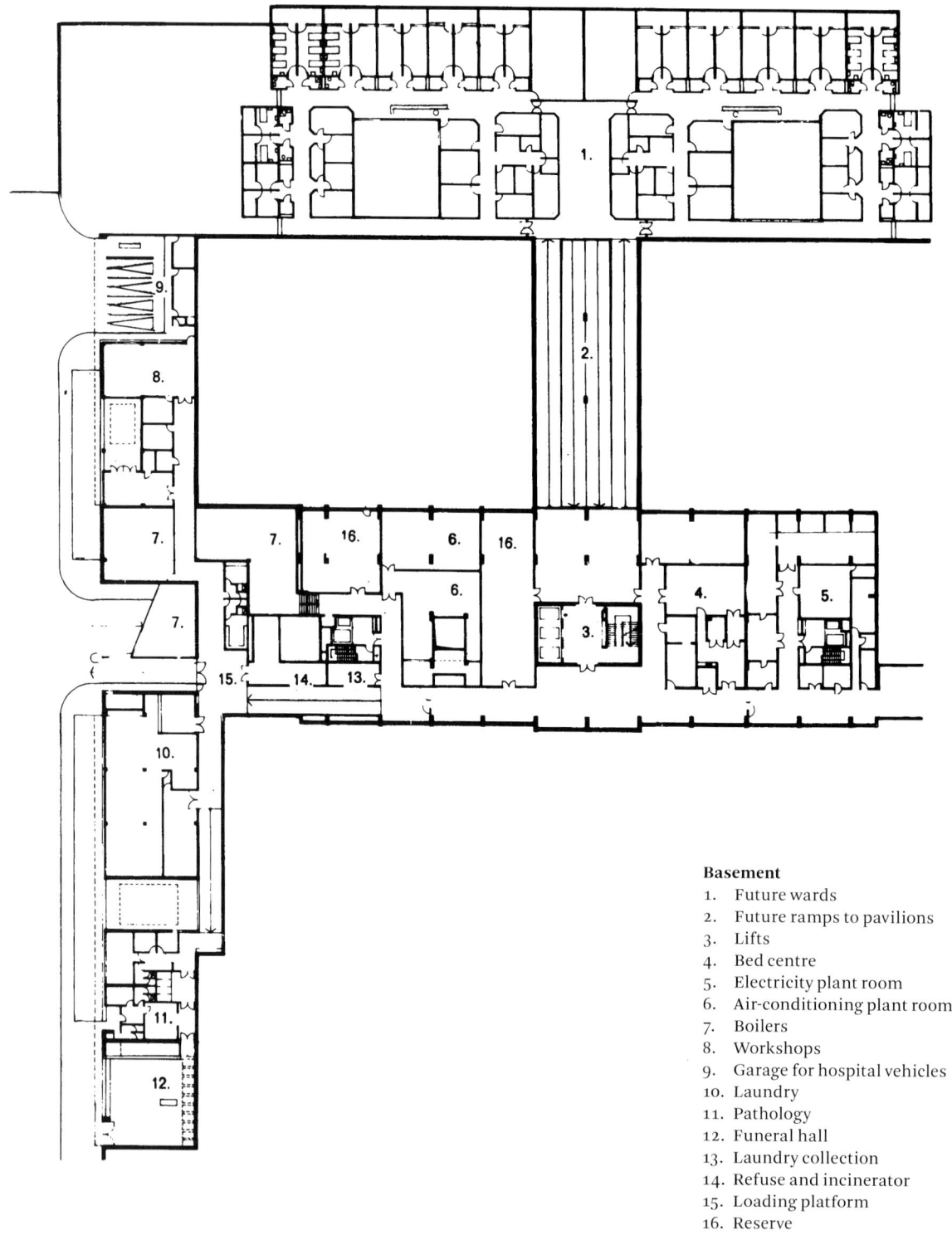

Basement

1. Future wards
2. Future ramps to pavilions
3. Lifts
4. Bed centre
5. Electricity plant room
6. Air-conditioning plant room
7. Boilers
8. Workshops
9. Garage for hospital vehicles
10. Laundry
11. Pathology
12. Funeral hall
13. Laundry collection
14. Refuse and incinerator
15. Loading platform
16. Reserve

5. The Hospitals and Health Facilities of Zarhy Architects

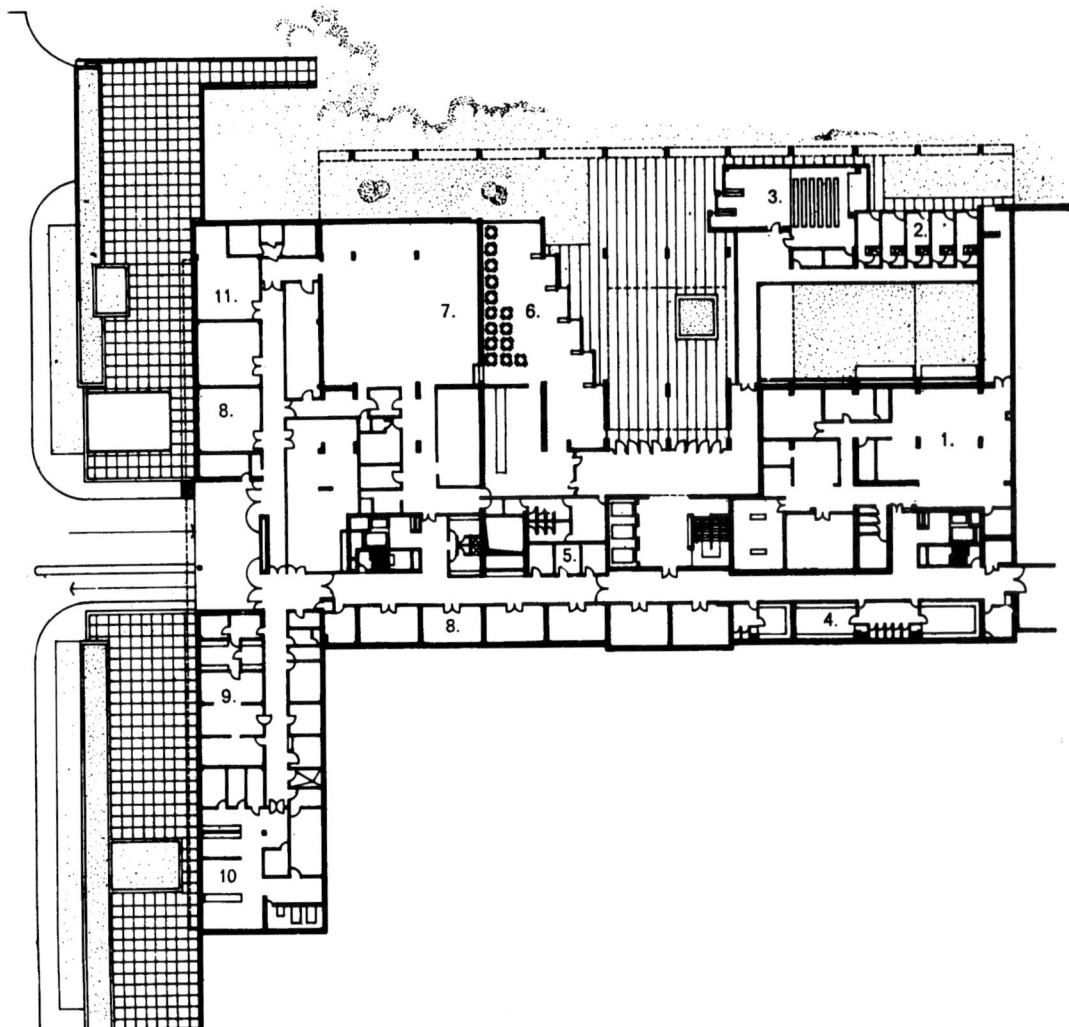

Service floor

1. Emergency hospital
2. Duty doctors' quarters
3. Medical library and auditorium
4. Staff locker room
5. Maintenance staff
6. Dining room
7. Kitchen
8. Technical and maintenance supply service
9. Pharmacy
10. Central sterile supply
11. Reserve store

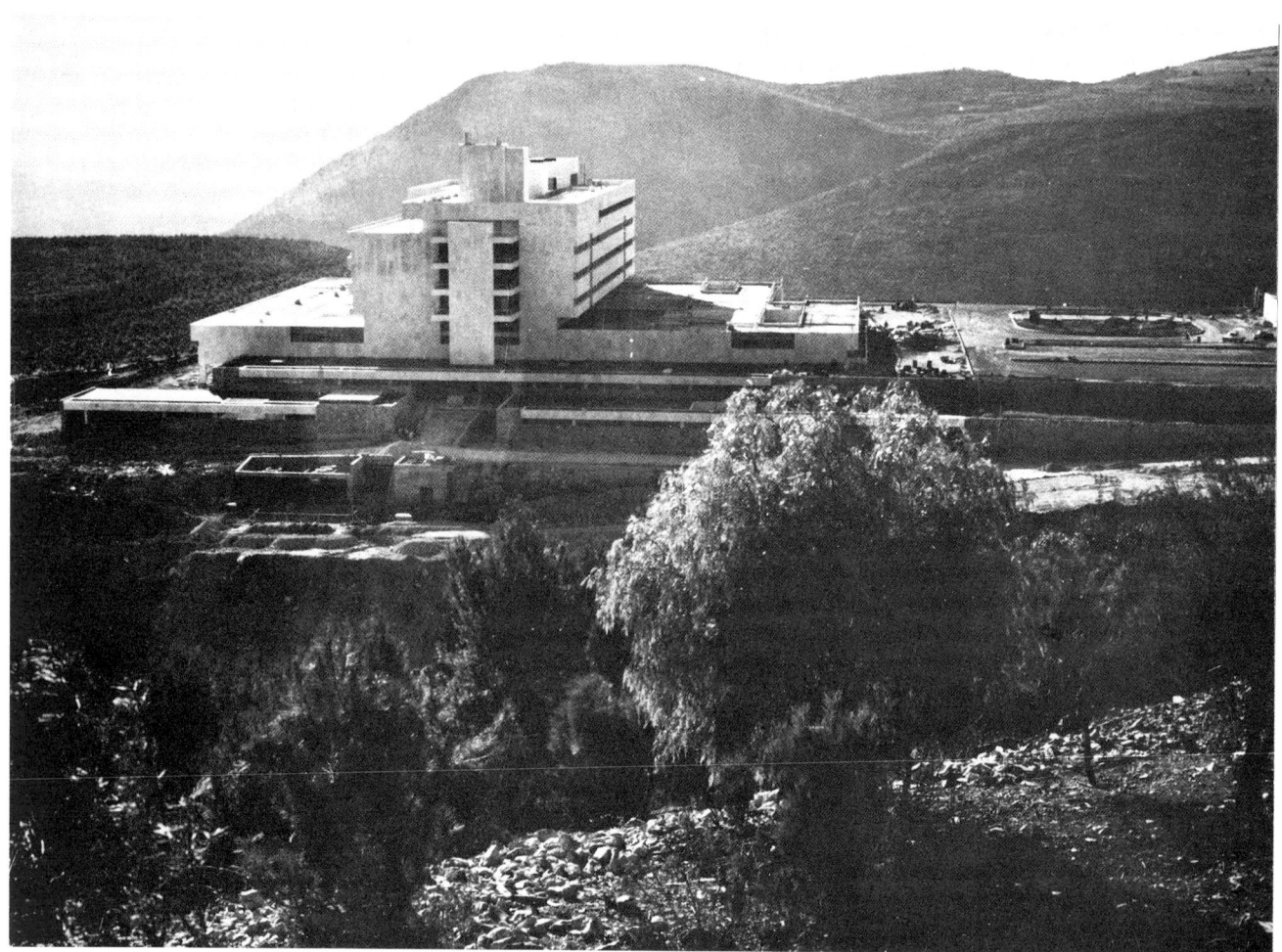

View from east

5. The Hospitals and Health Facilities of Zarhy Architects

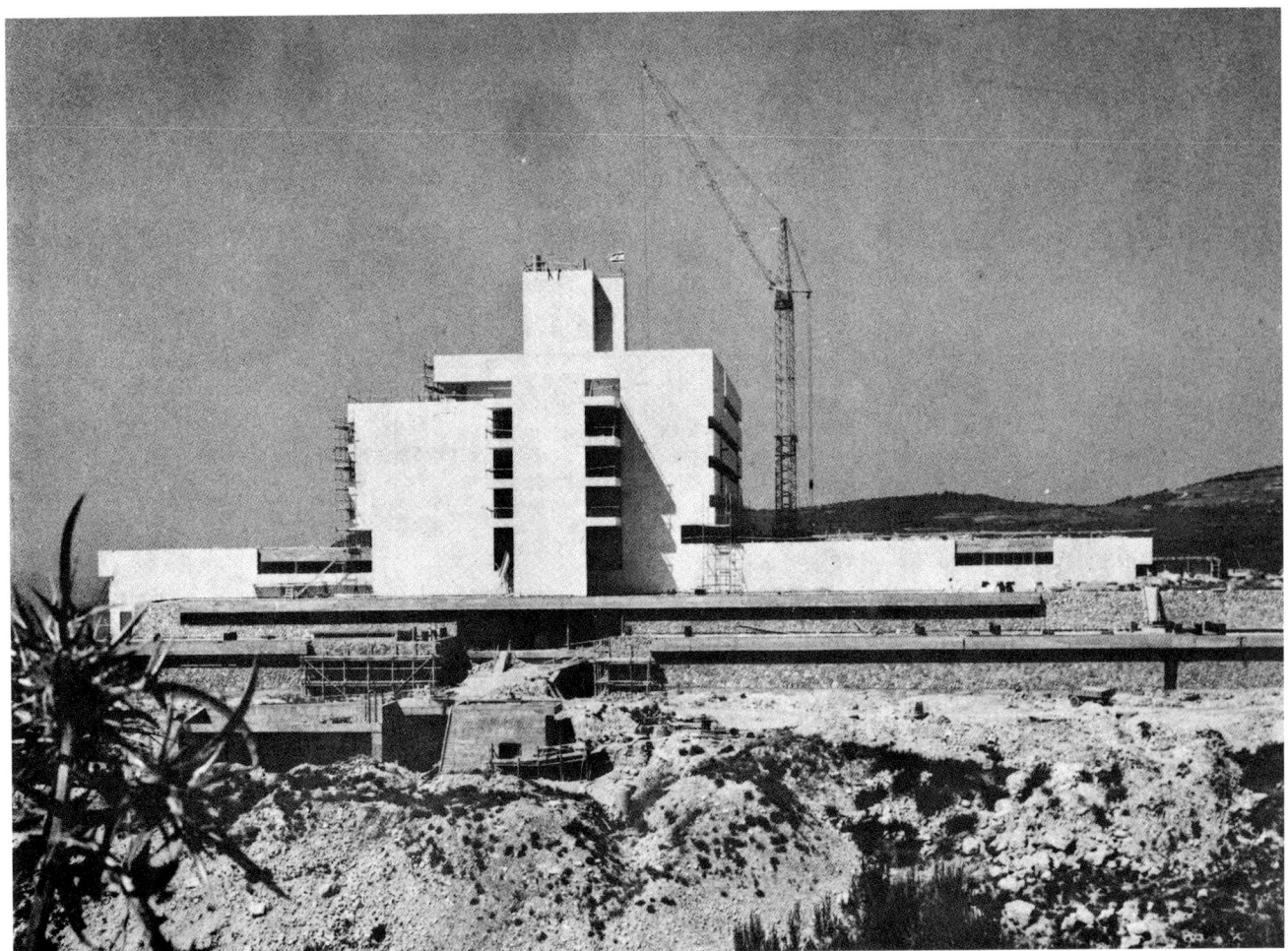

East elevation

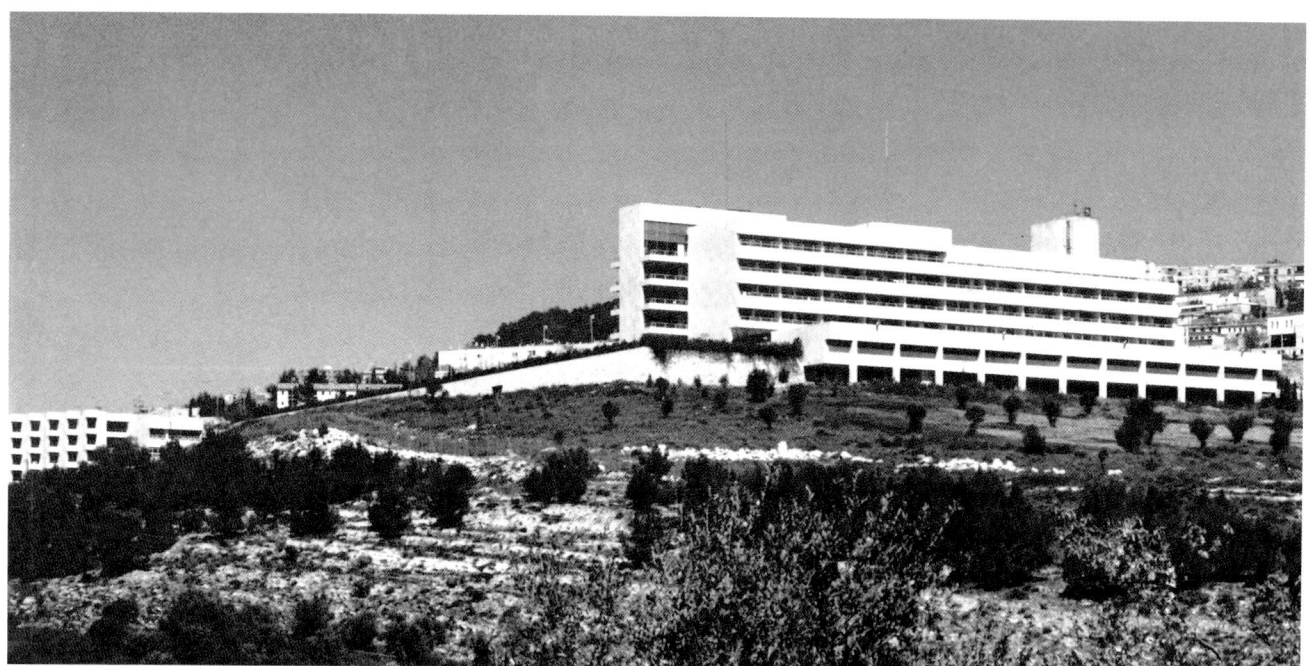

South west elevation

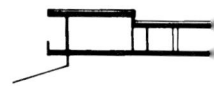

5. The Hospitals and Health Facilities of Zarhy Architects

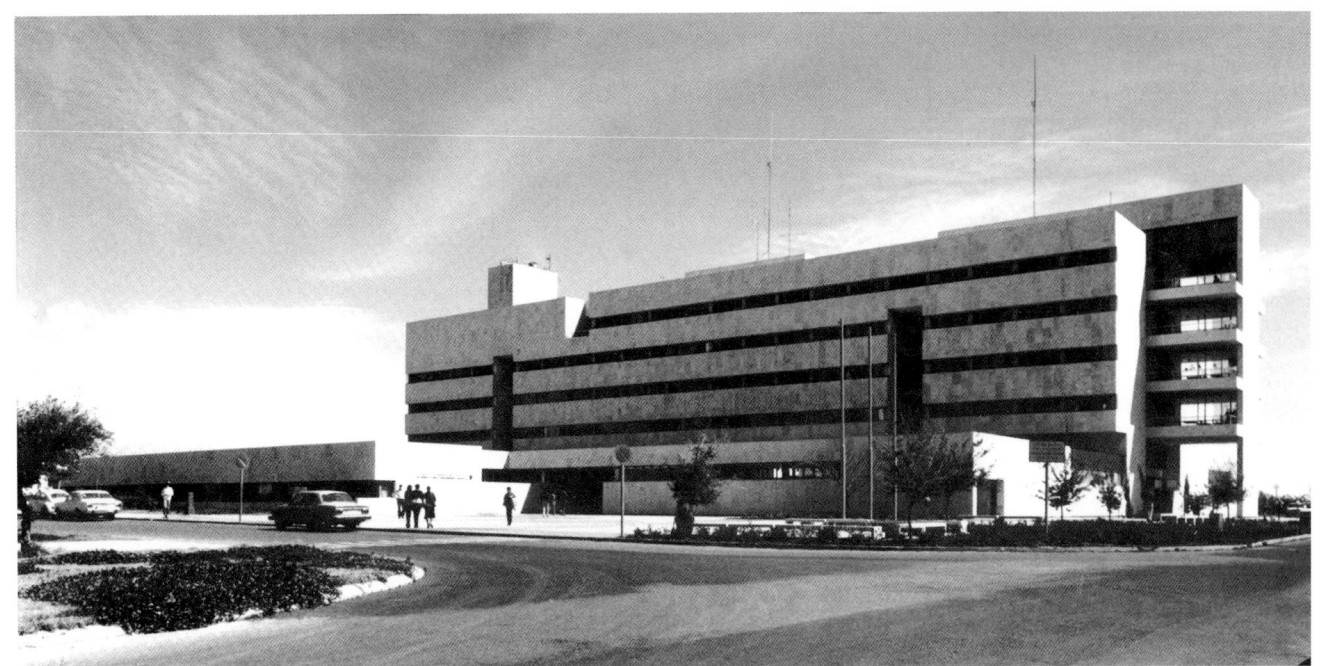

North elevation

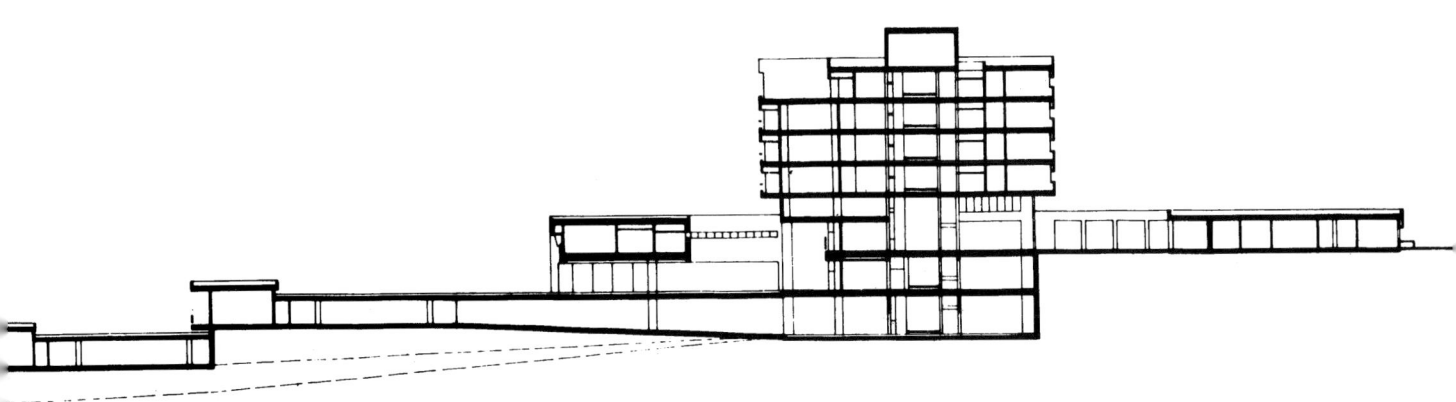

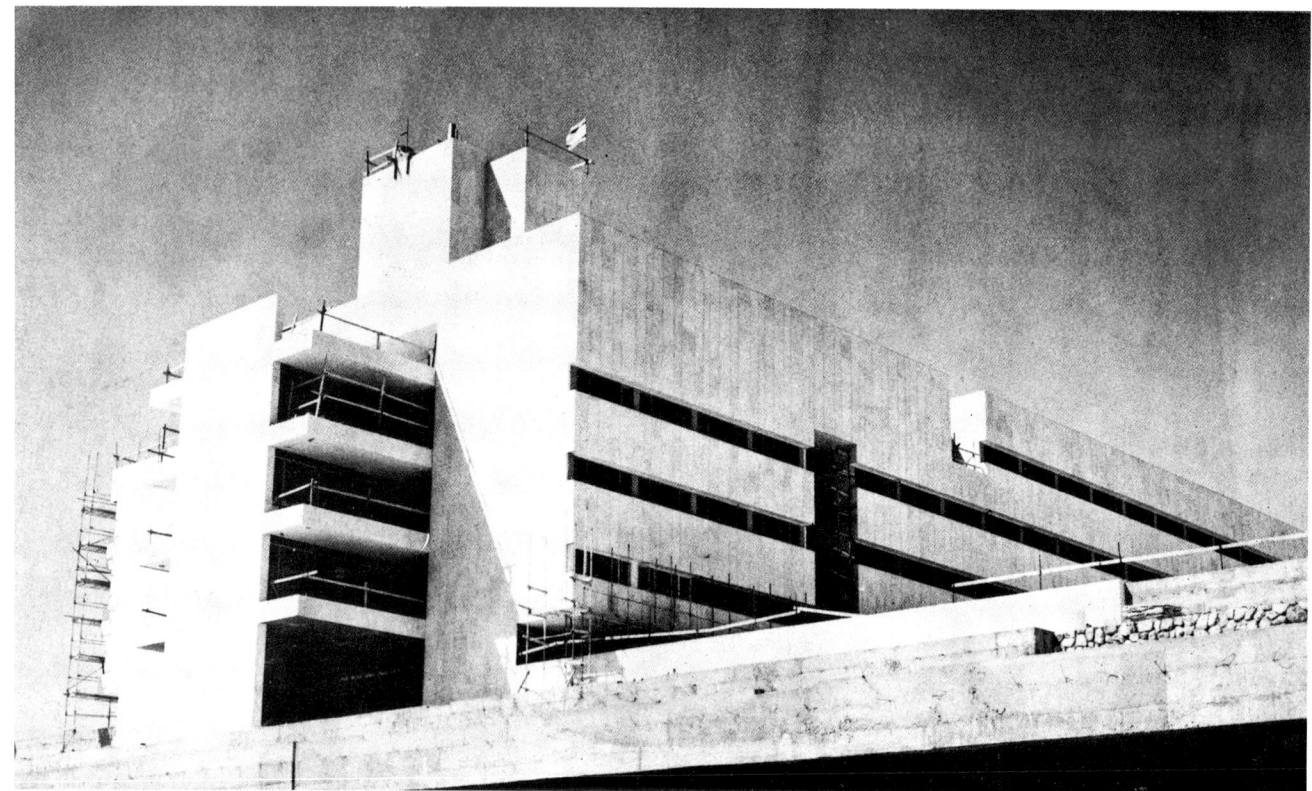

The following brief list of departments relates to the first stage, which is planned to go into operation in 1972.

North east corner

- Wards
- Casualty and admission section with facilities for emergency operations, plaster room and recovery room.
- Clinics, with examination and treatment rooms
- Radiology department, with four examination rooms and all the necessary services for a modern unit.
- Operating Theatre wing, with four operating theatre suites.
- Obstetrics section with four labour rooms, intervention theatre and all ancillary medical and technical services.
- Laboratory wing, including various laboratories, blood bank and a limited amount of space set aside for research.
- Physiotherapy and Occupational Therapy departments.
- Medical supplies wing, including central sterile supply and pharmacy.

5. The Hospitals and Health Facilities of Zarhy Architects

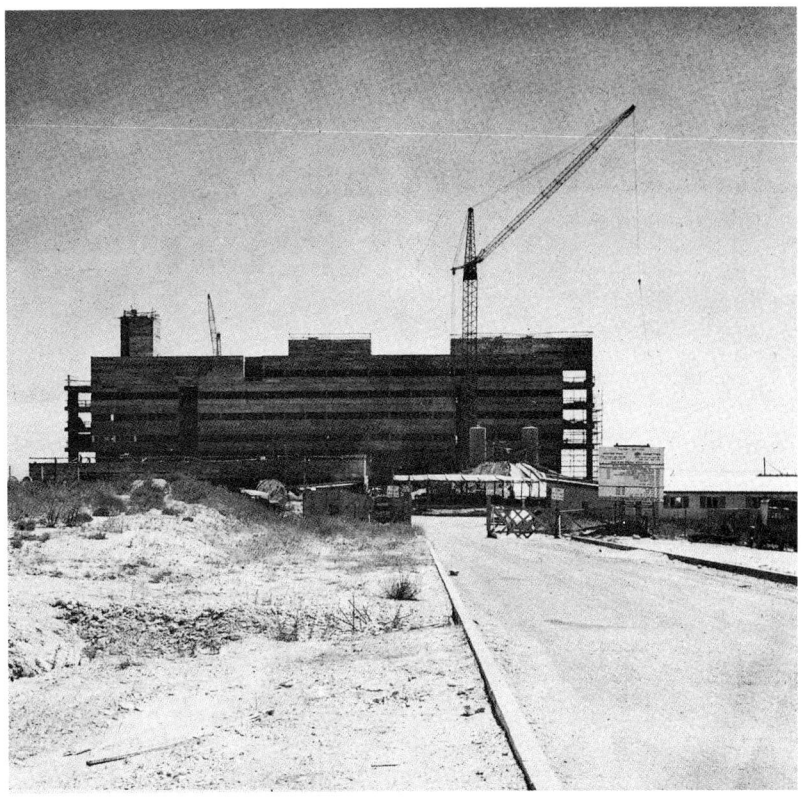

The hospital under construction

- A large emergency hospital in the basement shelter.
- Administration wing.
- Medical library, auditorium and duty-doctors' living quarters.
- Synagogue.
- Building and technical services, including kitchen, milk kitchen, staff dining hall, laundry, stores, staff locker rooms, workshops, plant rooms, telephone exchange and paging centre.
- Pathology section.
- Nurses' training college including teaching wing, professional library and living-in accommodation for 50 students.

The hospital will be centrally heated, with air-conditioning in the operating theatres, radiology department, labour rooms and intervention theatre. Medical gases and suction will be supplied from a central installation.

Construction of the building was commenced in 1967.

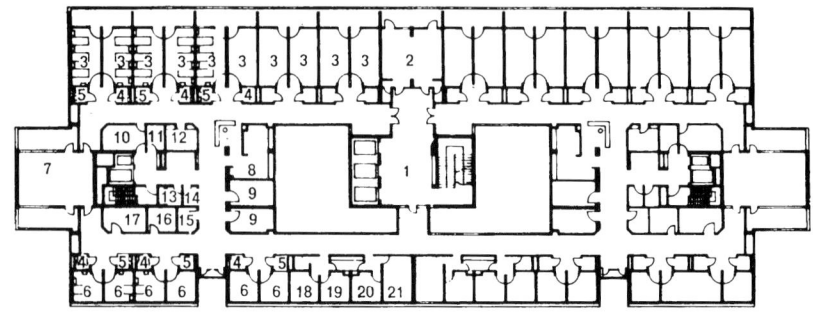

Ward floor
1. Lifts
2. Family room
3. 3 Bed ward
4. Shower
5. Toilet
6. Private ward
7. Day room
8. Nurses' workroom
9. Treatment room
10. Kitchenette
11. Patients' clothing store
12. Sluice room
13. Soiled linen store
14. Cleaners' cupboard
15. Linen store
16. General store
17. Bathroom
18. Senior nurse
19. Department manager
20. Doctors' room
21. Doctors' room

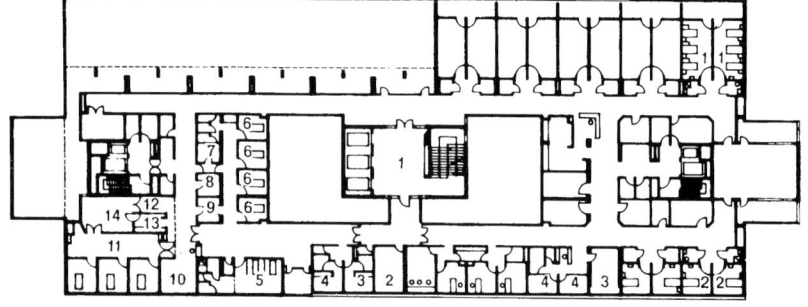

Maternity and obstetrics floor

Maternity department
1. 3 Bed maternity ward
2. Private ward
3. Nursery
4. Isolation room

Obstetrics department
1. Lifts
2. Family room
3. Doctors' locker room
4. Locker room
5. Preparation room
6. Labour room
7. Linen store
8. Sluice room
9. Kitchenette
10. Nurses' work room
11. Delivery room
12. Scrub-up
13. Sterilizing room
14. Operating theatre suite

5. **The Hospitals and Health Facilities of Zarhy Architects**

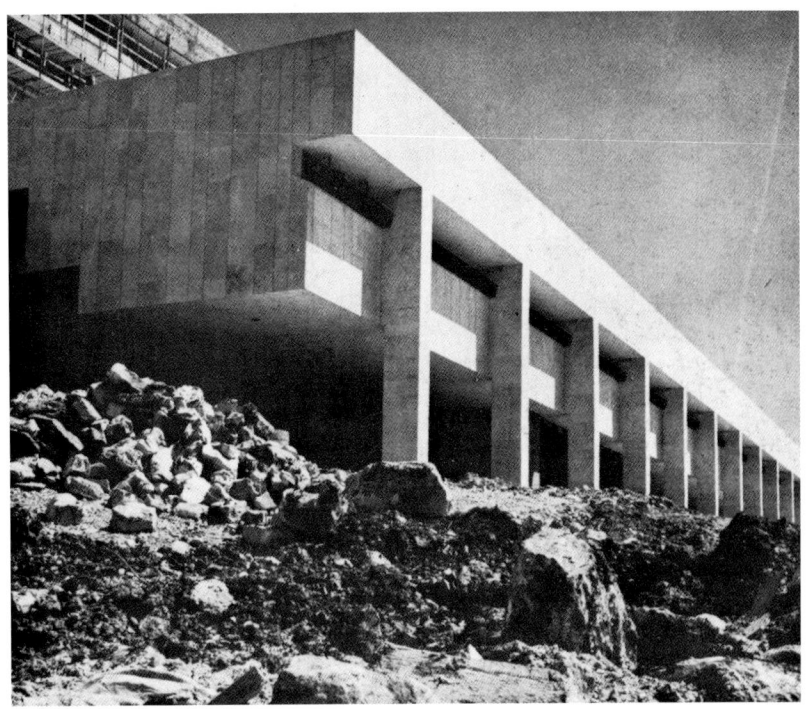

South-west corner of lower block

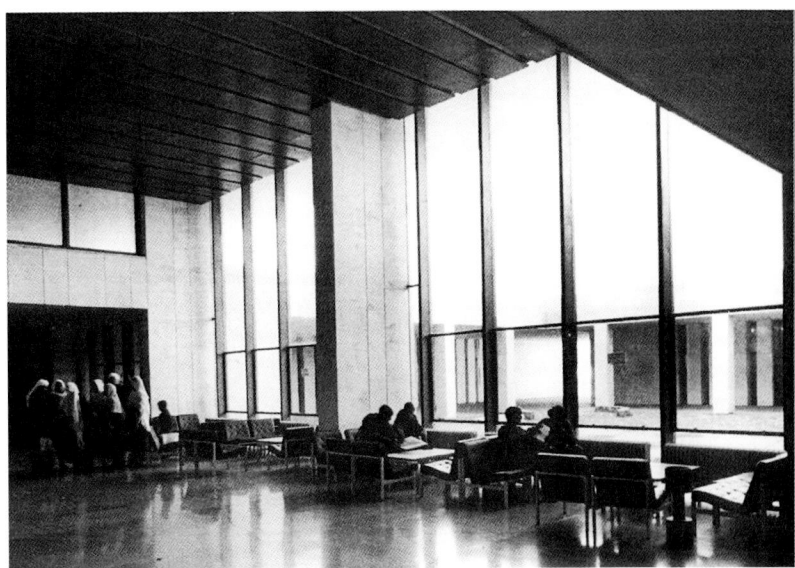

Waiting room

The Nurses Training School

1. Main entrance hall
2. Student's quarters
3. Kitchenette
4. Washing and ironing room
5. Sickroom
6. House mother's apartment
7. Sewing room
8. Clinic
9. Patio
10. Waiting hall
11. Secretary
12. Principals room
13. Instructors room
14. Seminary room
15. Classroom
16. Demonstration room
17. Air raid shelter
18. Machine room
19. Store room
20. Living room
21. Furniture store
22. Library

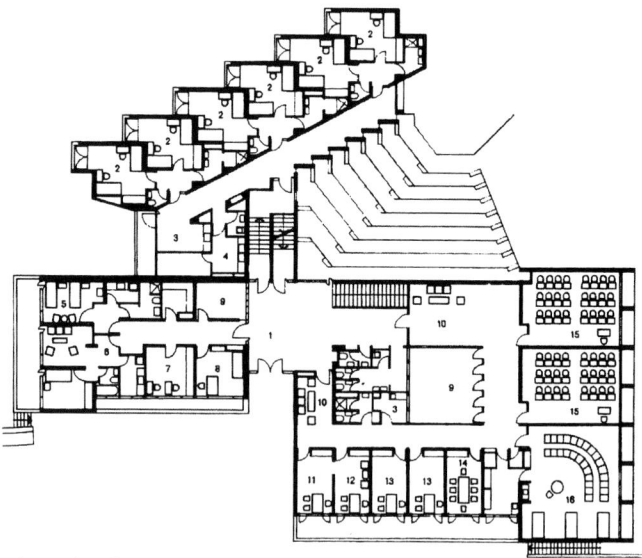

Plan at level -0.00, +1.39

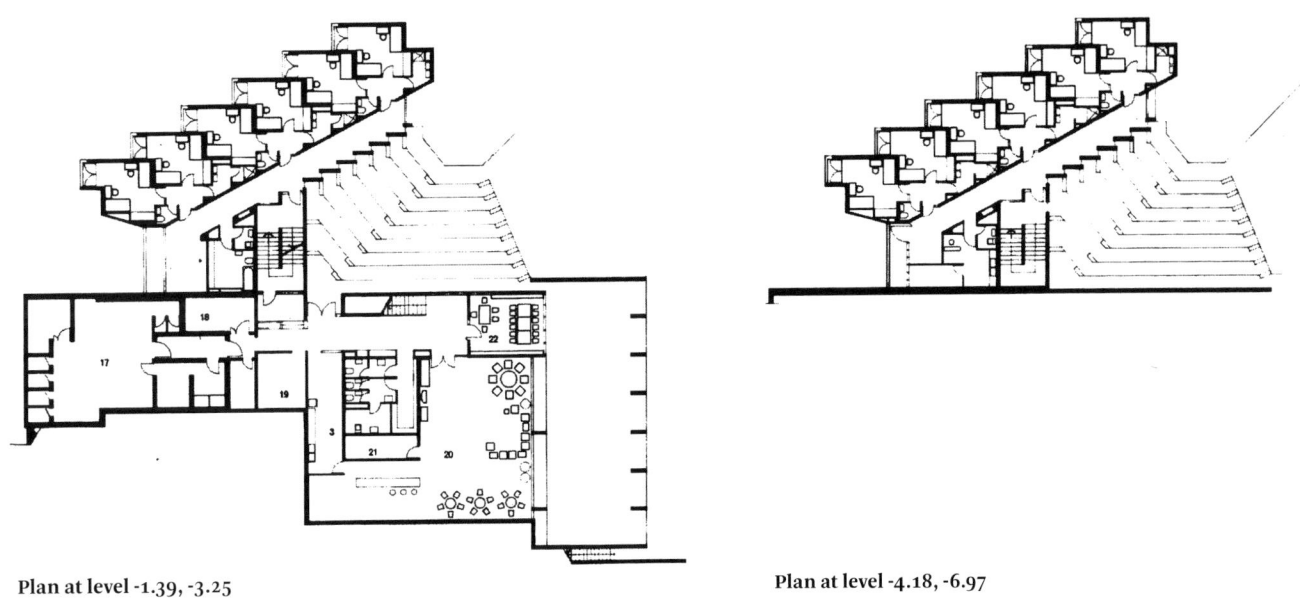

Plan at level -1.39, -3.25   Plan at level -4.18, -6.97

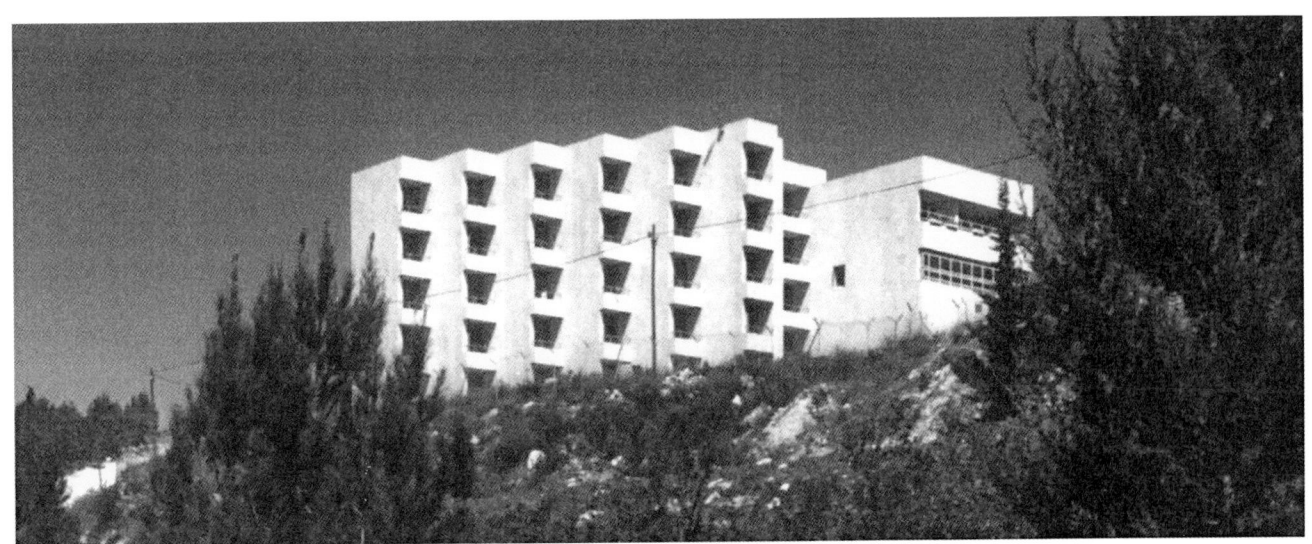

4. Tel Aviv University – School of Medicine

Clinics and School of Dental Medicine

Tel Aviv, 6,000 sqm, 1972–1975

The Sackler Faculty of Medicine is Israel's largest institute of higher medical education. The Sackler School of Medicine, the Goldschleger School of Dental Medicine and the School of Health Professions offer first professional degrees. In addition, the Faculty's School of Continuing Medical Education provides continuing medical education. The Graduate School offers further research studies towards MSc and PhD degrees.

Altogether, the Faculty includes approximately 1,000 teachers in preclinical departments and in affiliated clinical departments and institutes, located in 7 major medical centers, six psychiatric hospitals, and a large rehabilitation center. The clinics and the school of dental medicine have been built by Zarhy Architects.

Main view

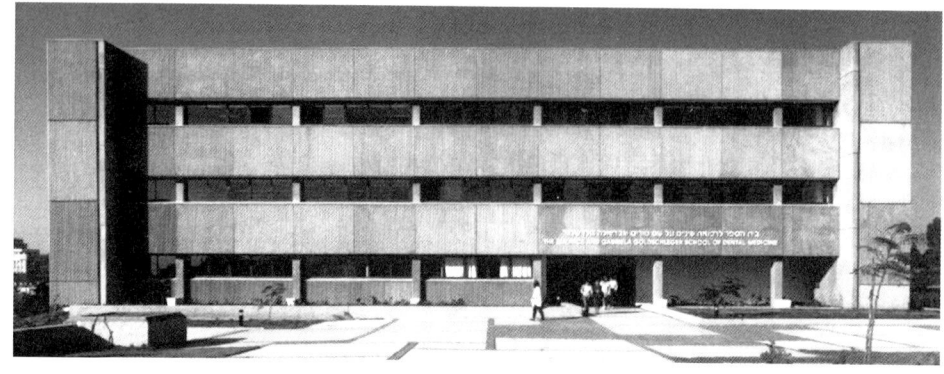

Entrance floor at level ±0.00
1. Entrance hall
2. Main auditorium
3. General reception
4. Records
5. Cafeteria
6. Kitchen
7. Waiting area
8. Clinics' director
9. Seminar room
10. Secretary

Oral medicine
11. Nurses station
12. Students operating room
13. Students operating room
14. T.V. demonstration room

Oral surgery
15. Nurses station
16. Recovery room
17. General anesthetics
18. Seminar room
19. Students operating room
20. Students operating room

Radiology
21. Waiting area
22. X-ray
23. X-ray demonstration
24. Dark room
25. Radiologist's office
26. Dark room
27. Panorex encephalometrics
28. Radiographer
29. Radiology reception

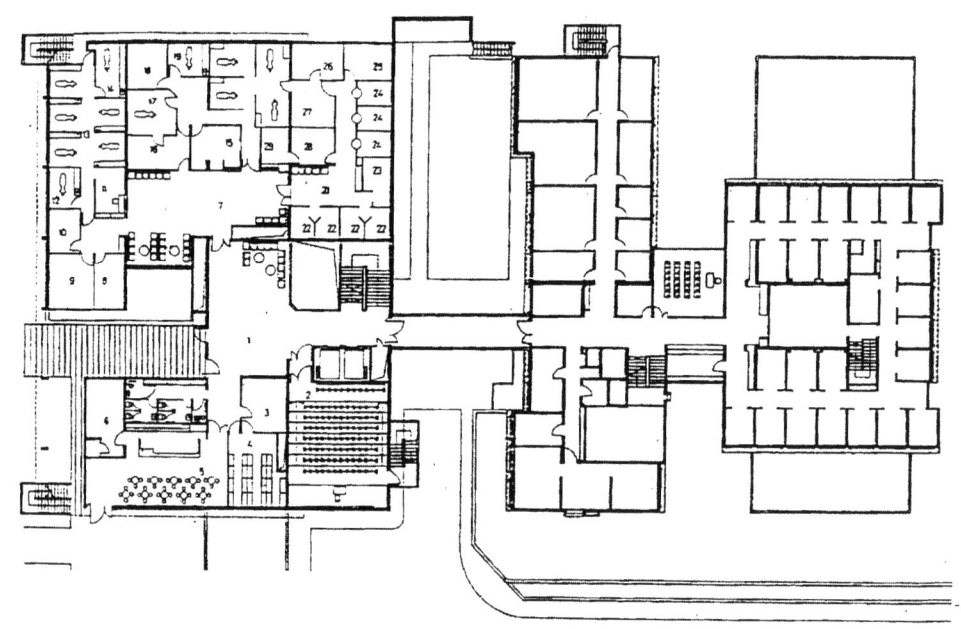

5. The Hospitals and Health Facilities of Zarhy Architects

View from south-west

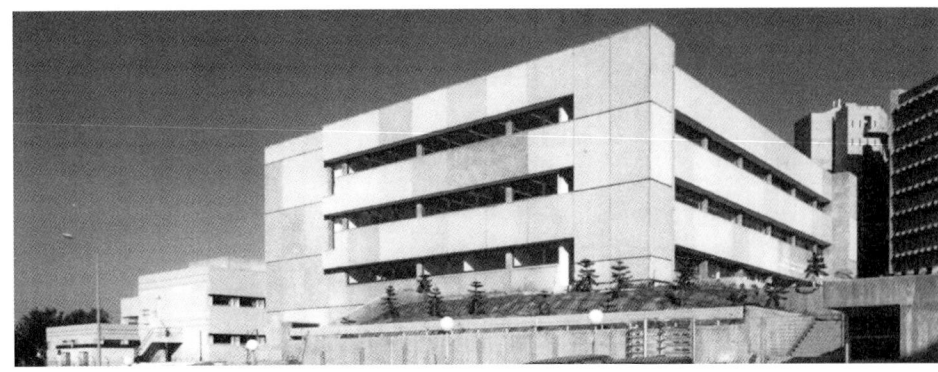

Lower ground floor
1. Elevators lobby
2. Central machinery
3. Students' microscope laboratory
4. Students' lounge
5. Technical laboratory
6. Acrylic processing room
7. Denture finishing
8. Plaster room
9. Porcelain laboratory
10. Metal coating room
11. Chief technician
12. Preclinical (phantom-head) laboratory
13. Central sterilization

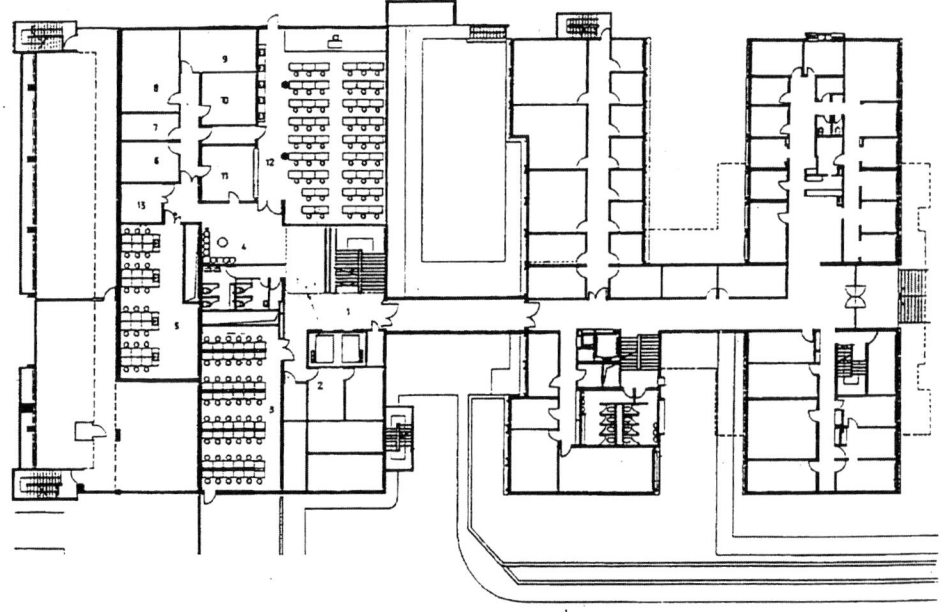

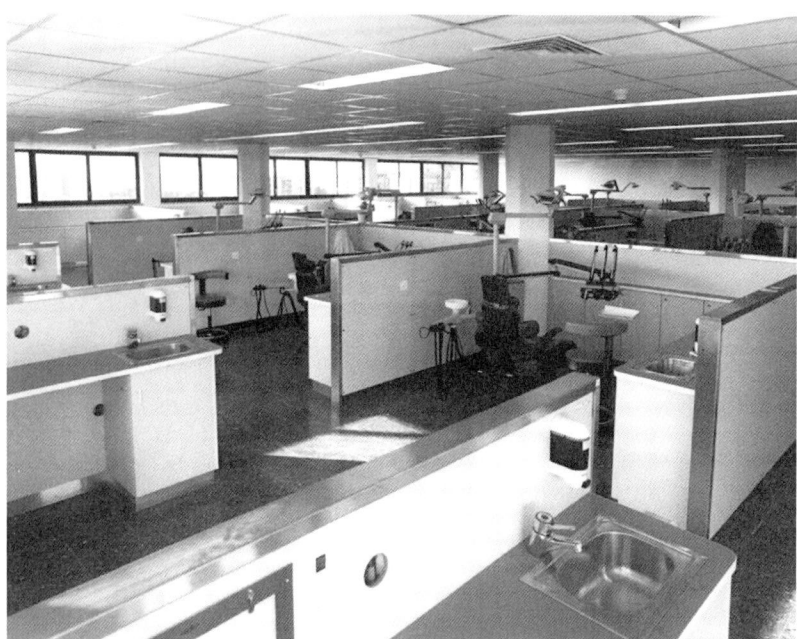

Students' clinic

5. The Hospitals and Health Facilities of Zarhy Architects

Second floor at level ±7.48

1. Elevators lobby
2. Class room
3. Class room
4. Seminar room
5. Waiting room
6. Dental assistants
7. Students' clinic
8. X-ray
9. Dark room
10. Technical laboratory
11. Instructions room

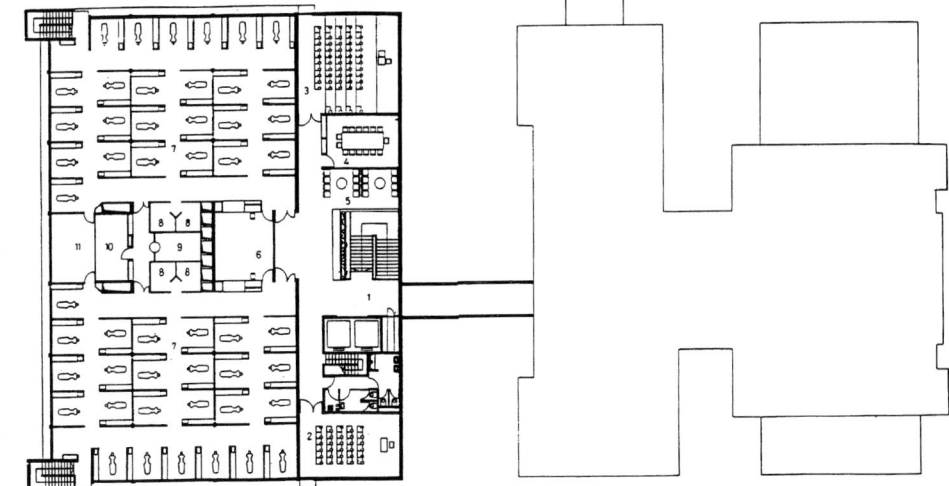

First floor at level ±3.74

1. Elevators lobby
2. Class room
3. Class room
4. Seminar room
5. Waiting room
6. Dental assistants
7. Students' clinic
8. X-ray
9. Dark room
10. Technical laboratory
11. Instruction' room

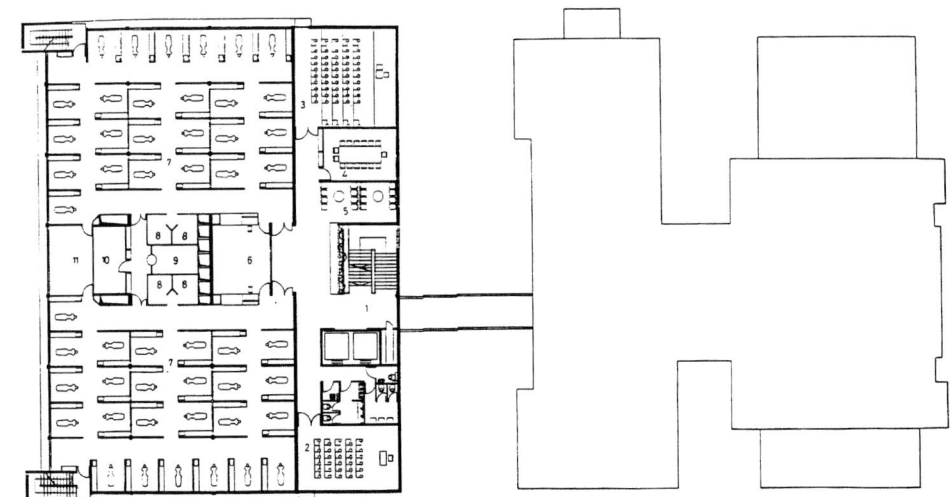

5. The Government Hospital Dimona

Dimona, 150 Beds, Planned 1965, not built

The Dimona Hospital will serve the town of Dimona and the surrounding area. Dimona is a development town, situated approximately midway between Beersheba and Sodom. The town was founded in the early 1950's and has grown progressively; today it has a population of approximately 20,000 inhabitants. The town and the region which it serves has become an important industrial centre, including the potassium plant on the Dead Sea, the phosphate mine at Oron, the Arad Chemical Industry (which will manufacture phosphoricacid for fertilisers) and the various textile plants in Dimona itself.

The new hospital has been planned to serve the needs of the whole region, including the minority – groups, which consist mainly of Bedouin.

The master plan for the new hospital takes into account the existing population, with provision for growth according to potential demands of the region. The first stage is planned for approximately 150 beds. These will include 72 general beds, 36 pediatric beds, and 36 maternity beds. (The birthrate in Dimona is amongst the highest in Israel).

The new hospital is located on a hill on the outskirts of the town, overlooking the Paula Ben-Gurion Park.

The building is at present under construction, with the service area due to be completed at the end of 1969. It covers approximately 5,000 sqm. of the ground floor, and includes the emergency hospital.

Set out hereunder are the different sections of the building forming the first stage:

1) Wards, including Pediatrics, Maternity Section and Delivery Rooms
2) Casualty and Admittance Sections
3) Operating Theatre Wing
4) Radiology Department
5) Clinics, Physiotherapy and Occupational Therapy
6) Laboratories
7) Main Entrance Hall, Administration Wing, Circumcision Hall, Circulation area, etc.
8) Medical Library and Auditorium and Duty Doctors' Living Quarters
9) Pathology Section
10) Services including:
    Milk Kitchen
    Medical supplies- Pharmacy, Central
    Sterile Supply, Medical Equipment Store
    Building and Maintenance Supply Services
    Cleaning Services
    Workshops
    Hospital Vehicle Garage
    Laundry Services
    Food Services
    Staff Dining Room
    Staff Lockers
    Bed-pan Centre
    Emergency Hospital Shelter
11) Nurses' Training School

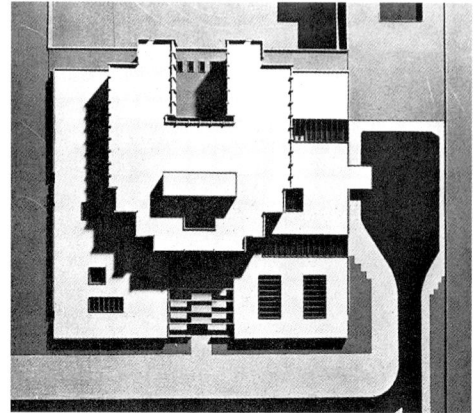

Model view from above

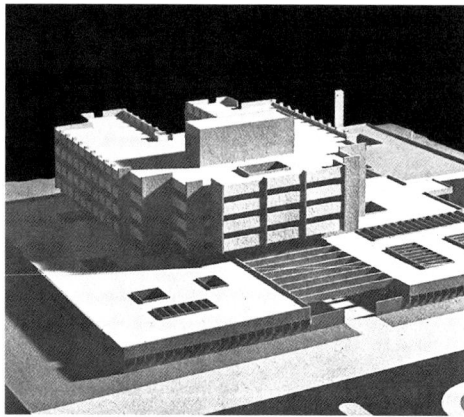

View from the southwest, model

This project of Zarhy Architects was not realized. In 1964, the construction of Dimona Hospital had begun. That hospital was never finished. Ever since, people of Dimona and the peripherals are dragged to Soroka hospital in Be'er-Shava for any medical issue especially after health services hours. These treatments, including emergency cases, are in 35 minutes ride to Be'er Sheva. The final project was planned by architect Shachar Tsentsiper.

Site plan
1. Main entrance
2. Casualty entrance
3. Service entrance
4. Main plant
5. Power plant
6. Pathology
7. School of nursing
8. Parking
9. Heliport

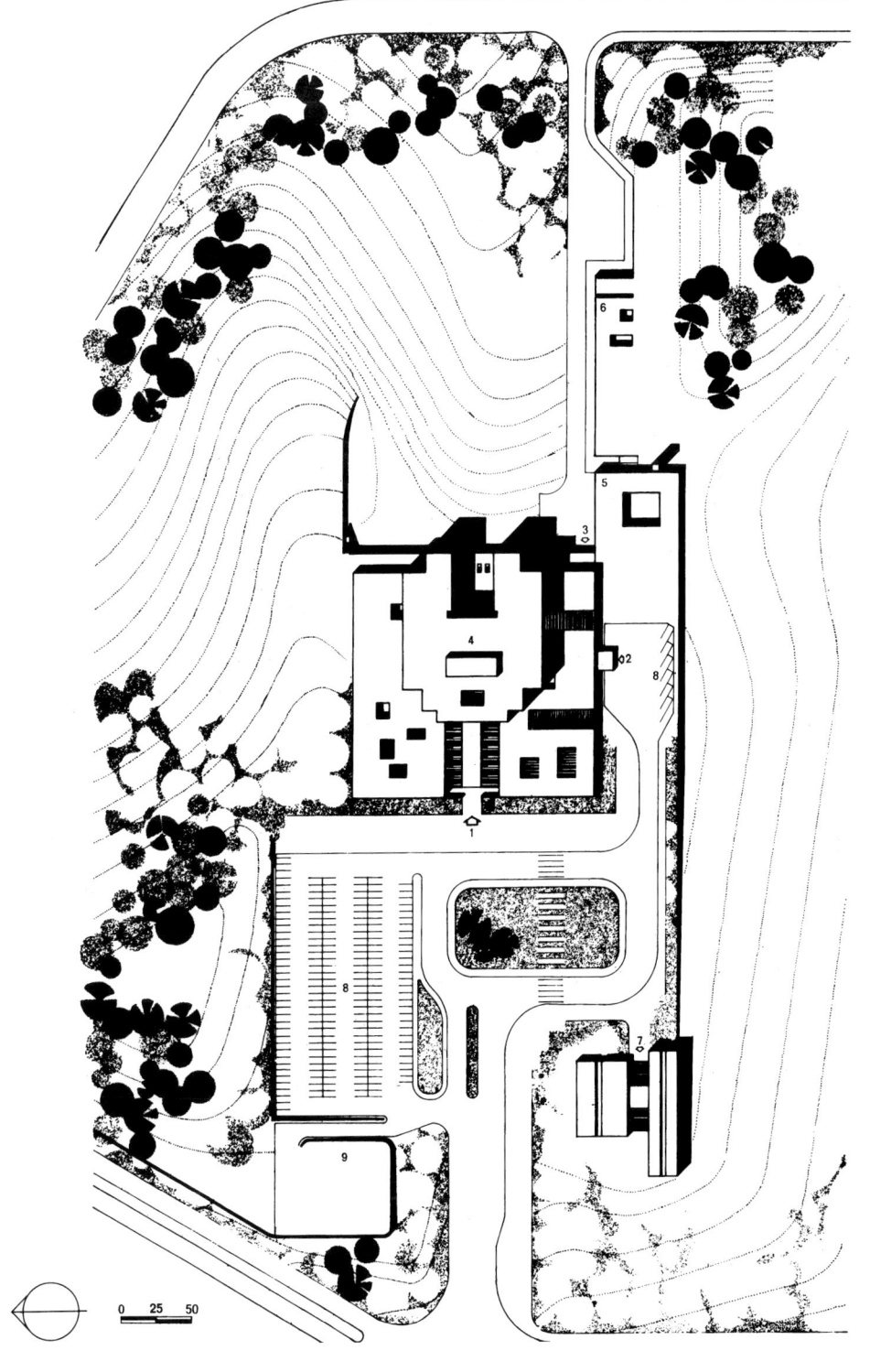

0 25 50

Ground floor medical services

A. Entrance hall
1. Service lifts
2. Visitor and patient lifts

B. Laboratory department
3. Histology, bacteriology, chemistry and haematology laboratories

C. Casualty department
4. Children's casualty ward
5. Casualty ward
6. Waiting
7. Treatment and plaster application rooms

D. Patient admission
8. Medical records

E. Administration

F. Religious facilities
9. Synagogue
10. Circumcision hall

G. Out-patients' department
11. Waiting
12. Cystoscopy and treatment rooms
13. Consulting and examination rooms
14. Opthalmology

H. Physiotherapy department
15. Waiting
16. Occupational therapy
17. Hydrotherapy
18. Gymnasium

I. Radiology
19. Waiting
20. X-ray work rooms
21. Dark room
22. Reception and X-ray files

J. Operating theatres
23. Entrance hall
24. Patient reception
25. Recovery room
26. Operating theatre
27. Lay-up room
28. Anaesthetic room
29. Scrub-up and gowning
30. Lift to central supply
31. Medical staff changing rooms

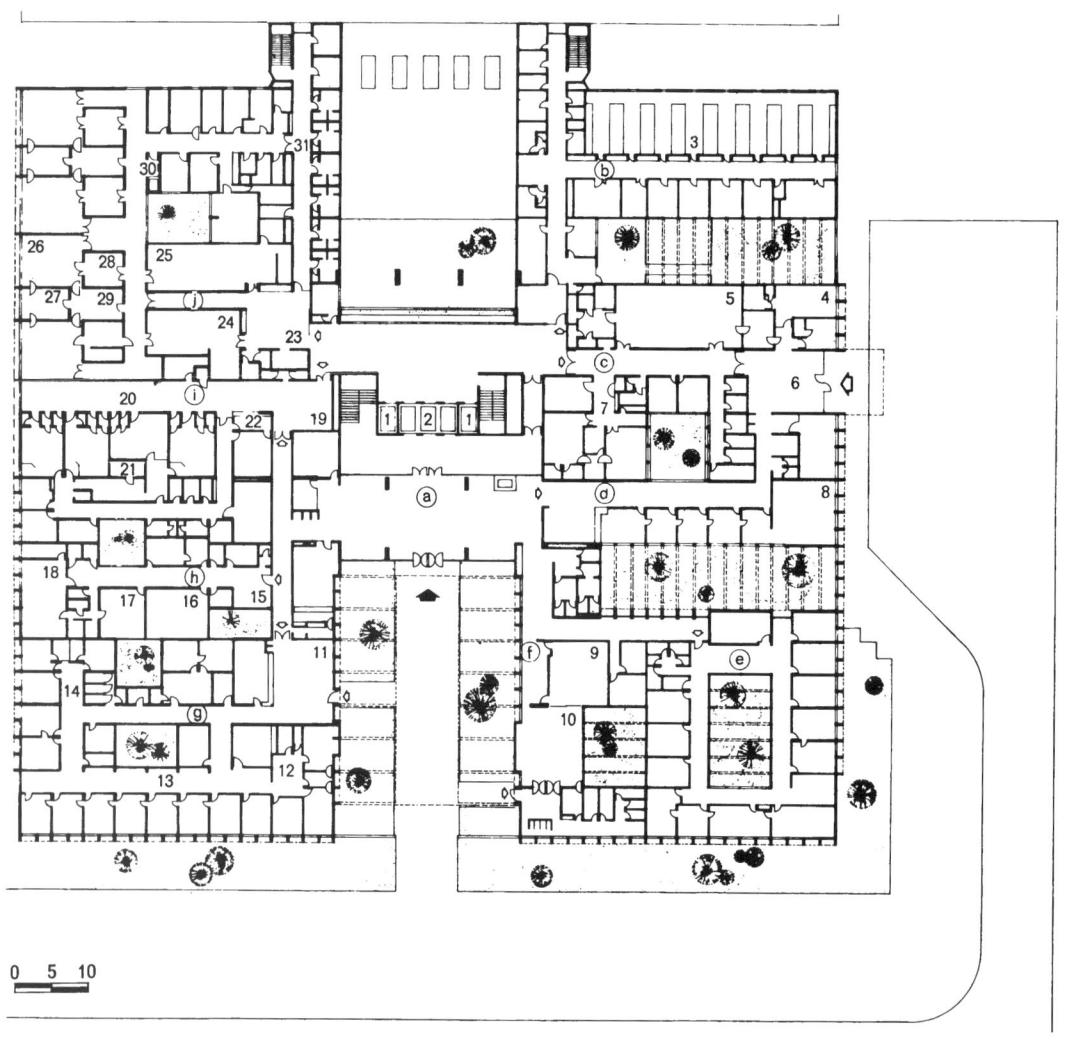

0   5   10

5. The Hospitals and Health Facilities of Zarhy Architects

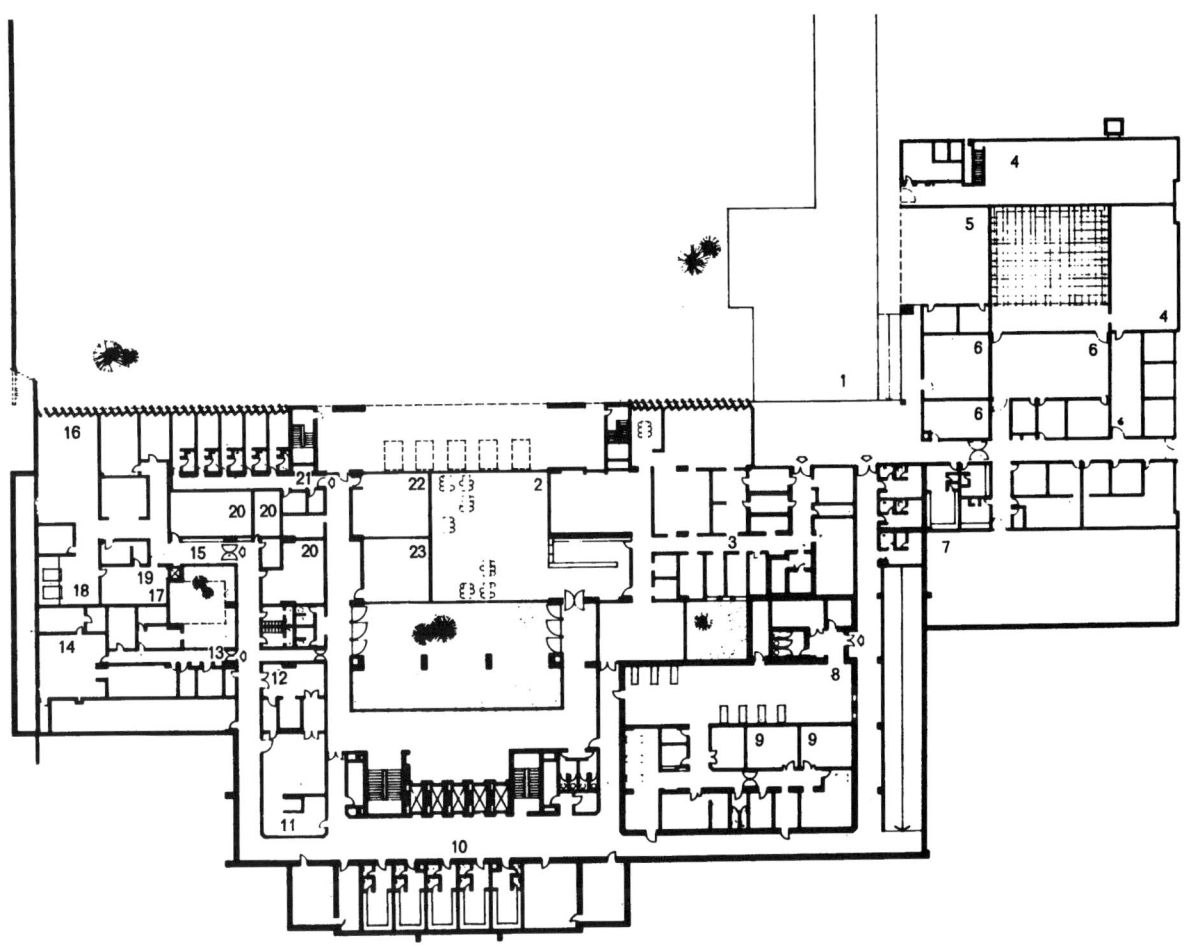

**Lower ground floor medical
Services and technical services**

1. Service road
2. Staff dining room
3. Kitchen
4. Plant room
5. Garage
6. Workshops
7. General storage
8. Underground casualty unit
9. Emergency operation
   theatres
10. Central cloakrooms
11. Kitchen utensils cleaning
12. Bed and mattresses cleaning
13. Pharmacy
14. Bulk preparation
15. Central sterile supply
16. Inspection and assembly
17. Sterile store
18. Autoclave room
19. Lift to operating theatres
20. Stores
21. Night duty staff rooms
22. Library
23. Lecture hall

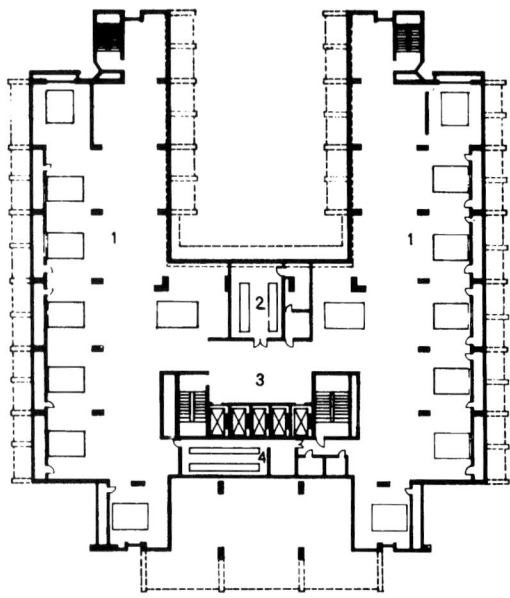

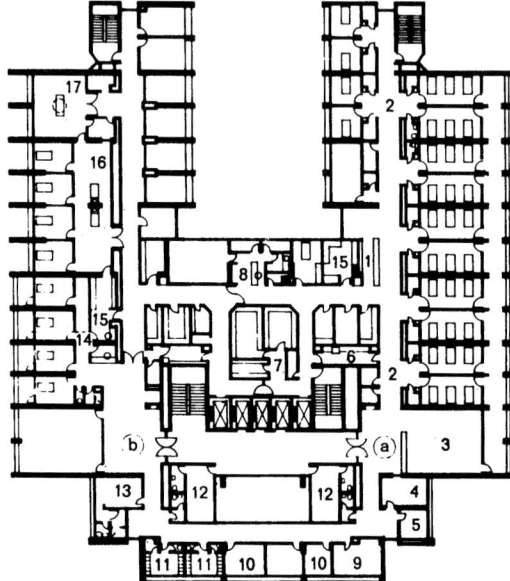

Mezzanine
A.C. power plant
1. A.C. Equipment
2. Electrical equipment
3. Maintenance shop
4. Communication equipment

First floor
Maternity
Delivery rooms
a. Maternlty
1. Nurses' station
2. Wards
3. Day room
4. Senior nurse
5. Laboratory
6. Kitchen
7. Nursery kitchen
8. Nursery

9. Doctors' room
10. Examination and treatment
b. Delivery rooms
11. Medical staff changing rooms
12. Visitors' room
13. Lay-up room
14. Labour rooms
15. Nurses' work room
16. Delivery room
17. Intervention room

Section
1. **Lower ground floor**
   Medical services and services
2. **Ground floor**
   Medical services
3. **Mezzanine**
   Power plant
4. **First floor**
   Maternity, delivery room

5. **Second floor**
   Children's ward department, typical ward department
6. **Third floor**
   Typical ward department

0   5   10

5. The Hospitals and Health Facilities of Zarhy Architects

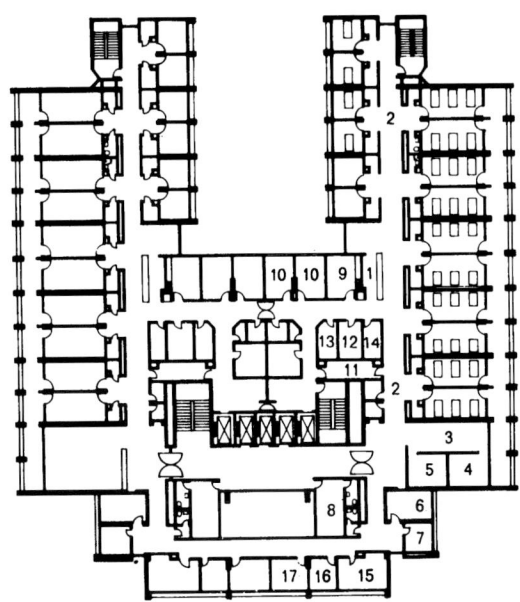

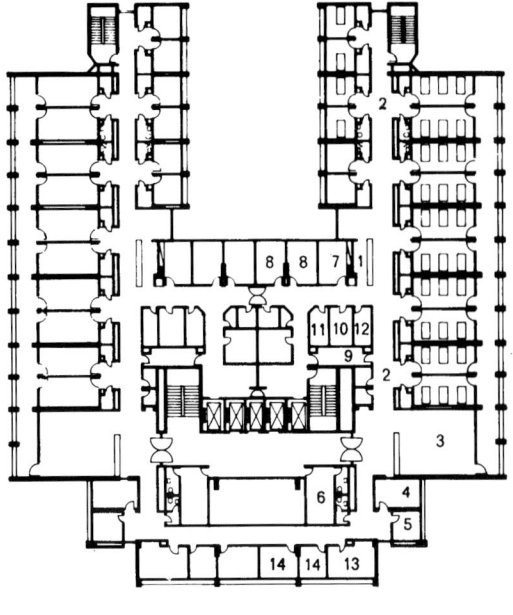

Second floor
Children's ward department

a. Children's ward department
1. Nurses' station
2. Wards
3. Day room
4. Kindergarten
5. Classroom
6. Senior nurse
7. Laboratory
8. Visitors' waiting room
9. Nurses' work room
10. Treatment
11. Kitchen
12. Bath room
13. Utility room
14. Linen store
15. Doctors' room
16. Examination and treatment
17. Head of department

Third floor
Typical ward department

1. Nurses' station
2. Wards
3. Day room
4. Senior nurse
5. Laboratory
6. Visitors' waiting room
7. Nurses' work room
8. Treatment
9. Kitchen
10. Bathroom
11. Utility room
12. Linen store
13. Doctors' room
14. Examination and treatment

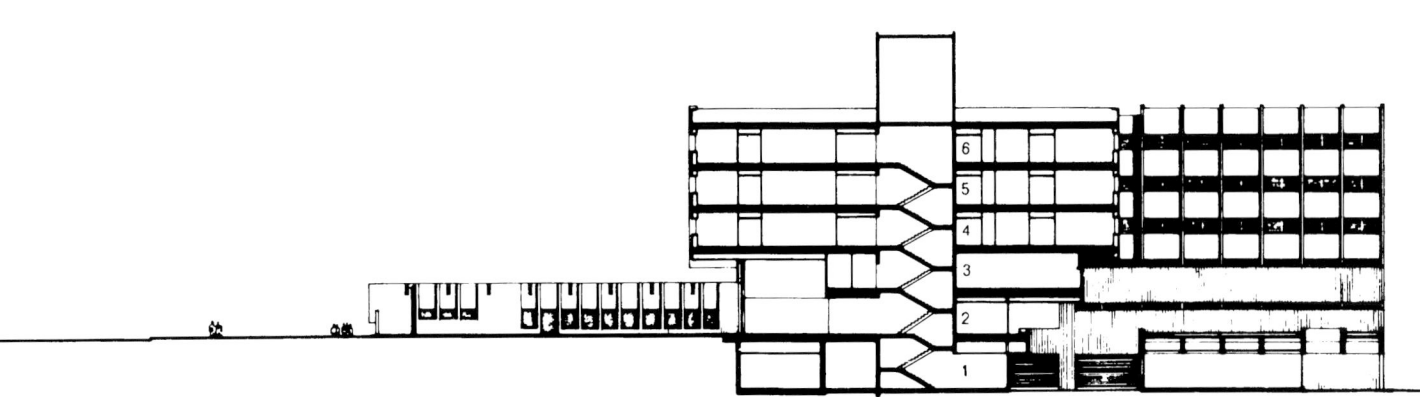

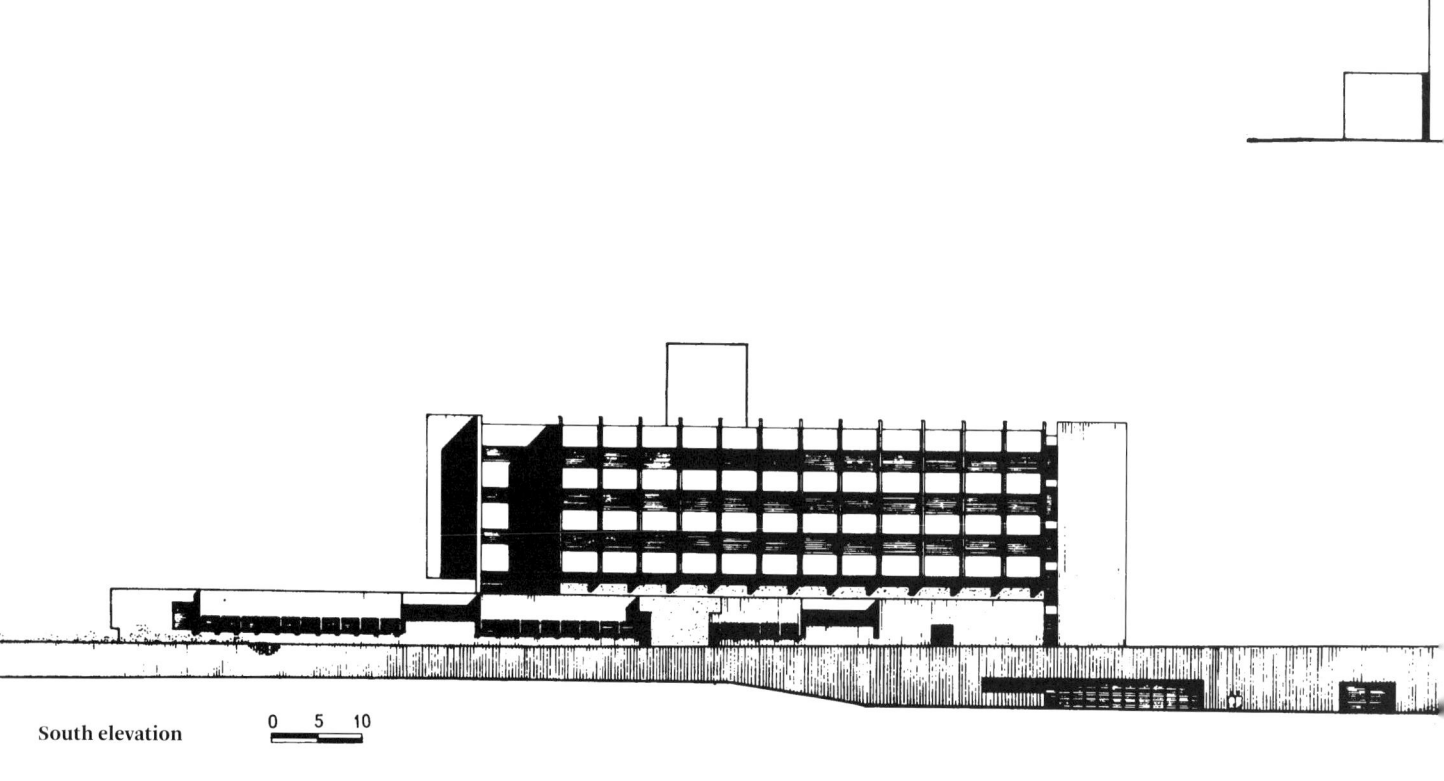

South elevation   0   5   10

5. The Hospitals and Health Facilities of Zarhy Architects

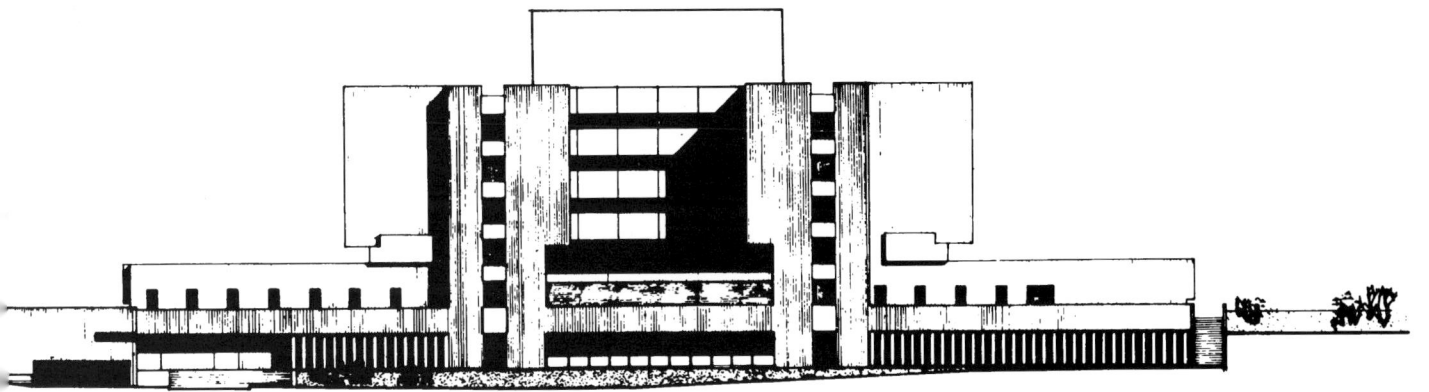

East elevation

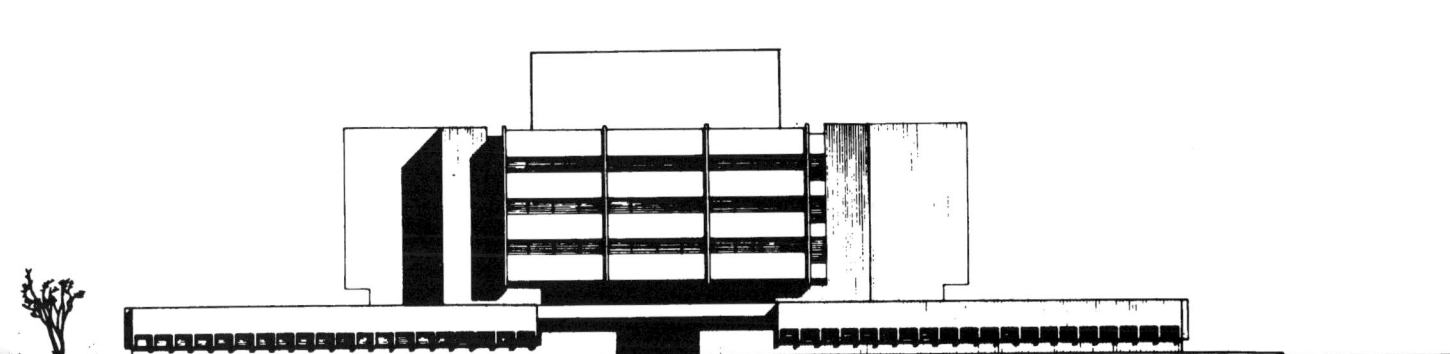

West elevation

6. Home for mentally retarded people

in Ramat Hasharon – Greater Tel Aviv Area
for AKIM Israel – National Association for the Habilitation
of the Mentally Handicapped in Israel

One out of every hundred children is born mentally retarded to some
degree. Some of these children grow up to become a part of society or
live at its edges, perhaps without the general public being aware of it.
Today, after years of relentless efforts and determination, AKIM
ISRAEL has become the National organization leading the campaign
that aims the changing the way the Israeli society and its authorities
see the mentally disabled person.

Nowadays AKIM serves a wide population: 19 social clubs for 2,000 adults,
59 sheltered workshops for 2,500 adults, summer camps for 2,000 teen-
agers and young adults, 24 group homes for 600 people, and 14 apartments in regular buildings with an average of 6 residents each.

Zarhy Architects have built a small home for mentally retarded people
in Ramat Hasharon in the greater Tel-Aviv area.

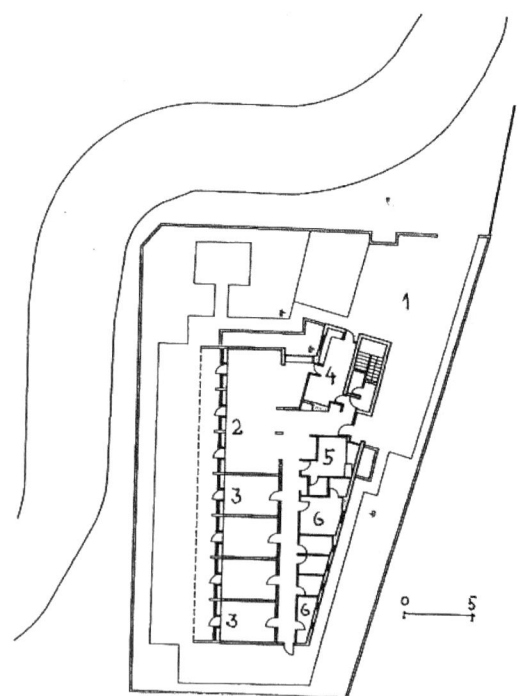

1. Entrance courtyard
2. Living room
3. Bed rooms
4. Kitchen
5. Directors room
6. Conveniences

5. The Hospitals and Health Facilities of Zarhy Architects

7. The private Clinics in central Tel Aviv

Tel Aviv, 45 clinics, 1960

1960 one of the first buildings housing private clinics in central Tel Aviv, Frishman street corner of Reines street was built by Zarhy Architects. At that time, most Health facilities in Israel were public facilities treating everyone. The Private Clinic Building enabled physicians to have private practice.

It consists of 6 floors of private clinics above ground floor, approximately 45 clinics in all.

The central core includes staircase, elevators and conveniences. The outer walls are "permanent", while the inner walls can be changed or removed according to demand.

The design and architecture of the building harmonizes with its neighboring buildings. The ground floor and the basement are used for parking. The entrance hall contains the information desk. The basement houses machinery room and the shelter.

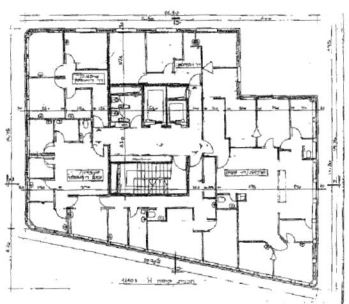

Typical floor plan

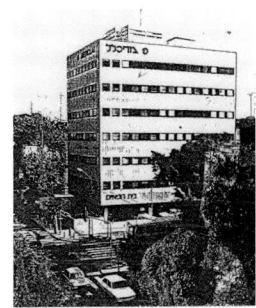

Main view

8. Home for autistic children and adults

"Autism is a lifelong neuro-developmental disorder, which typically appears during the first three years of a child's life. It occurs in approximately 1 out of every 250 births and is four times more prevalent in males than females. Autism affects a person's ability to communicate, form relationships with others, and respond appropriately to the surrounding environment. Autism affects families throughout the world of all racial, ethnic and social backgrounds. It is a complex developmental disability that typically results in a neurological disorder which affects the functioning of the brain. It impacts the normal development of the brain in the areas of social interaction and communication skills, resulting typically in difficulties in verbal and non-verbal communication, social interactions, and leisure or play activities. Some people with autism exhibit repeated body movements, unusual responses to people or attachments to objects, and resistance to changes in routine. They may experience sensitivities in the five senses. There are currently no therapeutic cures for autism, although early behavioral intervention dramatically improves outcome. With support and care, individuals with autism can realize at least some of their personal goals and dreams." www.alut.org.il

My intention in designing this project is to provide the inhabitants with LIVING CONDITIONS especially suitable for their needs and the possibility to improve and develop their artistic talents like painting, design and music. The lecture hall provides facility for meetings and activities with outsiders.

First floor

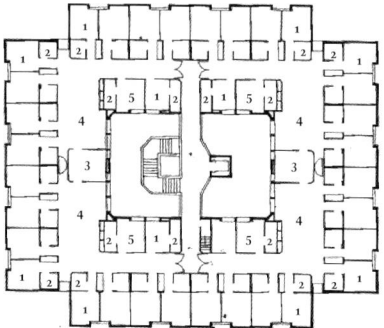

Dwelling accomodation

1. Bed room
2. Bathroom
3. Kitchen
4. Day and dining room
   for the group always consisting of members
5. Teachers room

Ground floor

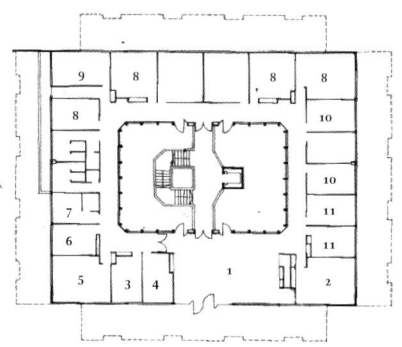

Main entrance to the building

1. Entrance hall
2. Office of management
   Office of the main supervisor on duty
3. Directors office
4. Office of secretaries
5. Teachers and meeting room and
   meeting of special problems
6. Nurses office for general treatment
7. Room for on duty staff
   for individual treatment
8. Workshop
   Art therapy
9. Music room, sound isolated
10. Individual work room for various disciplines
11. Room for creative workshop

Basement floor

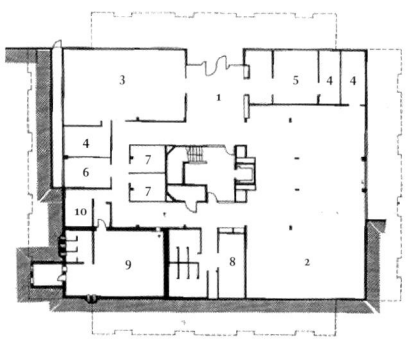

1. Entrance hall
   Additional entrance hall
   also used for meetings
2. Lecture hall
3. Gymnastic room
   Physical exercise room with equipment
4. Storage room
5. Central kitchen
   Receives pre prepared food for processing
6. Laundry room
   Providing facilities
   for machine and hand laundry
7. Clock room
8. Machinery room
9. Shelter
   Air raid shelter
   according to government rules
10. Generator room
    Emergency generator room

5. The Hospitals and Health Facilities of Zarhy Architects

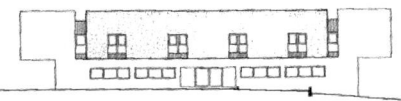

South elevation

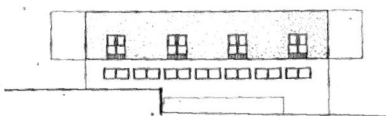

East elevation

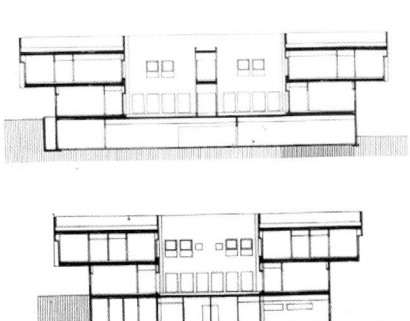

Sections

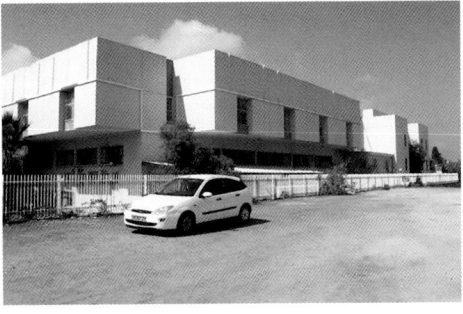

View from south-east

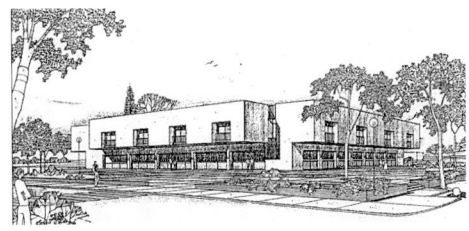

Sketch of the main view

In the three stored cubic building, training professionals provide assistance to families of people with autism. Autistic children and adults get special treatment for a better communication and social interaction.

People enter the building through the basement floor with the main entrance, a big lecture hall and a gymnastic room. In the ground floor we find the administration, teachers and meeting rooms. The top floor with the accommodations cantilevers over the ground floor.

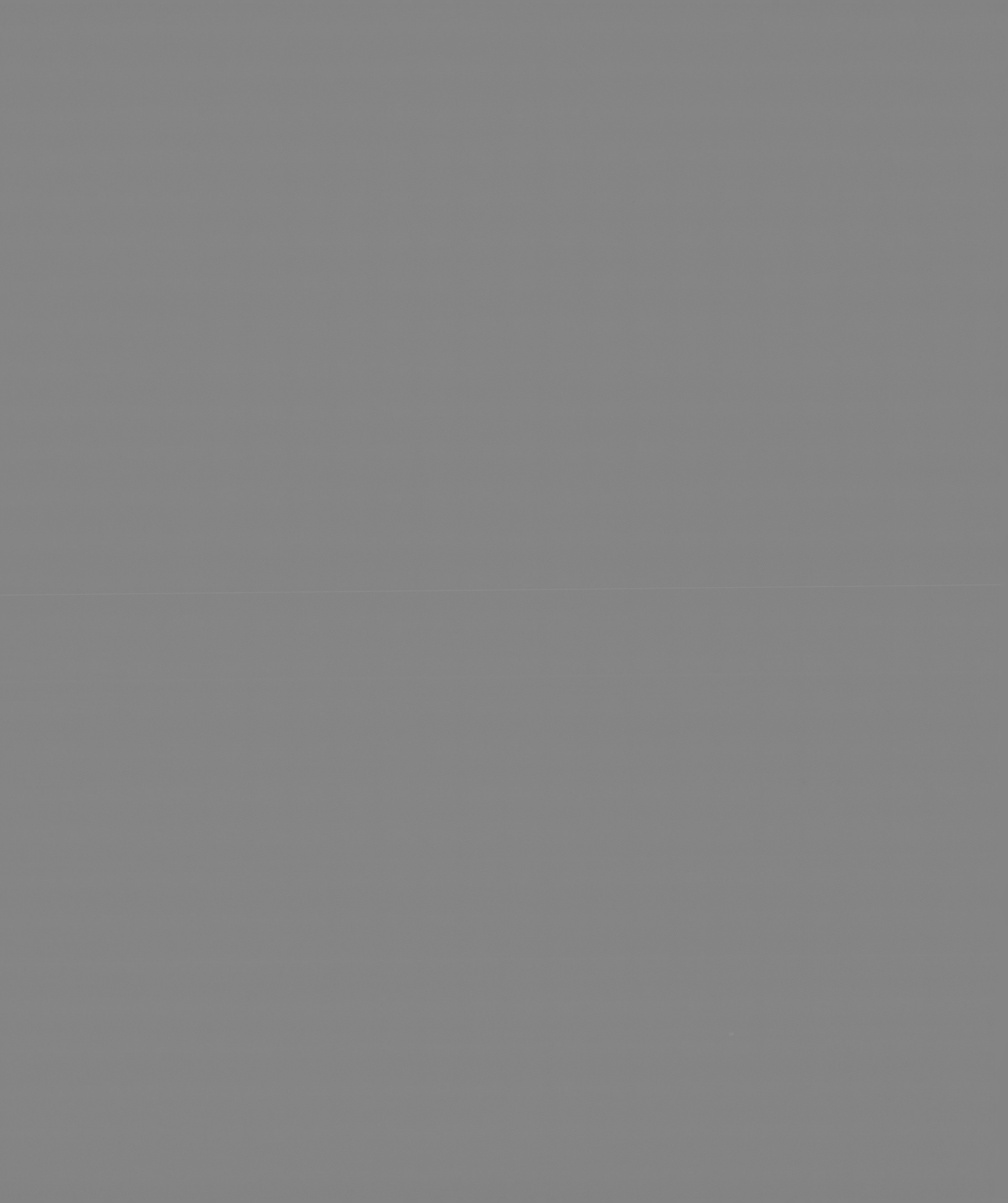

9. Tel Giborim Hospital

Competition projects

Tel Giborim, 600 Beds, 78,000 sqm

Two projects were submitted for the competition, which was commissioned by the Ministry of Health for the design of the Regional Hospital at Tel Giborim. The Regional Hospital is situated on the boundaries of the three Municipalities which it is designed to serve Tel Aviv, Bat Yam and Holon. Plan B was awarded the 2nd prize and Plan A was awarded the 3rd prize, which was subsequently cancelled in accordance with a specific rule which was in force at the time within the Association of Engineers and Architects in Israel, that a planning firm is entitled to one prize only. The hospital comprises 600 beds, grouped into 11 general hospitalization units made up of 36 beds each; one unit for chronic illnesses of 36 beds; a psychiatric unit of 36 beds; a maternity section of 60 beds; a section for premature babies of 15 beds and a children's section of 60 beds.

The medical services include: Admittance and casualty section, operating rooms. X-ray department, clinical and research laboratories and animal house, medical photography section, electroencephalography unit, cardiology department and pulmonary function department, physiotherapy and occupational therapy department, and outpatients' clinic.

General services include: Food services, laundry services, stores, cleaning services, workshops and power centre. Also included in the project in addition to the above, are administration services, nursing school and residential quarters for staff.

In both projects the general hospitalization units were planned as a superblock, two departments per floor, with a vertical connection joining the wards to entrances and medical and other services. Additional beds would be obtained by the addition of more storeys. The medical and other services are spread out horizontally. This planning principle allows for organic growth, additions and changes in the medical and general services. Planning emphasis was placed on circulation, keeping it as simple as possible, with logical separation between the different types of circulation; patients and staff, supply, visitors, etc., as expressed in the schematic diagram. This was made possible due to maximum utilization of the natural topography and placing of the supply services on one level lower than the entrance level.

Plan A

Main Building (Wards)

Obstetrics

Night Duty Staff_____

Delivery Rooms_____

Laboratories_____

Outpatient Department_____

Pediatrics

Psychiatric Department_____

Lecture Room_____

Premature Babies_____

Administration_____

Main Entrance Hall_____

Main Entrance_____

Entrance to Outpatient Department_____

Outpatient Department_____

To Psychiatric Outpatient Department_____ _____

Medical Services

Operating Theatres_____

Casualty Department_____

Radiology_____

Casualty Entrance_____

Outpatient Department_____

Supply Services

Machine Room_____

_____

Main Kitchen_____

Pathology_____

Workshop_____

Laundry_____

5. The Hospitals and Health Facilities of Zarhy Architects

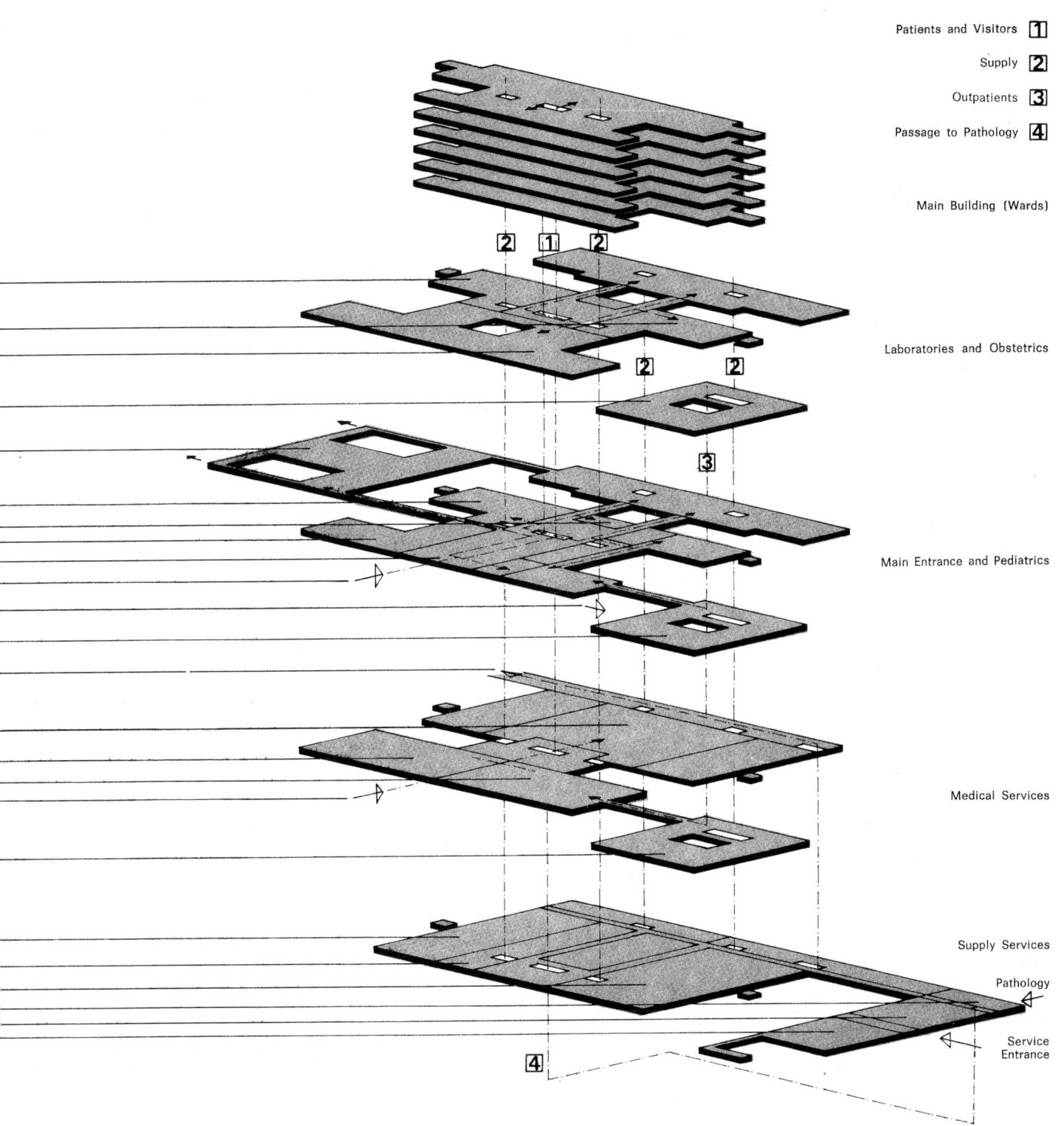

Patients and Visitors **1**

Supply **2**

Outpatients **3**

Passage to Pathology **4**

Main Building (Wards)

Laboratories and Obstetrics

Main Entrance and Pediatrics

Medical Services

Supply Services

Pathology

Service Entrance

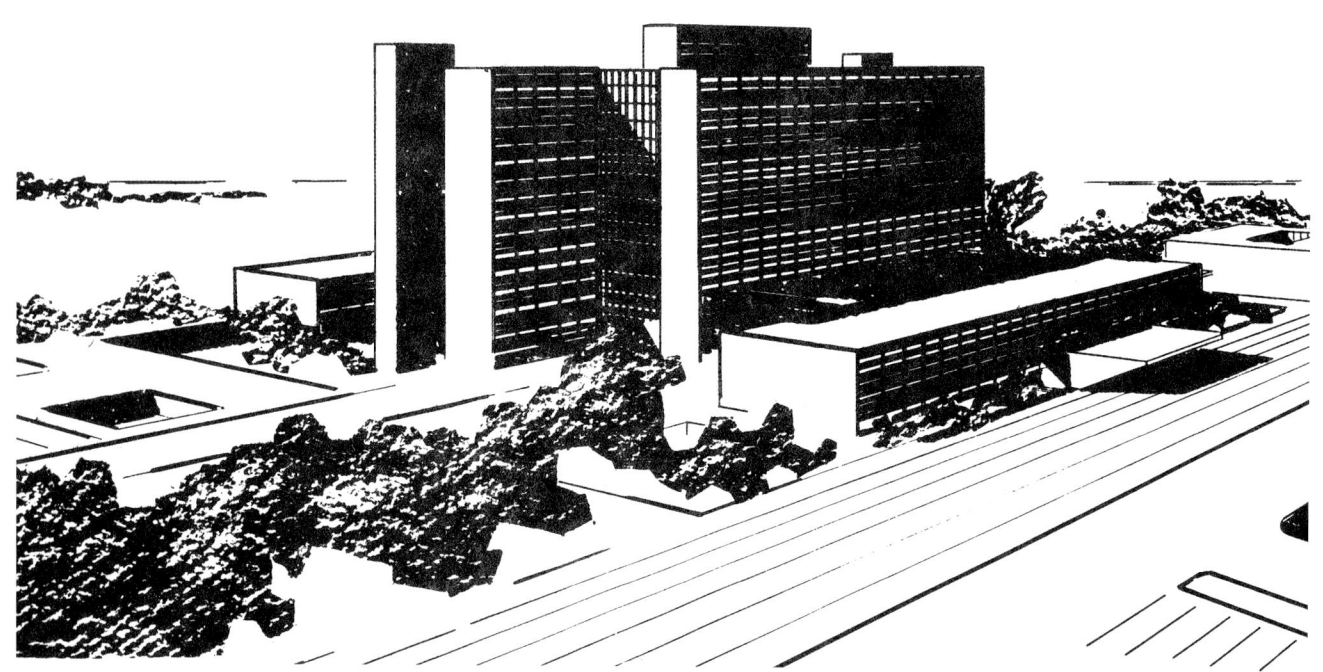

In Plan A special emphasis was placed on the planning of efficient wards, with shortest possible paths for passage and treatment of the patient from the moment of his entry into the hospital until his departure. Similar attention was given to provision of efficient medical services from the point of view of the patient.

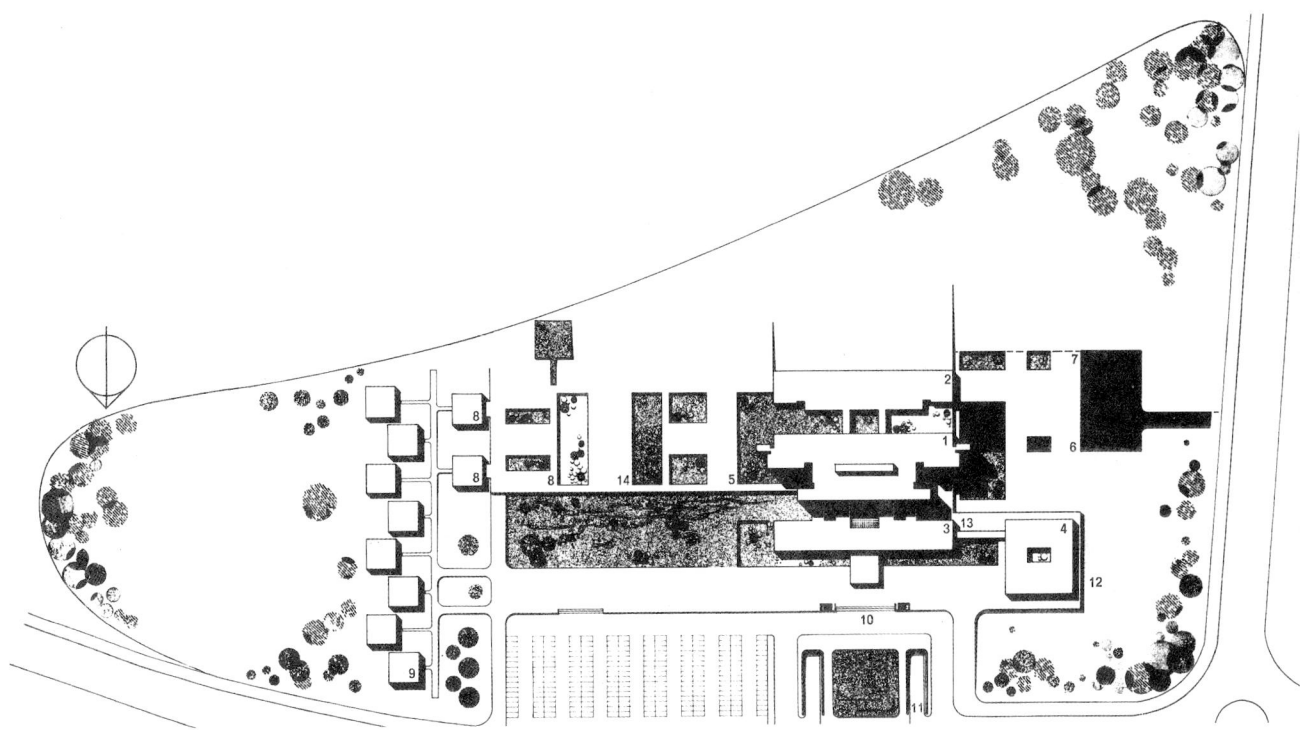

Site plan

1. Main building (wards)
2. Pediatrics and obstetrics
3. Medical services
4. Outpatient department
5. Psychiatric department
6. Supply services
7. Pathology
8. School for nurses
8a. Living quarters for students
8b. Living quarters for students
(future expansion)
9. Living quarters for personnel
10. Main entrance
11. Admission and casualty entrance and
access to underground parking
12. Access road to service, yard and pathology
13–14. Extension areas

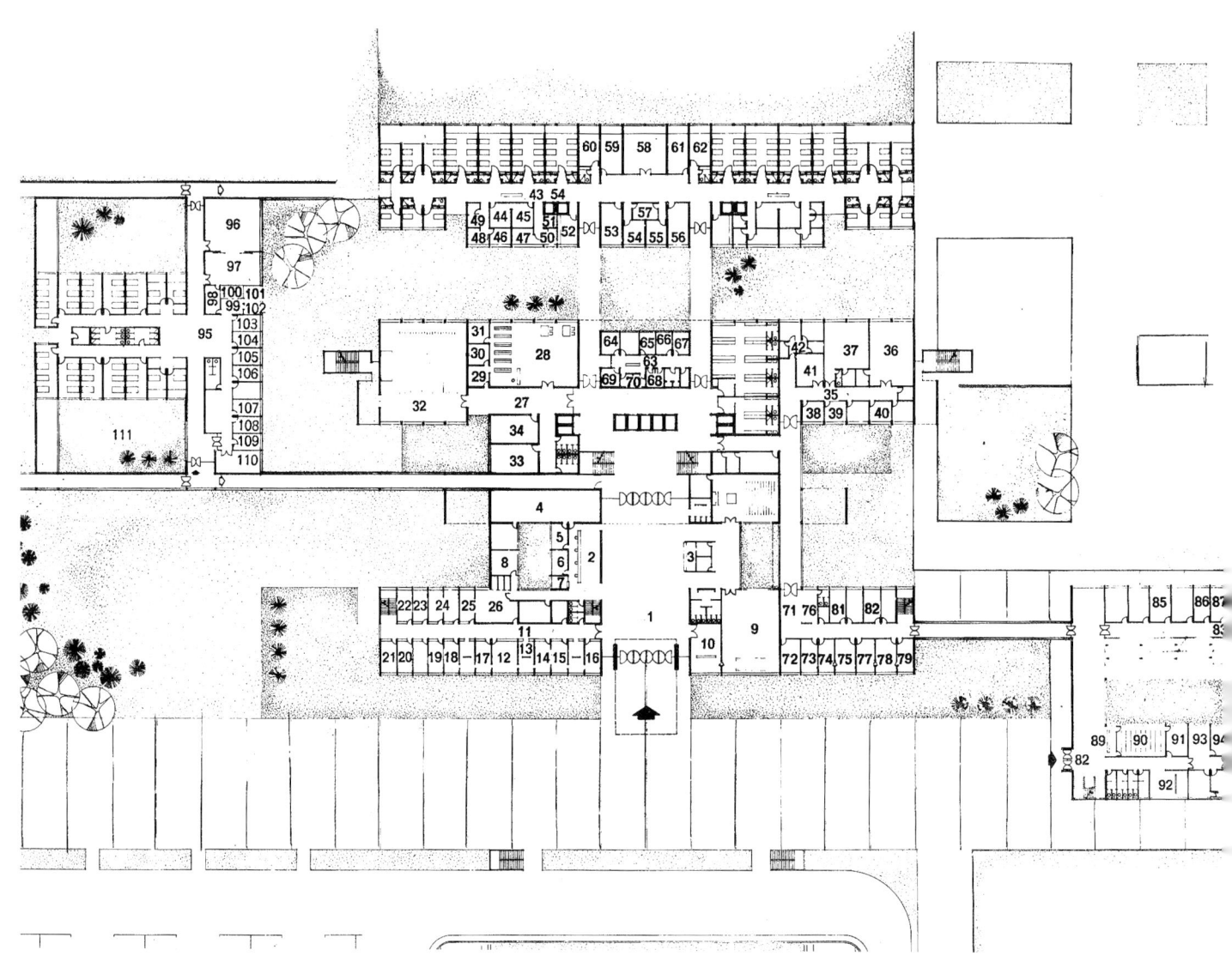

5. The Hospitals and Health Facilities of Zarhy Architects

A. Entrance level
1. Entrance hall and admission
2. Entrance hall
3. Patients admission office
4. Information
5. Archives
6. Clerical office
7. Clerical office
8. Cashier
9. Chief admitting office
10. Circumcision hall
11. Cafeteria

B. Administration
12. Administration
13. Director's office
14. Waiting and director's secretary
15. Deputy director
16. Matron's office
17. Deputy matron
18. Administrator
19. Chief assistant administrator's office
20. Social worker
21. Personal manager
22. Records store
23. Library
24. Women volunteers
25. Accounting
26. Chief accountant
27. Central general secretariat

**C. Library, (med.),
     museum and lecture halls**
27. Entrance to library and lecture hall
28. Library and main reading area
29. Librarian's office
30. Projection room
31. Store
32. Lecture hall
33. Museum (med)
34. Seminar room

**D. Physiotherapie and
     occupational theraphy**
35. Entrance to physiotherapy and
     occupational therapy
36. Occupational therapy room
37. Gymnasium
38. Physiotherapist's office
39. Examination
40. Treatment
41. Hydrotherapy
42. A.D.I.

E. Children's department
43. Nurses' station
44. Nurses clean utility room
45. Treatment room
46. Nurses' office
47. Bathroom
48. Dirty utility and sluice room
49. Clean linen
50. Store
51. Soiled linen
52. Kitchenette
53. Seminar room
54. Room for chief of department
55. Physician's room
56. Physician's room
57. Laboratory
58. Dining- and day room
59. Kindergarten
60. Parent's room
61. Cleanroom
62. Rest room for nurses

F. Premature babies ward
63. Nurses' station
64. Premature babies room
65. Incubators
66. Feeding room
67. Demonstration room
68. Linen store
69. Nurses' workroom
70. Isolation

**G. Cardiology department,
     pulmonary functions etc.**
71. Waiting room
72. Office
73. Neurologist
74. Control room
75. Consulting and examination room
76. Reception and records
77. Cardiologist
78. Consulting and examination room
79. Electrocardiography
80. Pulmonary function room
81. Laboratory

H. Outpatient department
82. Entrance hall and general waiting
83. Children's O.P.D.
84. Waiting
85. Consulting and examination room
86. Nurses' room
87. Office
88. Women's O.P.D.
89. Information and registration
90. Records
91. Office
92. Cafeteria
93. Waiting for jaw O.P.D.
94. Radiology

I. Psychiatric department
95. Nurses' station
96. Occupational therapy room
97. Dining hall
98. Kitchenette
99. Dirty utility and sluice room
100. Soiled linen
101. General store
102. Clean linen
103. Nurses' workroom
104. Nurses' office
105. Treatment room
106. Physician's room
107. Psychologist
108. Room for chief of department
109. Social worker
110. Group therapy
111. Patio

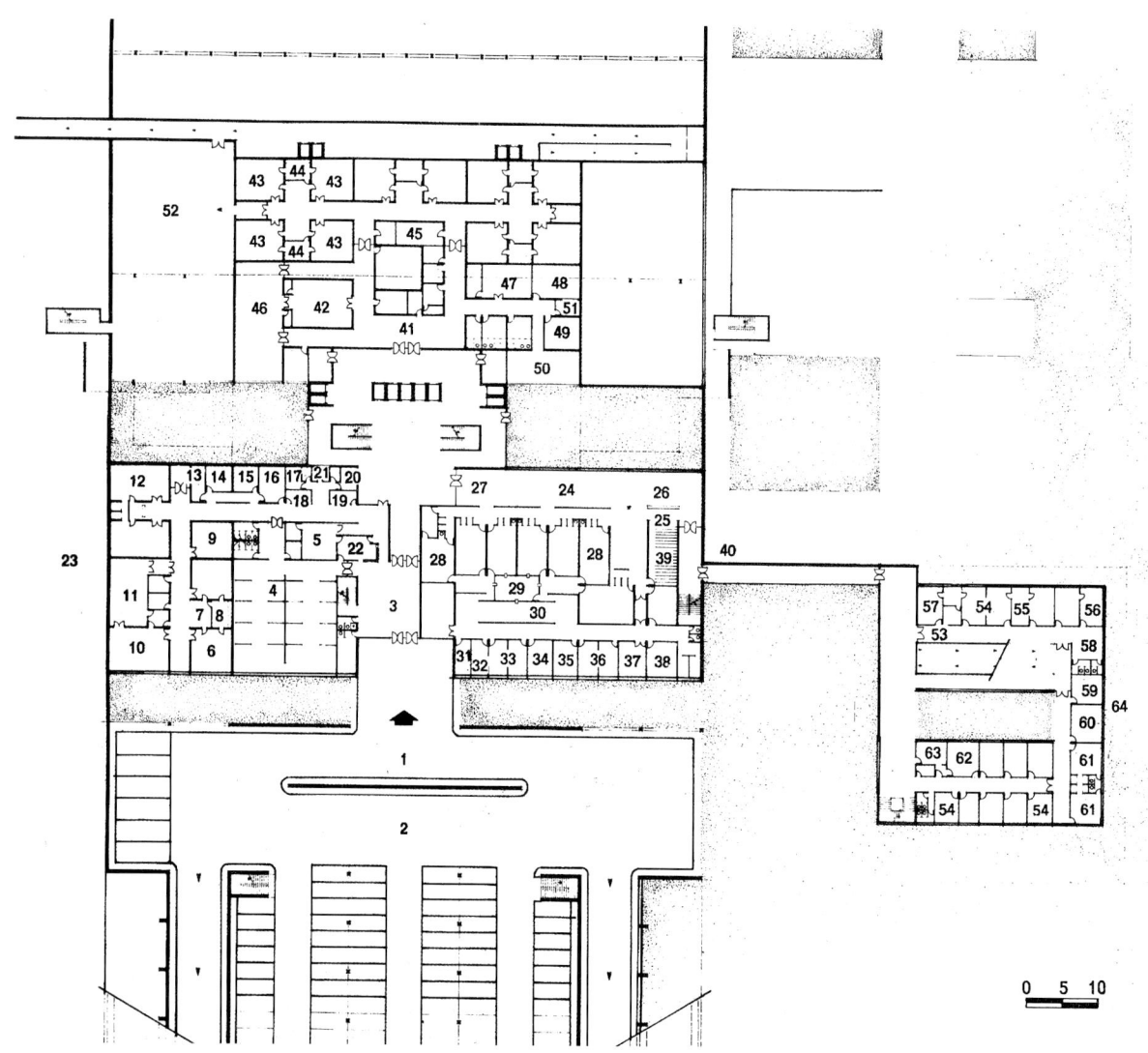

5. **The Hospitals and Health Facilities of Zarhy Architects**

Medical services level

1. Casualty entrance
2. Underground parking

A. Medical services level
3. Casualty entrance hell
4. Cubicles for examination
5. Examination room for children
6. Treatment room
7. Scrub-up
8. Sub-sterile room
9. General treatment room
10. Preparation and post-operation recovery room
11. Room for treatment shock
12. Observation room
13. Laboratory
14. Medical examination
15. Physician's room
16. Blood taking room
17. Linen room
18. Kitchenette
19. Cubicle for stretchers and wheel chairs
20. Store for various equipment
21. Stores
22. Nurses' station
23. Extension area for casualty department

B. Radiology
24. Radiology waiting room
25. Reception
26. Outpatient's waiting
27. Inpatient's waiting
28. General purpose radio diagnostic
29. Processing room
30. Immediate viewing and sorting room
31. Film store
32. Workshop
33. Junior radiologists' room
34. Chief of department
35. Secretary
36. Senior radiologists' room
37. Senior radiologists' room
38. General store
39. Filing and film archives
40. Extension area for radiology

C. Operating theatres
41. Entrance hall
42. Admission, and reception
43. Operating theatres
44. Lay-up rooms
45. Nurses' work room
46. Recovery room (short stay)

47. Surgeon's office and room for report writing
48. Rest room for surgeons
49. Rest room for nurses
50. Store
51. Kitchenette
52. Extension area, for operating theatres

D. Outpatients' department (o.P.D)
53. E.N.T. and ophthalmology waiting room
54. Consulting and examination room
55. Dark room
56. Nurse's room
57. Examination room for e.N.T.
58. Waiting
59. Recovery room
60. Plaster room
61. Cystoscopy
62. Treatment room
63. Nurse's room
64. Extension area for O.P.D

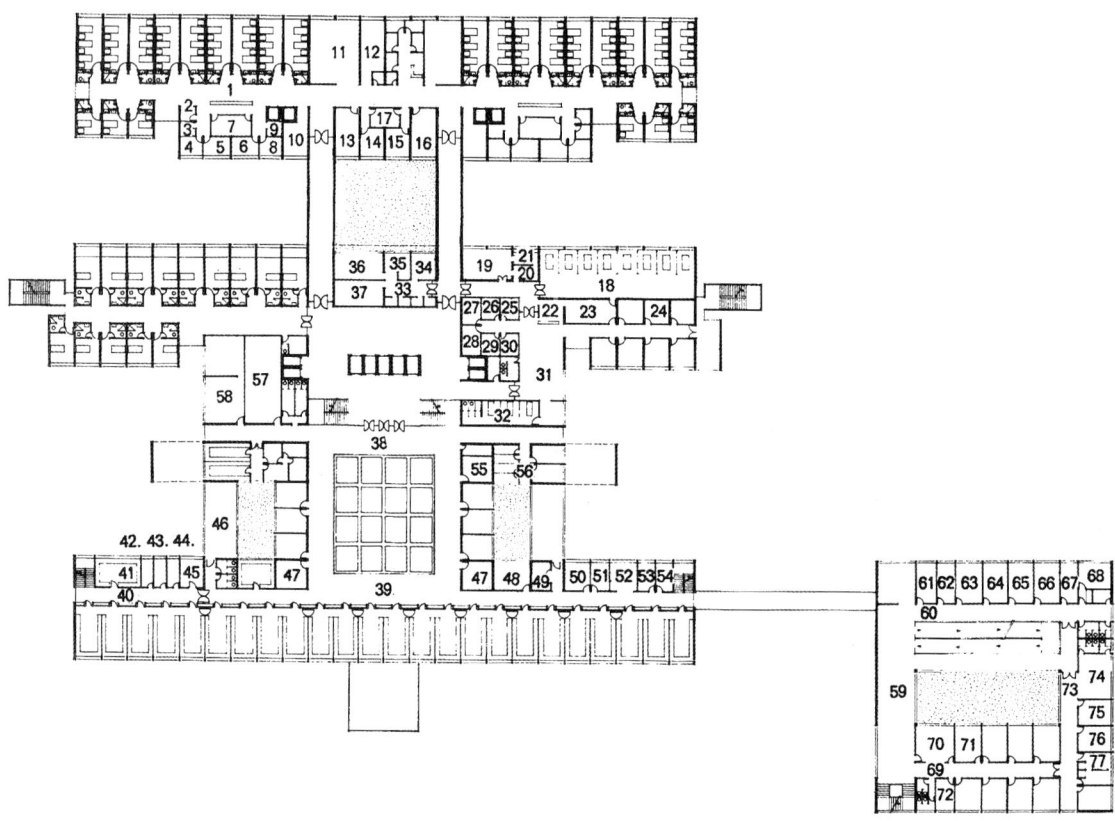

5. The Hospitals and Health Facilities of Zarhy Architects

Obstetrics and laboratories level

A.   Obstetrics
1.   Nurse's station
2.   Store for various equipment
3.   Clean linen
4.   Nurses' office
5.   Dirty utility and sluice room
6.   General store
7.   Nurse's clean utility room
8.   Kitchenette
9.   Soiled linen
10. Demonstration room
11. Day room
12. Treatment room
13. Seminar
14. Chief of department
15. Physicians' room
16. Physicians' room
17. Laboratory

B.   Delivery rooms
18. Delivery room
19. Intervention room
20. Scrub
21. Sub-sterile cubicle
22. Nurses' station
23. Clean utility room
24. Labour rooms
25. Kltchenette
26. Clean linen
27. Dirty utility and sluice room
28. Soiled linen
29. General store
30. Clothes store
31. Waiting
32. Preparation room

C.   Dairy kitchen
33. Dairy kitchen
34. Office
35. Store
36. Solutions preparation
37. Room for bottles wash-up

D.   Laboratories wing
38. Laboratories wing
39. Clinical laboratories
40. Research laboratories
41. Laboratory
42. Store
43. Cold room
44. Wash-up room
45. Instruments room
46. Rest room and library
47. Director's room
48. Tissue culture "bank"
49. Constant temperature rooms
50. Laboratory kitchen
51. Office
52. Waiting
53. Examination room
54. Blood taking room
55. Change room
56. Radio isotopes laboratory
57. General store
58. Instruments store

E.   O.P.D.
59. Waiting
60. Psychiatric O.P.D.
61. Office
62. Nurse
63. Consulting and examination rooms
64. Psychologist
65. Consulting and examination rooms
66. Social worker
67. Clean linen
68. General store
69. Internal medicine O.P.D.
70. Treatment room
71. Consulting and examination room
72. Nurse
73. Dermatology treatment suite
74. Waiting
75. Nurse
76. Consulting and examination room
77. Treatment room

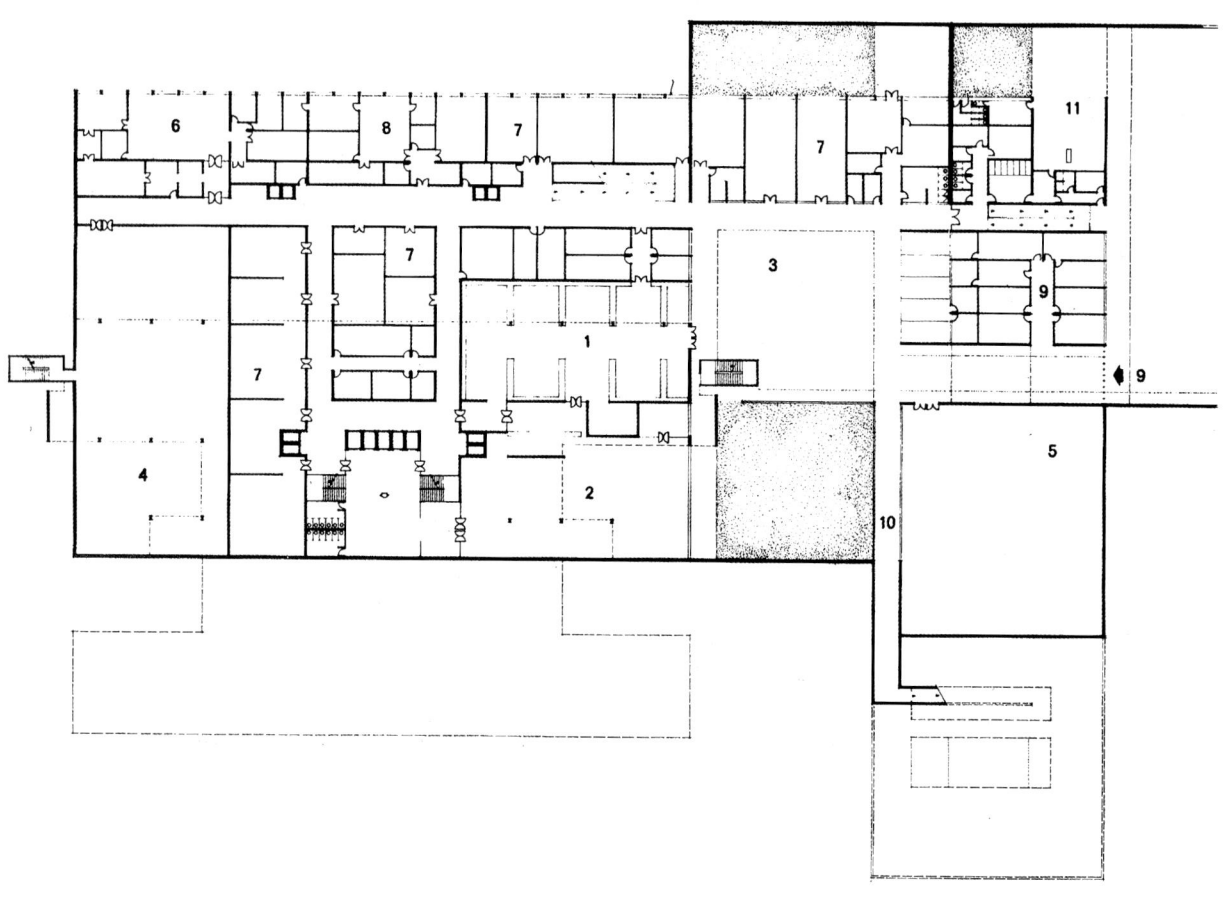

5. The Hospitals and Health Facilities of Zarhy Architects

Service level

1. Main kitchen
2. Dining hall
3. Service yard
4. Machine room
5. Laundry
6. Central supply
7. Stores
8. Pharmacy
9. Service entrance
10. Service connection to O.P.D.
11. Pathology

School of nurses

1. Entrance hall
2. Living quarters
3. Secretary
4. Archives
5. Instructors room
6. Director's room
7. Deputy director's room
8. Conference room
9. Teaching laboratory
10. Classroom
11. Seminar
12. Reading room
13. House mother

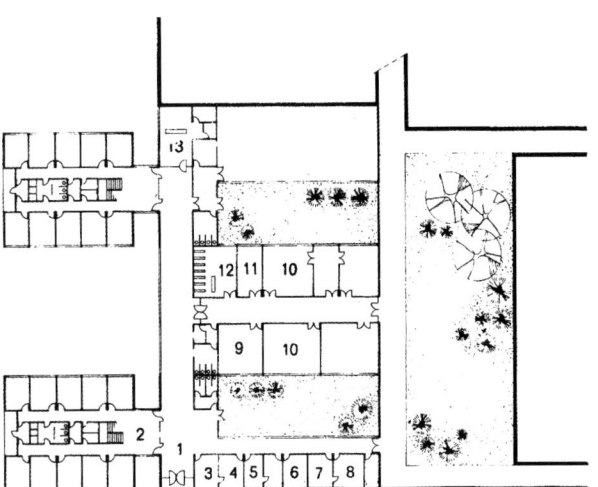

Typical floor

1. Nurses' station
2. Day room and dining hall
3. Nurses clean utility room
4. Kitchen
5. Treatment
6. Soiled linen
7. Cubicle for stretchers and wheelchairs
8. Store for various equipment
9. Dirty utility and sluice room
10. Linen store
11. Store
12. Bathroom
13. Physician's room
14. Room for chief of department
15. Physician's room
16. Laboratory
17. Nurses' office
18. Staff restroom
19. Seminar room

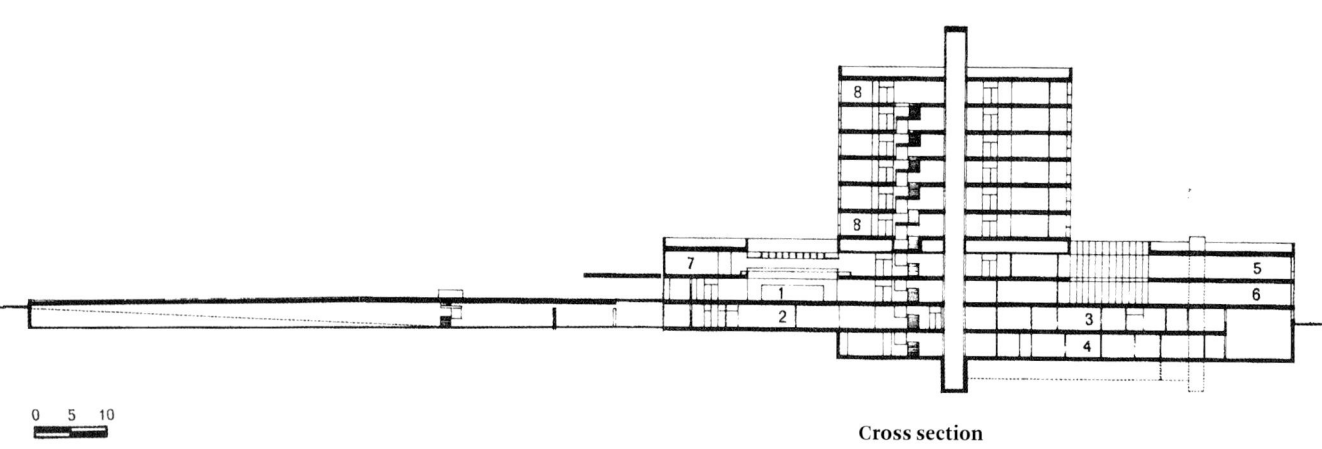

0 5 10

Cross section

5. The Hospitals and Health Facilities of Zarhy Architects

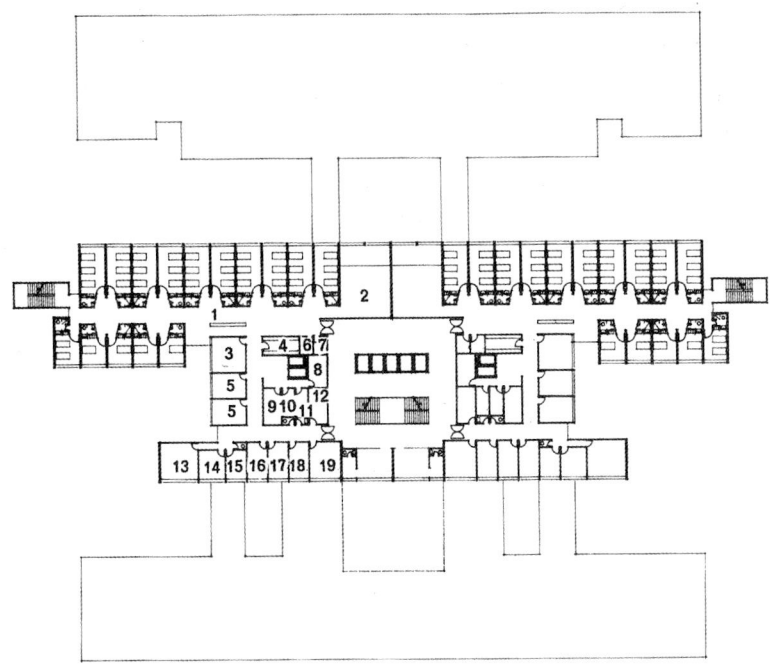

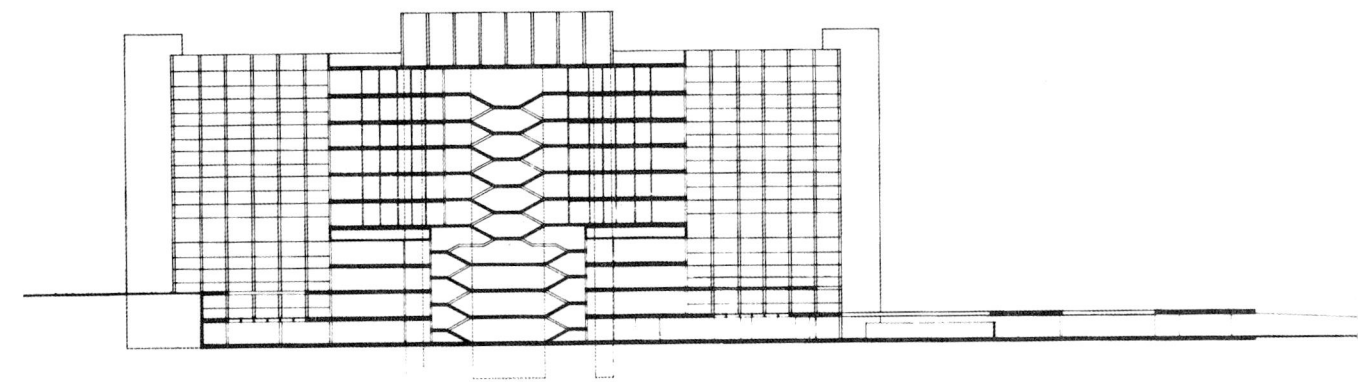

Longitudinal section

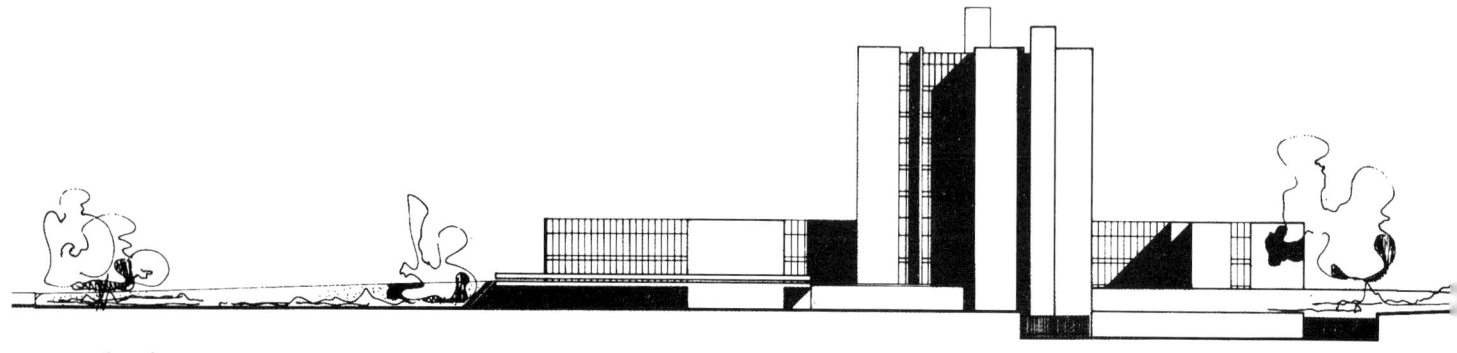

West elevation

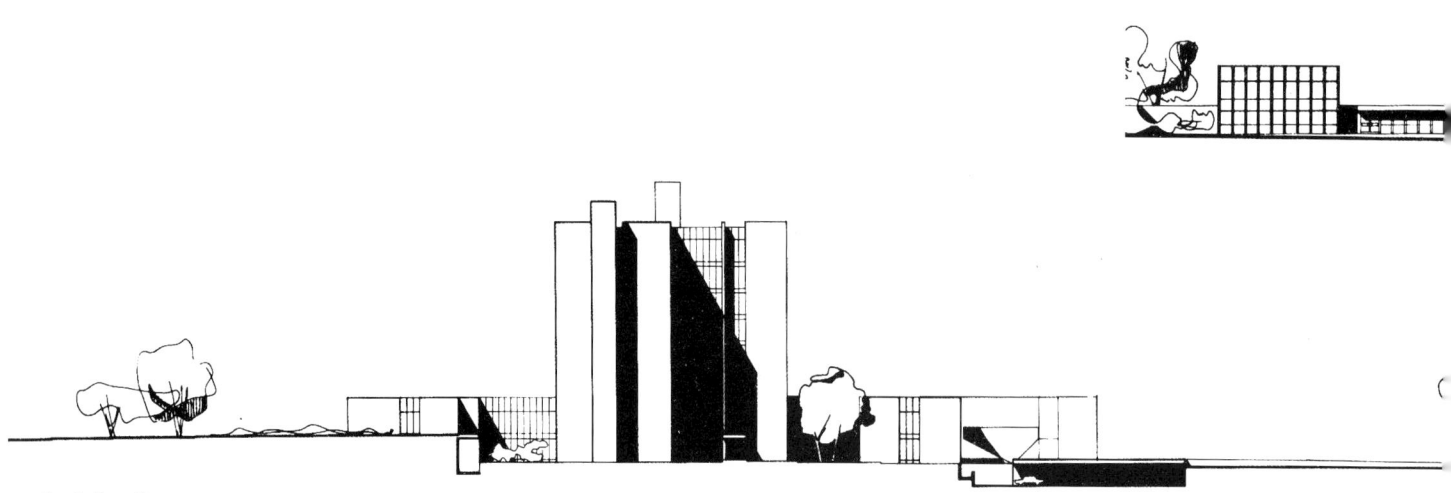
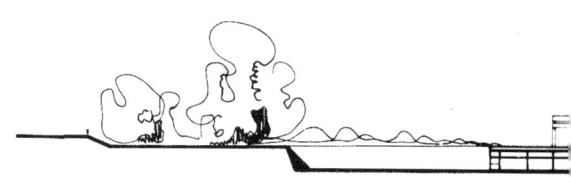

East elevation

5. The Hospitals and Health Facilities of Zarhy Architects

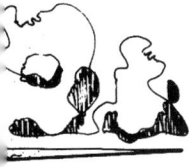

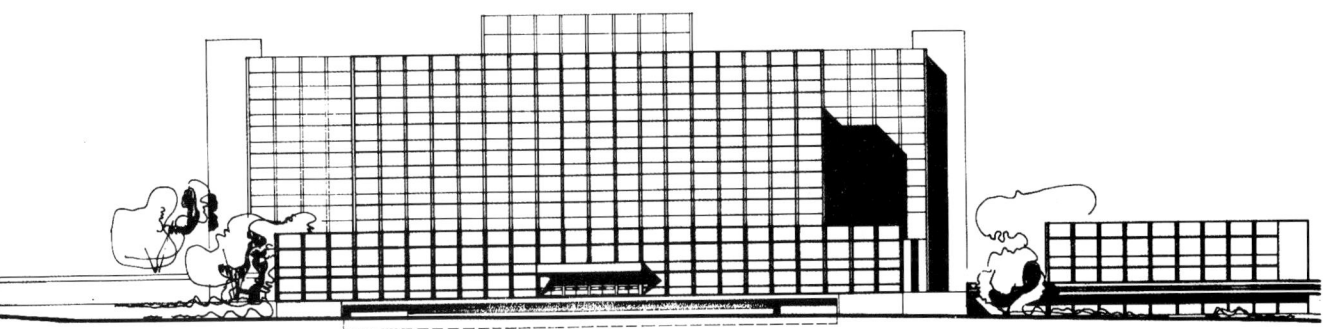

North elevation

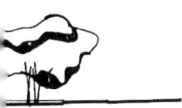

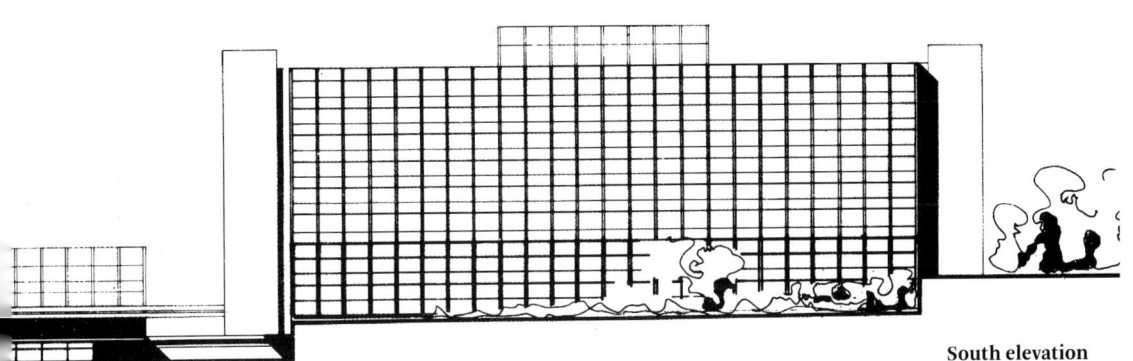

South elevation

Plan B

TYPICAL FLOOR _____

Outpatient Department _____

Psychiatric Department _____

Delivery Room _____
Clinical Laboratories _____

Research Laboratories _____

Lecture Hall _____
Outpatient Department _____
Pediatrics and Obstetrics _____

Casualty Entrance _____
Radiology _____
Psychiatric Outpatient Department _____

Casualty Department _____

Administration _____
GROUND FLOOR _____
Main Entrance _____
Children's Outpatient Department _____

Underground Parking _____

Underground Casualty Department _____

Operating Theatres _____

Central Supply _____

Pharmacy _____

Circumcision Hall _____
Dining Room _____

Cafeteria _____
Machine Room _____
Passage to Pathology _____
Supply Services _____
Laundry _____

Supply Entrance _____

5. The Hospitals and Health Facilities of Zarhy Architects

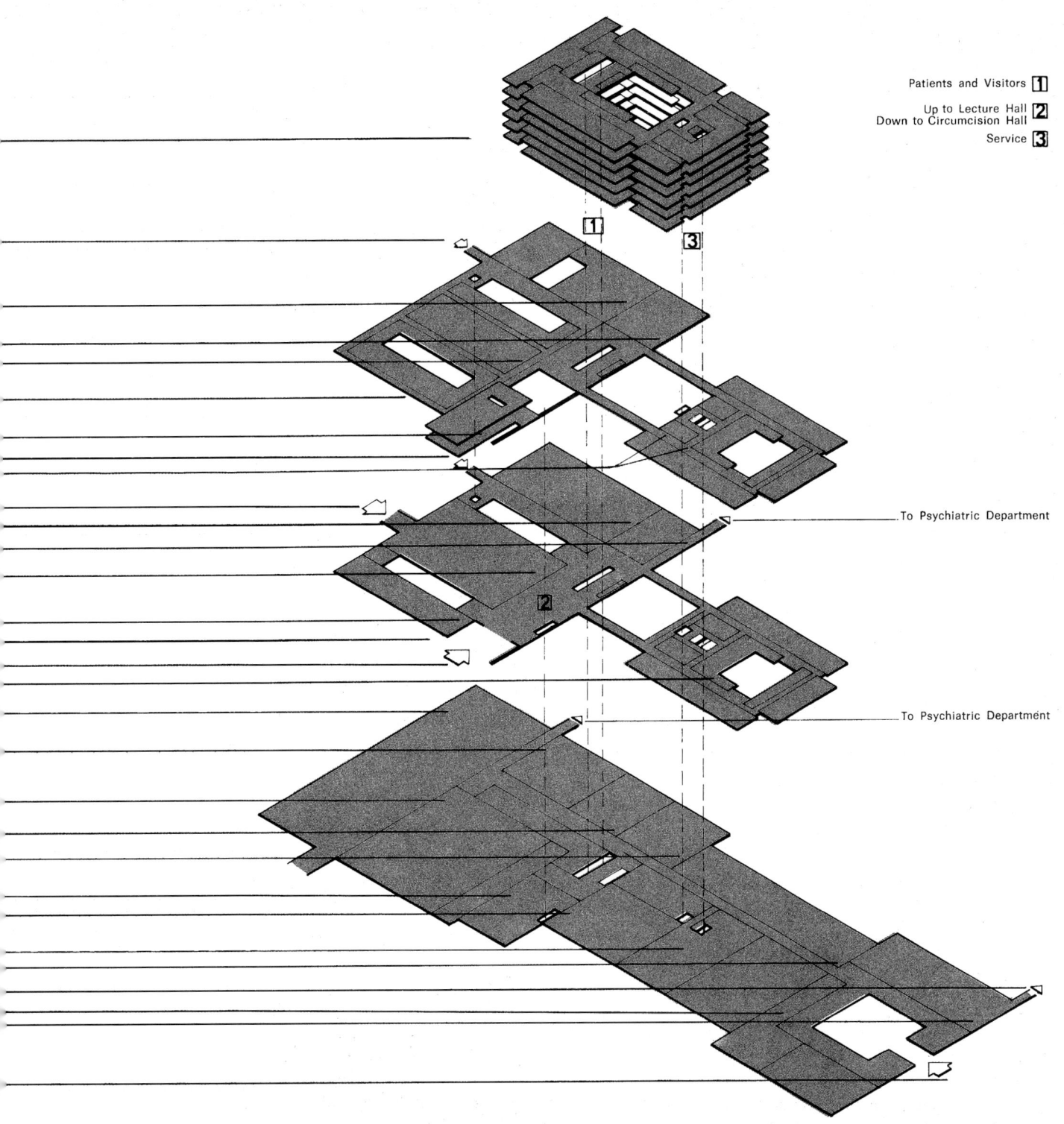

Patients and Visitors **[1]**

Up to Lecture Hall **[2]**
Down to Circumcision Hall

Service **[3]**

To Psychiatric Department

To Psychiatric Department

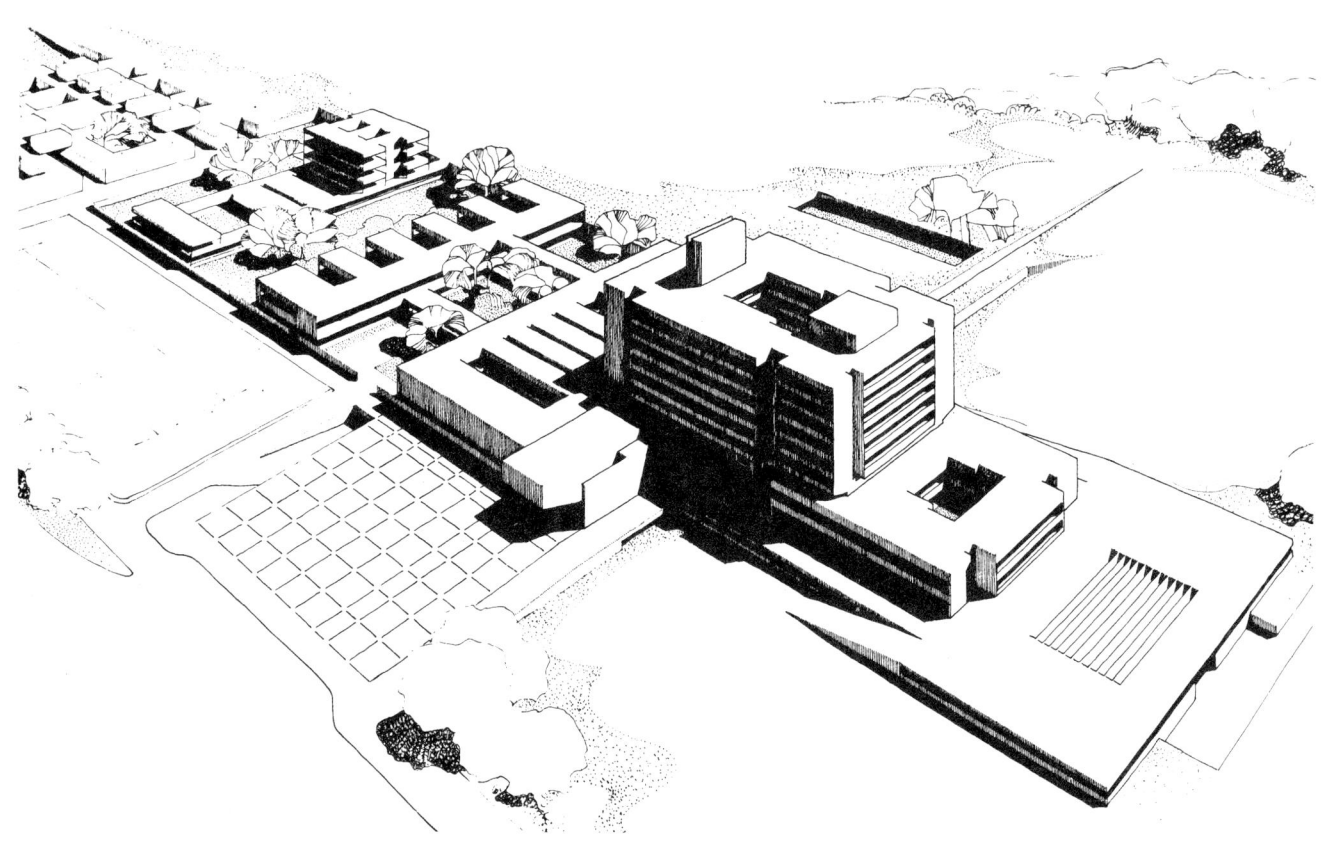

In Plan B emphasis was placed on balance and harmony between the
many different and sometimes conflicting functions of a hospital.
This project was not built.

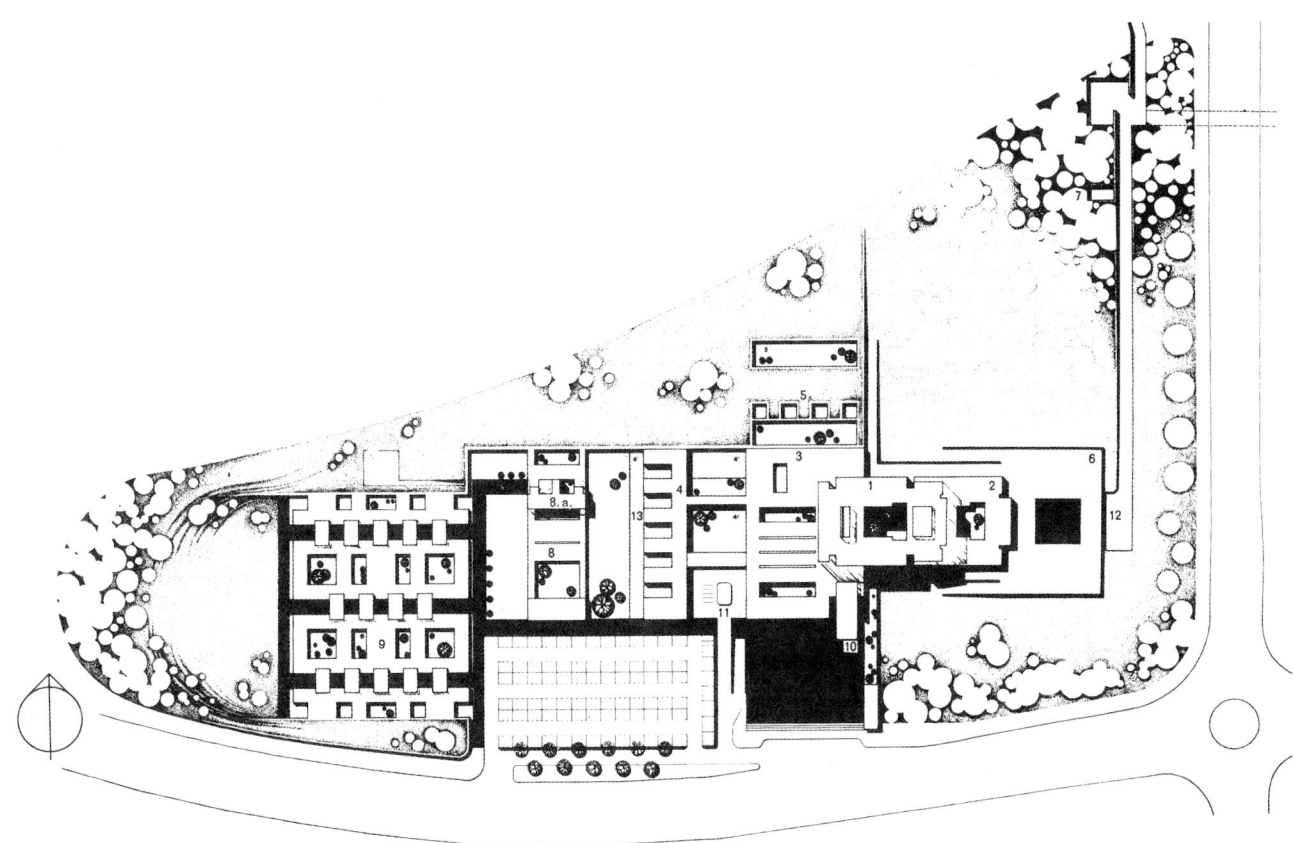

Typical floor

1. Main building (wards)
2. Pediatrics and obstetrics
3. Medical services
4. Outpatient department
5. Psychiatric department
6. Supply service
7. Pathology
8 School for nurses
8a. Living quarters for students
8b. Living quarters for students
   (Future expansion)
9. Living quarters for personnel
10. Main entrance
11. Admission and casualty entrance and access
   to underground parking
12. Access road to service yard and pathology
13–14. Extension area

Entrance level

A. Entrance hall and admission
1. Entrance hall
2. Patients admission office
3. Information
4. Archives
5. Clerical office
6. Clerical office
7. Cashier
8. Chief admitting office
9. To circumstance hall and synagogue
10. Cafeteria

B. Administration
11. Administration
12. Director's office
13. Waiting and director' secretary
14. Deputy director
15. Matron's office
16. Deputy metron
17. Administrator
18. Chief assistant administrator's office
19. Social worker
20. Personnel manager
21. Records store
22. Library
23. Women volunteers
24. Accounting
25. Chief accountant
26. Central general secretariat

C. Children's department
27. Nurse's station
28. Nurse's clean utility room
29. Treatment room
30. Nurse's office
31. Bathroom
32. Dirty utility and sluice room
33. Clean linen
34. Store
35. Soiled linen
36. Kitchenette
37. Seminar room
38. Room for chief of department
39. Physician's room
40. Physician's room
41. Laboratory
42. Dining and day room
43. Kindergarten
44. Parent's room
45. Classroom
46. Rest room for nurses

F. Premature babies ward
47. Nurses' station
48. Premature babies room
49. Incubators
50. Feeding room
51. Demonstration room
52. Linen store
53. Nurses work room
54. Isolation

G. Psychiatric department
55. Nurse's station
56. Occupational therapy room
57. Dining hall
58. Kitchenette
59. Dirty utility and sluice room
60. Soiled linen
61. General store
62. Clean linen
63. Nurses work room
64. Nurses' office
65. Treatment room
66. Physicians room
67. Psychologist
68. Room for chief of department
69. Social worker
70. Group therapy
71. Patio

School for nurses
72. Entrance hall
73. Up to living quarters
74. Secretary
75. Archives
76. Instructors' room
77. Director's room
78. Deputy director's room
79. Conference room
80. Teaching laboratory
81. Classroom
82. Seminar room
83. Reading room
84. House mother

Radiology
85. Radiology waiting room
86. Reception
87. General purpose radio diagnostic
88. Processing room
89. Immediate viewing and sorting room
90. Radiologists' room
91. Chief of department

Casualty department
92. Casualty entrance hall
93. Cubicles foe examination
94. Treatment room
95. Preparation and post-operation recovery room
96. Observation room
97. Physician's room

Outpatients' department (O.P.D.)
98. Entrance hall end general waiting
99. Information and registration
100. Records
101. Consulting and examination room

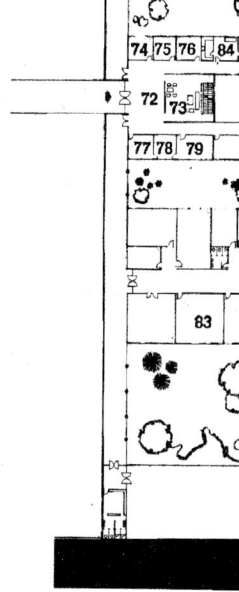

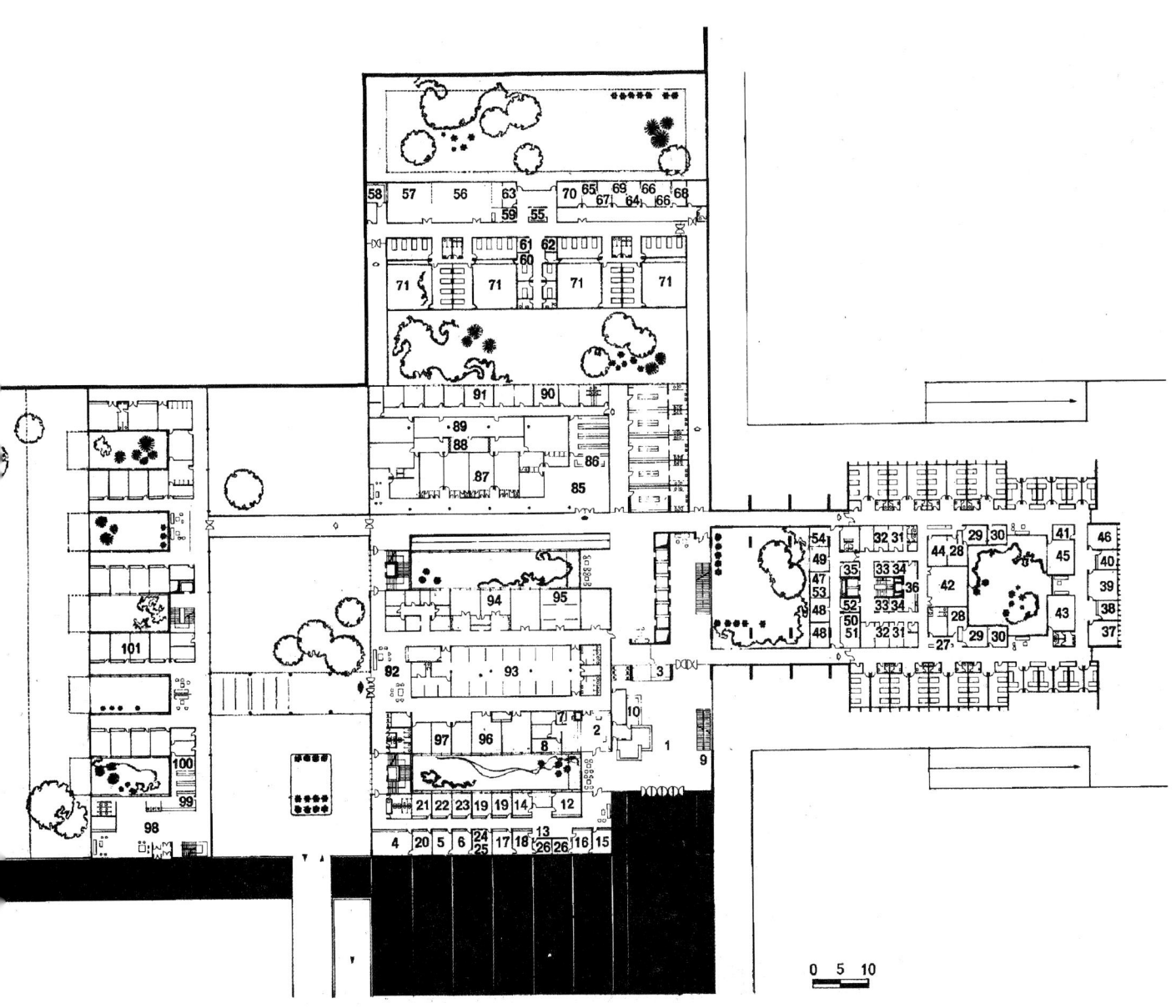

Obstetricis and laboratories level

A. Delivery rooms
1. Delivery room
2. Intervention room
3. Scrub-up
4. Substerile cubicle
5. Nurses station
6. Clean utility room
7. Labour room
8. Kitchenette
9. Clean linen
10. Dirty utility and sluice room
11. Soiled linen
12. General store
13. Clothes store
14. Waiting
15. Preparation room

B. Dairy kitchen
16. Dairy kitchen
17. Office
18. Store
19. Solutions preparation
20. Room for battles wash-up

C. Laboratories wing
21. Laboratories wing
22. Clinical laboratories
23. Research laboratories
24. Laboratory
25. Store
26. Cold room
27. Wash up room
28. Instruments room
29. Rest room and library
30. Director's room
31. Tissue culture "bank"
32. Constant temperature rooms
33. Laboratory kitchen
34. Office
35. Waiting
36. Examination room
37. Blood taking room
38. Change room
39. Radio isotopes laboratory
40. General store
41. Instruments store
42. Animals room

D. O.P.D
43. Waiting
44. Psychiatric O.P.D
45. Office
46. Nurse
47. Consulting and examination room
48. Consulting and examination room
49. Psychologist
50. Social worker
51. Cleen linen
52. General store
53. Internal medicine O.P.D
54. Treatment room
55. Consulting and examination room
56. Nurse
57. Dermatology treatment suite
58. Waiting
59. Nurse
60. Consulting and examination room
61. Treatment room

Obstetrics
62. Nurses' station
63. Store for various equipment
64. Clean linen
65. Nurses' office
66. Dirty utility and sluice room
67. General store
68. Nurses clean utility room
69. Kitchenette
70. Soiled linen
71. Demonstration room
72. Day room
73. Treatment room
74. Seminar
75. Chief of department
76. Physicians' room
77. Physicians' room
78. Isolation

School for nurses
79. Living quarters
80. Utility rooms

Psychiatric department
81. Nurses' station
82. Occupational therapy room
83. Dining hall

84. Treatment room
85. Physicians' room
86. Psychologist
87. Home for chief of department
88. Social worker
89. Group therapy

Lecture hall
90. Lecture hall

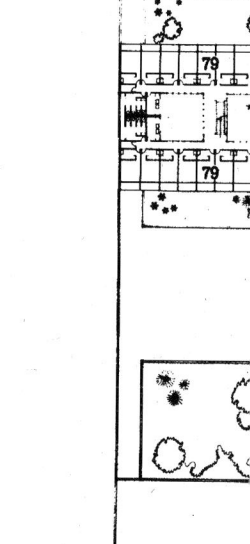

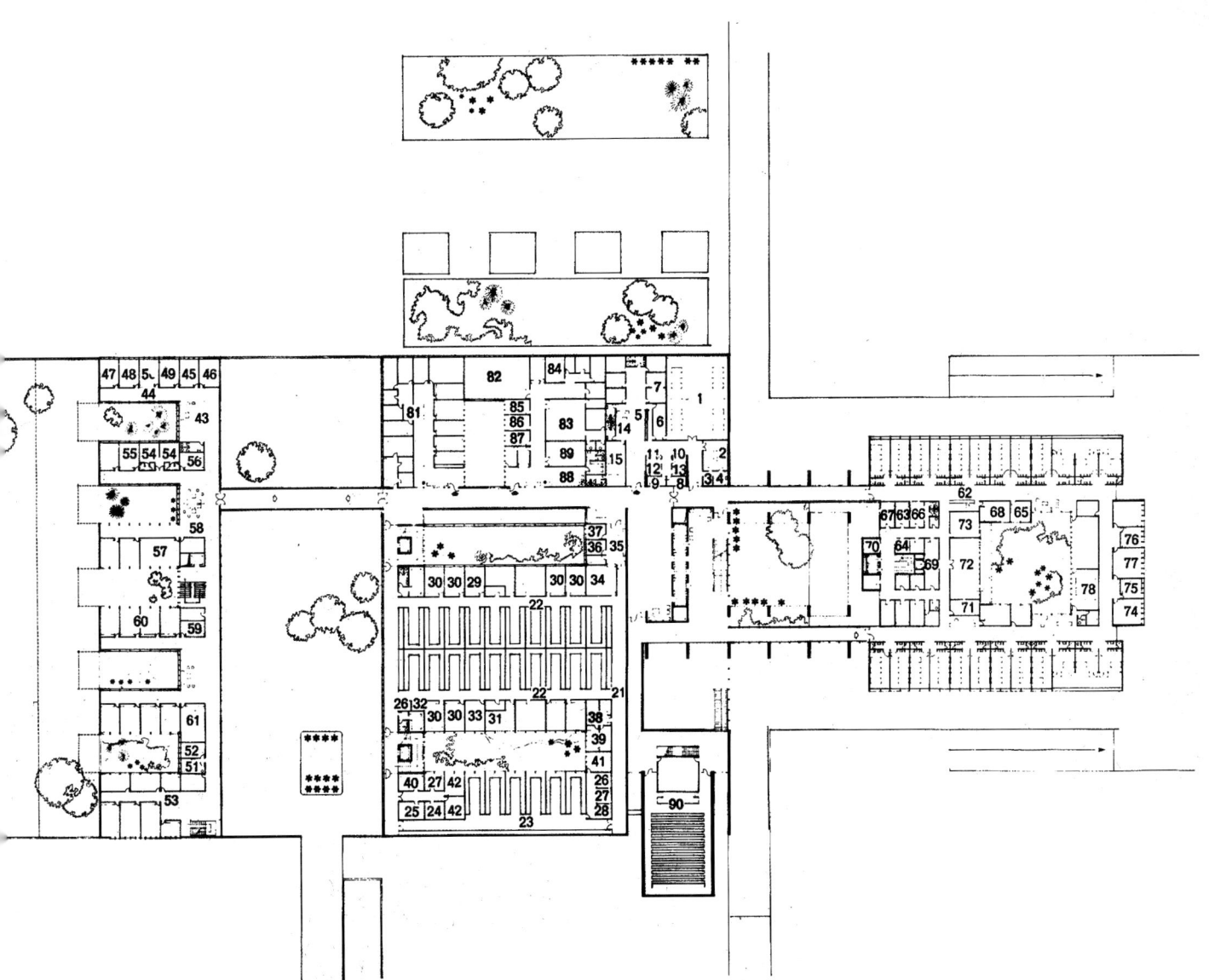

Service level

1. Main kitchen
2. Dining hall
3. Service yard
4. Machine room
5. Laundry
6. Central supply
7. Stores
8. Pharmacy
9. Service entrance
10. Service connection to O.P.D.
11. Pathology
12. Underground parking

Operating theatres

13. Entrance hell
14. Admission and reception
15. Operating theatre
16. Lay-up room
17. Nurses' work room
18. Recovery room (short stay)
19. Surgeon's office and room for report writing
20. Rest room for surgeons
21. Rest room for nurses
22. Store
23. Kitchenette

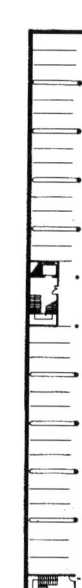

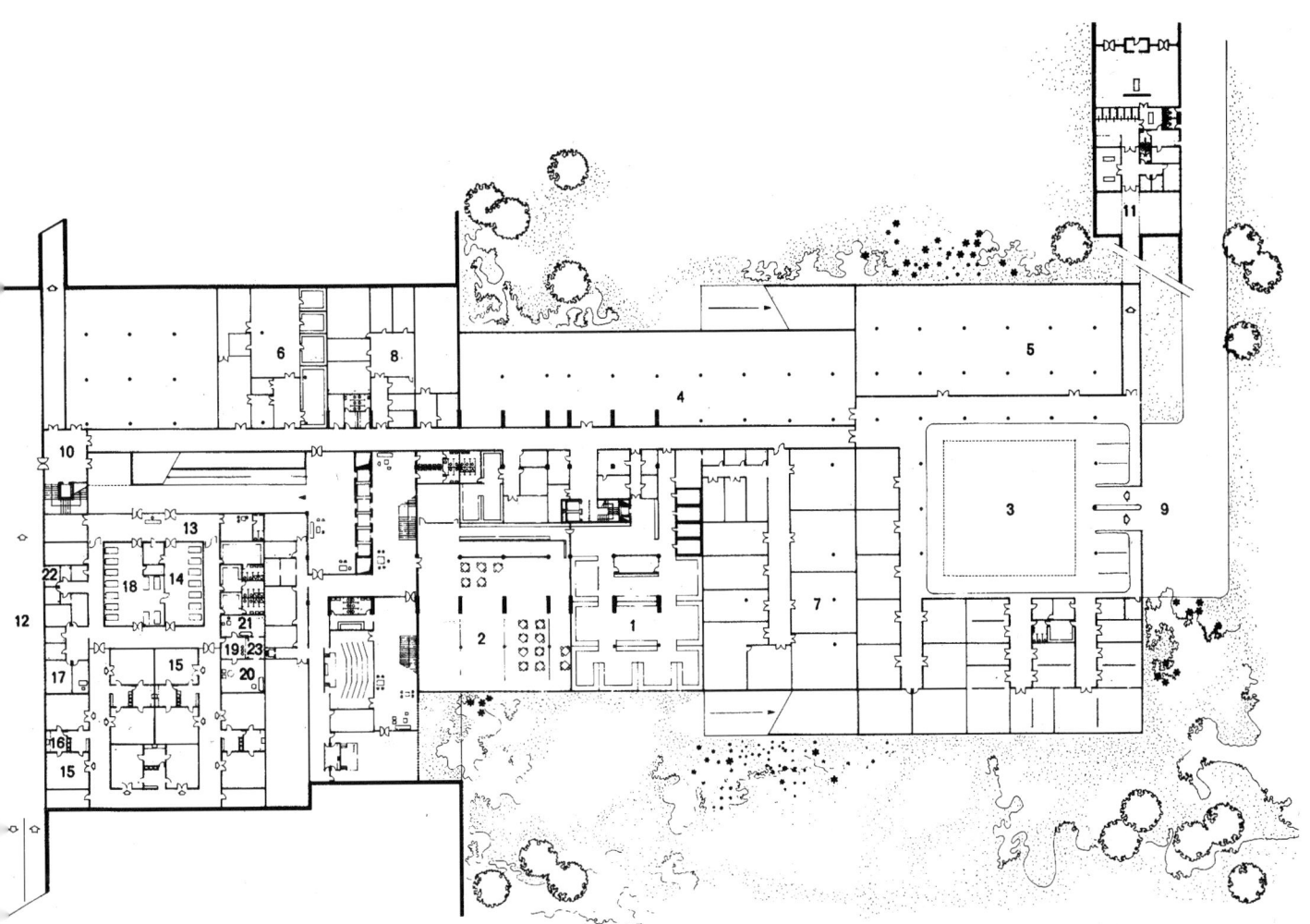

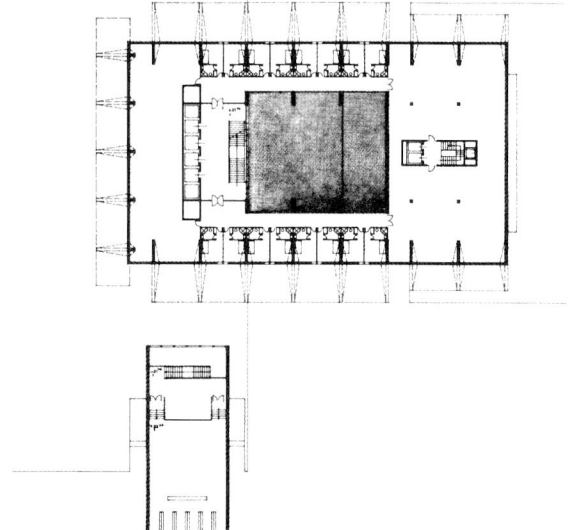

Mezzanine

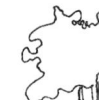

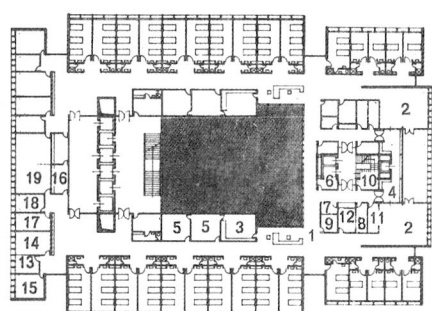

Typical floor
1. Nurses' station
2. Day room and dining hall
3. Nurses clean utility room
4. Kitchenette
5. Treatment
6. Soiled linen
7. Cubicle far stretchers and wheelchairs
8. Store for various equipment
9. Dirty utility and sluice room
10. Linen store
11. Store
12. Bathroom
13. Physicians' room
14. Room for chief of department
15. Physicians' room
16. Laboratory
17. Nurse's office
18. Staff rest room
19. Seminar room

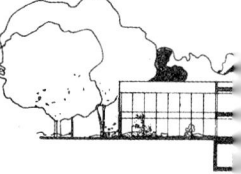

5. The Hospitals and Health Facilities of Zarhy Architects

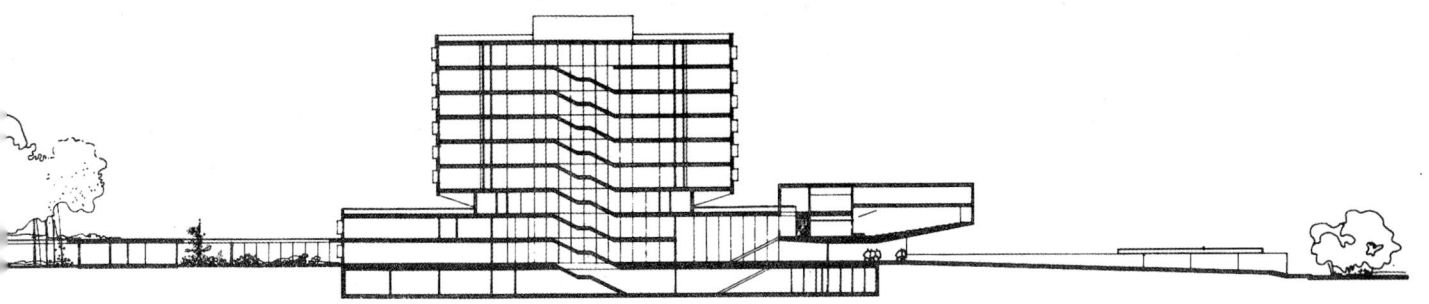

Cross section

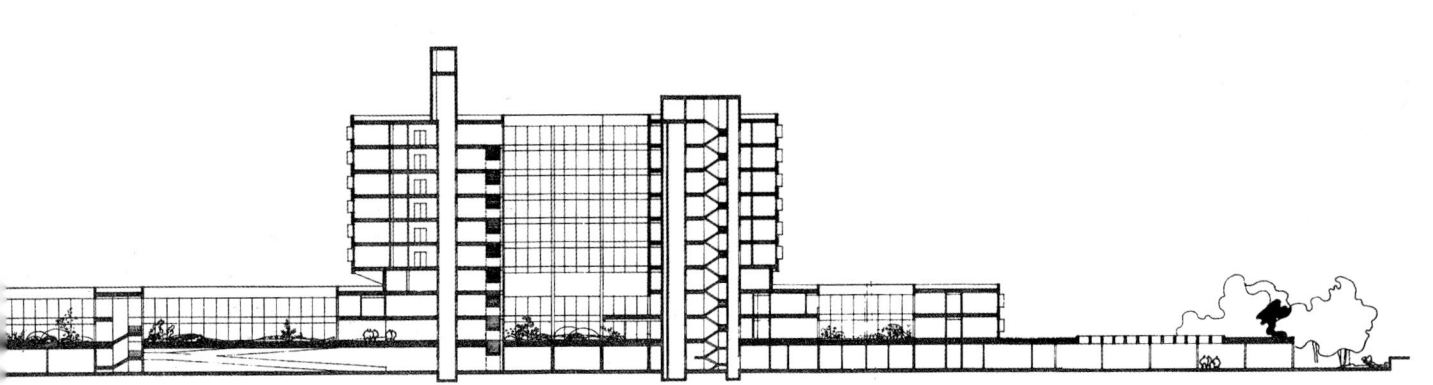

Longitudinal section

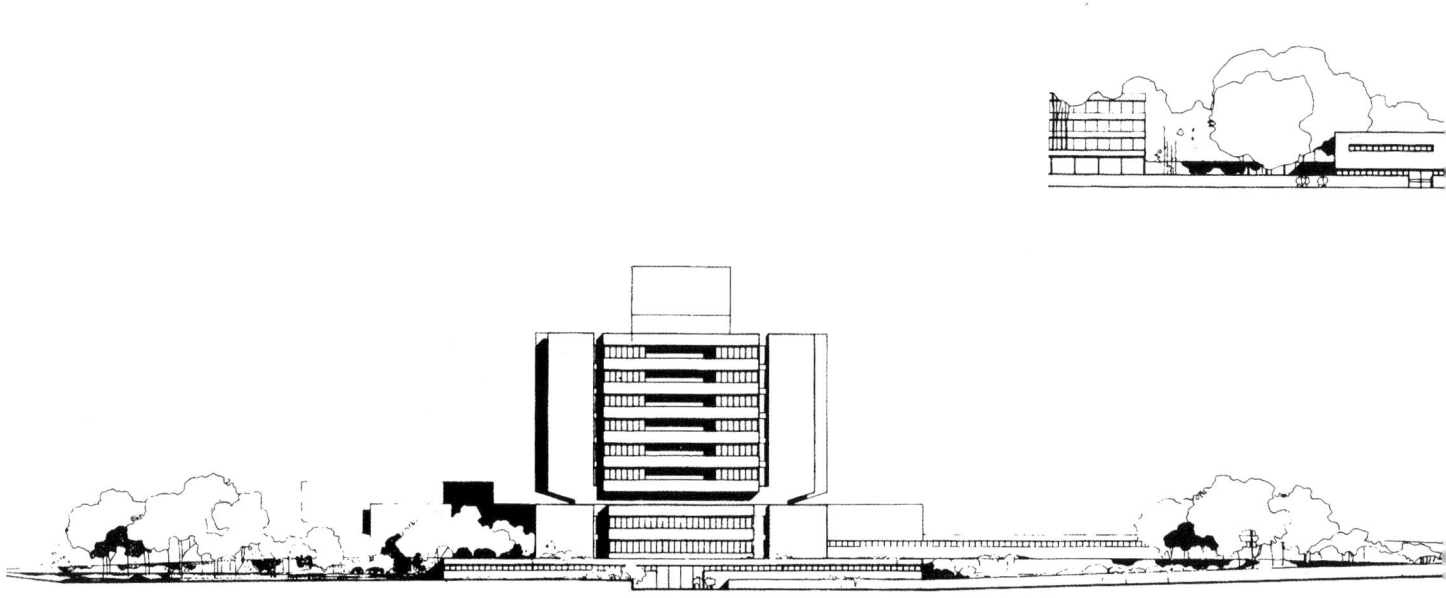

West elevation

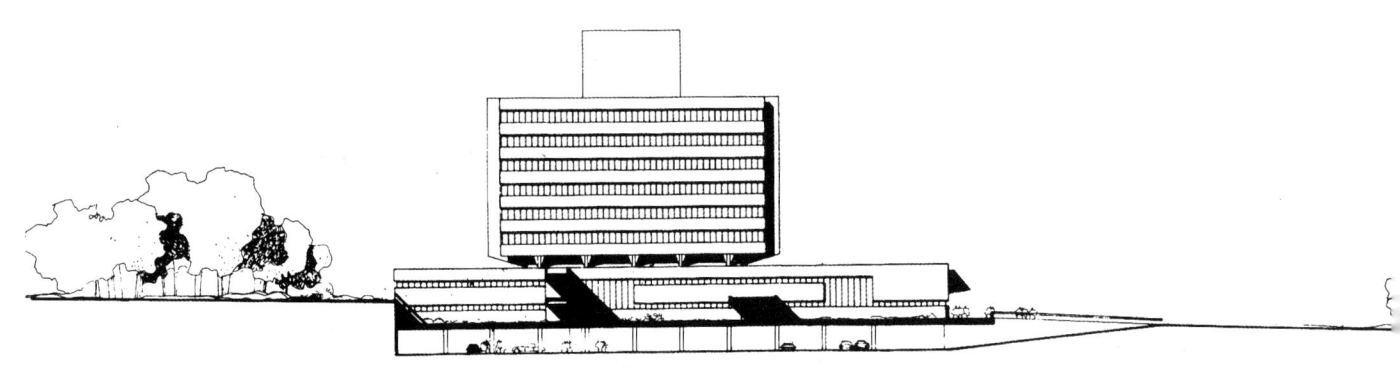

East elevation

5. The Hospitals and Health Facilities of Zarhy Architects

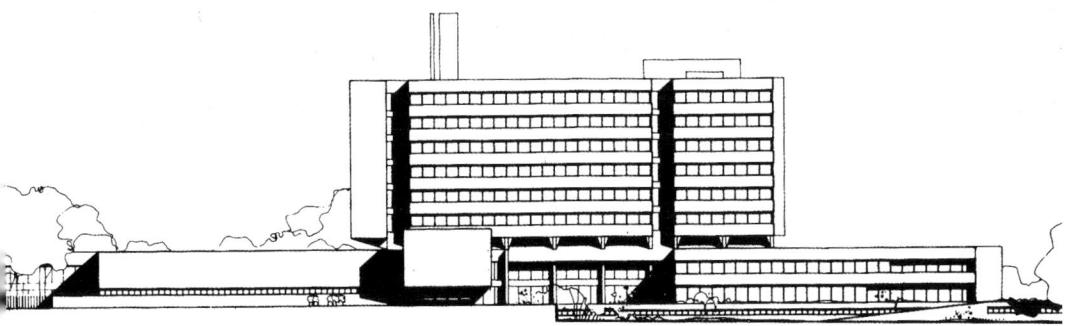

North elevation

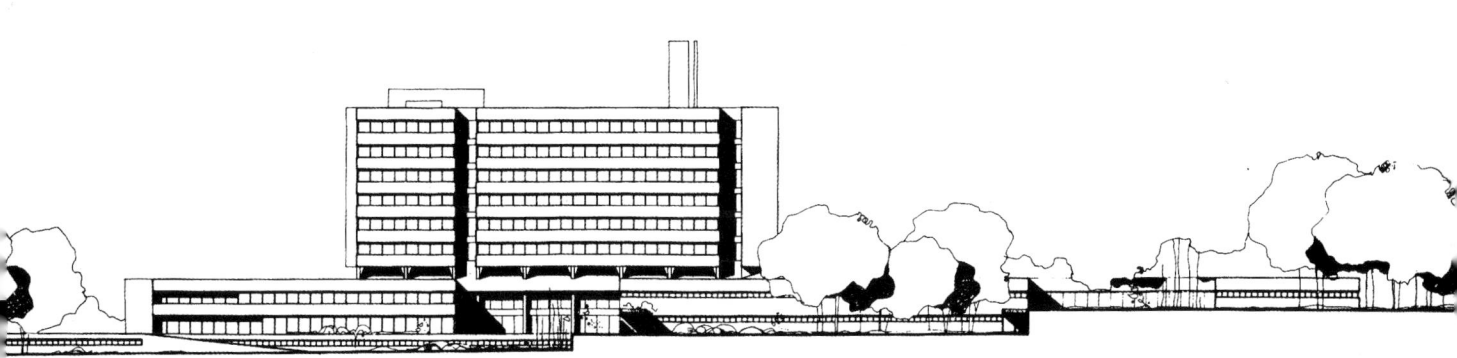

South elevation

6

Other Projects of Zarhy Architects

Residential

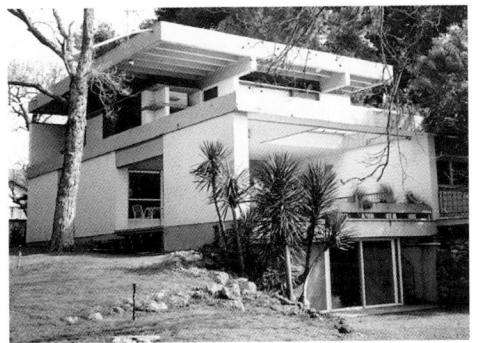

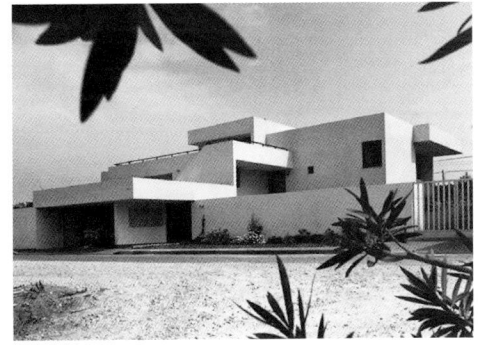

Moshe Zarhy has left his architectural marks in all areas of accommodation, from private homes to housing estates in the construction of whole neighbourhoods. In doing so he always achieved projects that were rational as well as functional. His sculpturesque buildings are avant-garde. His cubist private homes, partly built for leading figures of Israeli society, make Zarhy's commitment to rectilinear, unadorned structures visible. An architect's attitude is clearly expressed when he builds a house for himself. In the field of private homes, only two examples from Moshe Zarhy's oeuvre are to be presented in the photos beside, his own residence in Ramat Hasharon, a three-storey concrete masonry building with an angular single-storey extension, and the residence for Stef Wertheimer, an Israeli entrepreneur and philanthropist of German origin, founder of ISCAR, an industrial enterprise, for which Moshe Zarhy was also employed as architect in Upper Galilee. Moshe Zarhy built his own home as early as 1953; Stef Wertheimer's residence was constructed in 1980. Both buildings feature timeless modernity.

One project must not be omitted from this book, the present office of Zarhy Architects, at the same time the residence of Moshe Zarhy and Vera Ronnen-Zarhy:

Arlozorov 150, Tel Aviv
The building's new program includes a mix of uses; Zarhy Architectural office is located on the first floor, while the residential units are above it. The main concept and programmatic organization were drawn from the unique existing reference – Arlozrov street section, where Ficus trees are planted along unique and dense architectural sequences. In the new design, a small urban plaza was created, eliminating the clear separation between the building and the street. The new plaza is also used as a divider between the office main entrance on the right, and the residential main entrance to the left. The location of the office on the first floor, under the banyan trees, strengthens contact with pedestrians and allows them a glimpse into the backstage of architecture as a main event.

Top: Moshe Zarhy's Residence in Ramat Hasharon, a three-storey concrete masonry building, 1953
Ramat Hasharon, 300 sqm, 1953

Bottom: Stef Wertheimer Residence in Naharia, 1980
Naharia, 300 sqm, 1980

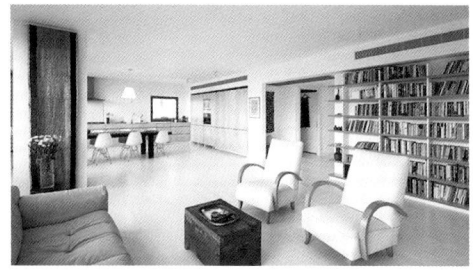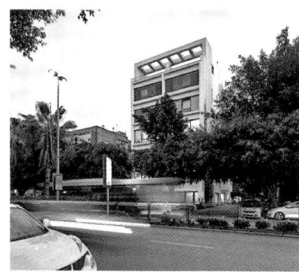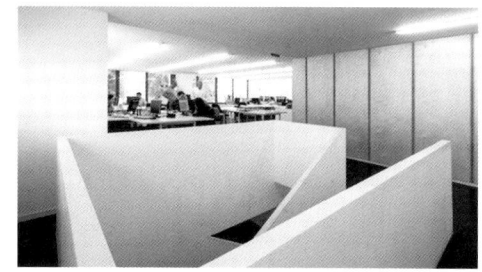

The building was created as a simple clear white box. The north facade facing Arlozorov street is transparent, thereby maintaining and strengthening the relationship with the street, while all other facades were riddled with openings, emphasizing the volume of the building. Woven into the urban fabric of the building on the one hand, and creating a unique architecture that integrates into and identity the street on the other, the design offers a new paradigm for the architecture of residential buildings in the city. The project was finished in 2011.

Housing Estates
Rather than satisfying the individual residential needs of wealthy clients, however, Israel depended on creating living quarters in great numbers for a continually growing population. It is above all in the foundation of new towns that rationally, planning with suitable materials and industrial prefabrication were necessary to provide affordable housing for all. Together with the Israeli concrete industry Moshe Zarhy developed the "Modul Beton Israel Building System" in the early 1960s. This System is a result of a continuing joint development effort by CLAL's Building Division, Architect Moshe Zarhy and TAMAT Ltd. In 11 different places in Israel, new neighbourhoods with 4,600 dwelling units were created, in Maoz Aviv, Ramat-Aviv, Beit Hakerem (Jerusalem), Mitzpe Ramon in Negev, Acre, Naharia, Tsur Shalom (Haifa), Nazareth, Givat Savyon, Carmiel in Upper Galilee and Ein Sarah in Western Galilee. The following text is taken from a catalogue with different types of buildings and completed examples:

"Modul Beton Israel was formed in 1964. Since then it has built thousands of flats on numerous sites, using a wide variety of dwelling unit prototypes. The sites on which the Company operates vary in size, as does the number of flats, averaging some 300 dwellings per project.

The office of Zarhy Architects and home of Moshe Zarhy and his wife Vera Ronnen-Zarhy in Arlozorov Street 150 in Tel Aviv.
Photos: Aviad Bar Ness
Tel Aviv, Israel, 1,500 sqm, 2011

6. Other Projects of Zarhy Architects

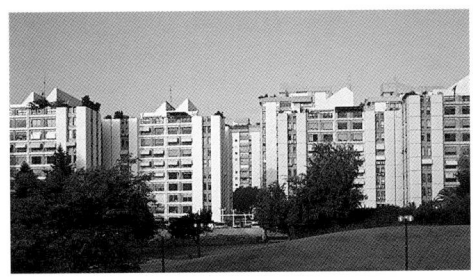

Six Residential Blocks in Ramat Aviv for 350 units
Photo: Amit Geron
Tel Aviv, 6,400 sqm, 1991

Modul Beton Israel has developed, by now, a wide variety of dwelling unit prototypes ranging in size from 1/2-bedroom up to 3-bedroom apartments, and two basic types of vertical transportation cores. The plan design of the dwelling unit was improved to make maximum use of the flat's area, for the benefit of the dweller. The attempt was made to provide dwelling schemes that would suit families of different socio-economic backgrounds and life styles. The plan design of the dwelling units permits multiple arrangements of two, three and four apartments of any size around the cores in a manner that forms a continuous building.
The Modul Beton design system allows for complete freedom of the creative mind and offers the opportunity to create a large variety of spaces, so as to overcome the monotony which is usually inevitable, when a site plan is composed solely from freestanding buildings."

The system of prefabricated parts is based on ideas that had been developed in Denmark at the same time. But building industries in all industrial countries in Europe, in the USA, and also in the Eastern Bloc then developed these systems of prefabricated parts from concrete, which set off a building boom. From a catalogue of ground plans different types of buildings could be assembled according to sizes of the building sites.

Six Residential Blocks Ramat Aviv
The project is located in an affluent residential area called Ramat Aviv in northern Tel Aviv. The complex is composed of 2 clusters of six residential blocks, each one rising 8 stories high and facing a lush park.
The buildings with 350 units are made of elegant pre-fabricated concrete elements and house relatively large apartments with 3–4 bedrooms, designed to suit various lifestyles. It was built in 1991.

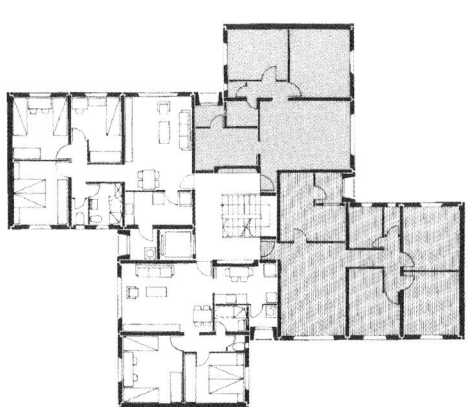

Example of X-Form-Type, with a lift. Type of flats: 2 and 3 bedrooms. Floor area: 323 sqm.

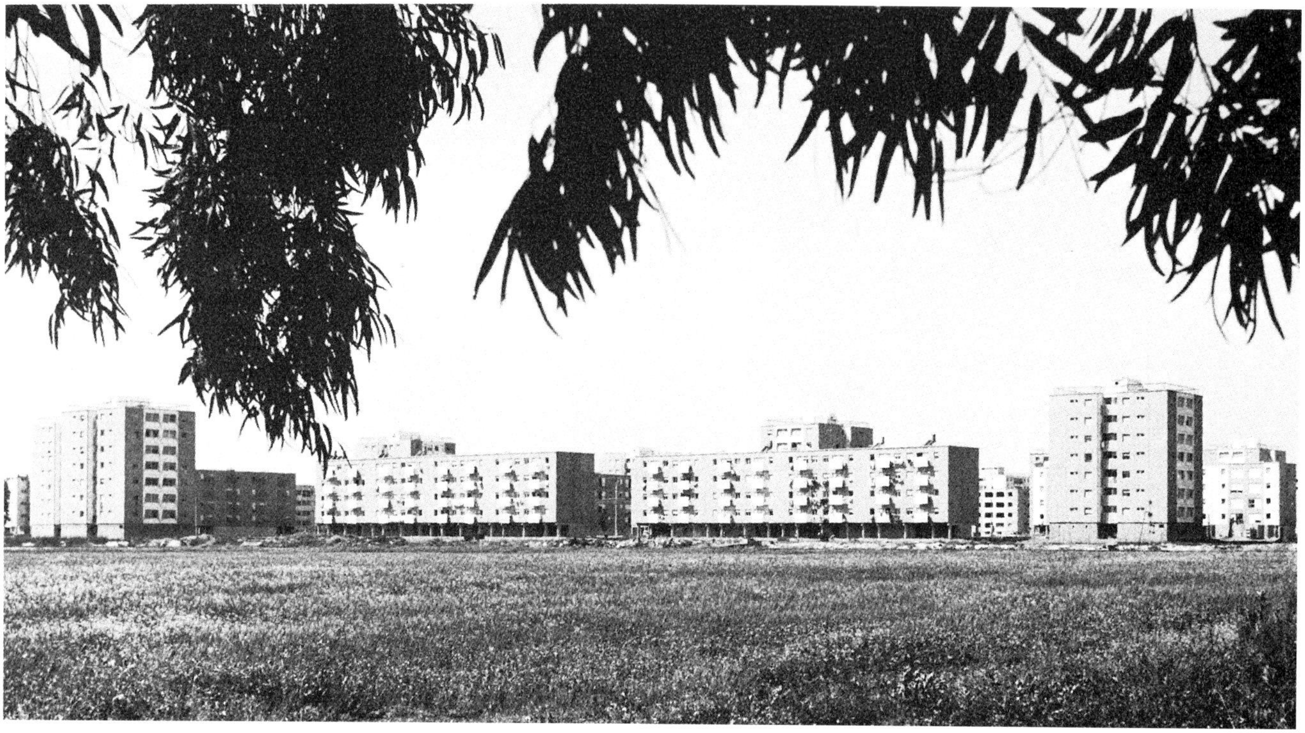

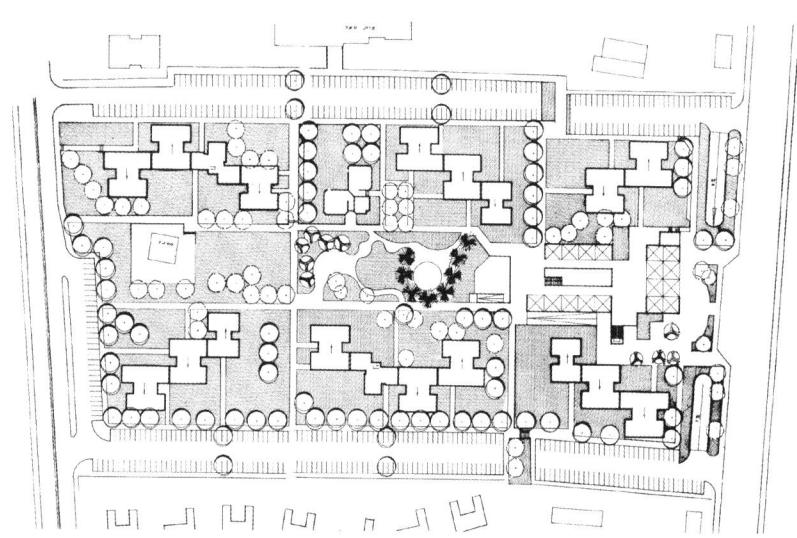

Location Acco, main view
Tel Aviv, Israel, 1,500 sqm, 2011

**Location Acco: 4 different building prototypes
for 392 flats**

6. Other Projects of Zarhy Architects

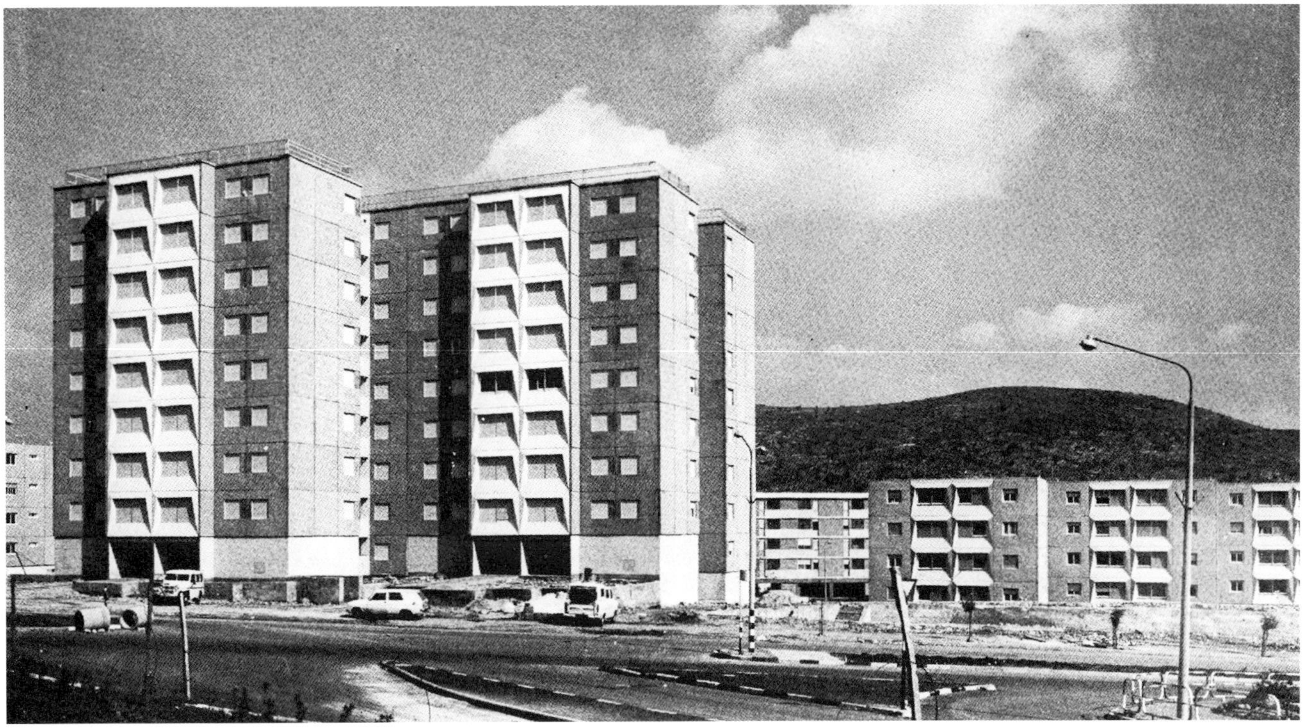

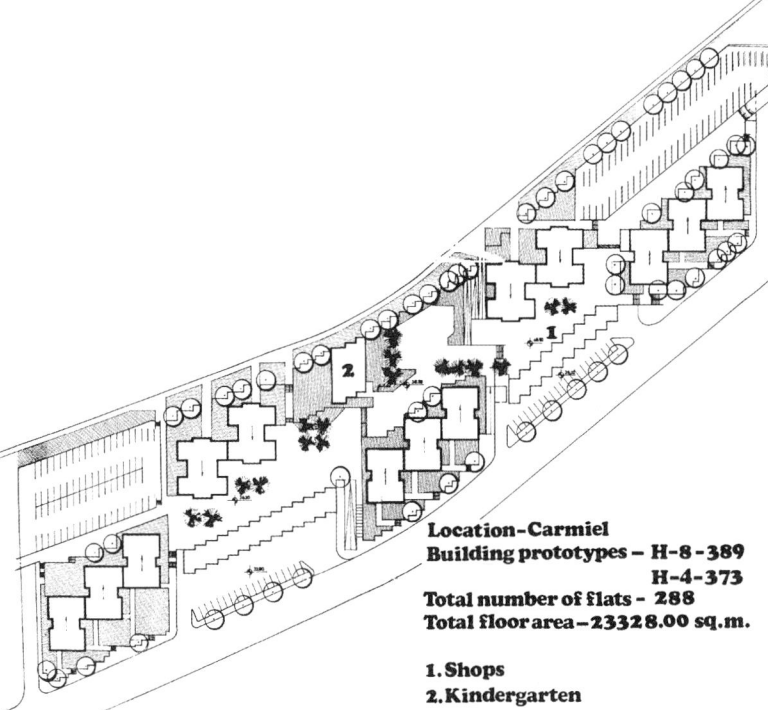

Location Carmiel: main view
Carmiel, 23,328 sqm for 288 flats, 2011

Location Carmiel: 2 different building prototypes for 288 flats

Location-Carmiel
Building prototypes – H-8-389
H-4-373
Total number of flats - 288
Total floor area – 23328.00 sq.m.

1. Shops
2. Kindergarten

Public and Education

Hebrew University of Jerusalem, The Institute of Life Sciences
Jerusalem, 25,000 sqm, 1973–1977

Background
The Institute of Life Sciences consists of the following departments: Biochemistry, Genetics, Botany, Zoology, Entomology. These departments are spread out today over five main centres, which are distant from each other. The Board of Governors gave its approval to transfer all the Life Sciences into one complex, which will be located on the campus of the Hebrew University at Givat Ram. In accordance with the above mentioned decision, a project has been prepared.

The Project
The site chosen for this project is located to the south of the campus between the Philadelphia and Geography buildings. A master plan of all the Life Sciences building has been prepared on an area of 23,000 square meters at the present planning stage, with provision for future expansion. The first stage of actual building is 13,000 square meters. The master plan has been conceived as a complex of inter-connected wings woven together according to their respective functions, which fall into four categories: (a) Research Laboratories (b) Lecture Halls, Library and Administration (c) Teaching Laboratories (d) Services and Maintenance. Research (a) and Teaching Laboratories (c) run from east to west forming' as it were the warp of a richly textured pattern, with

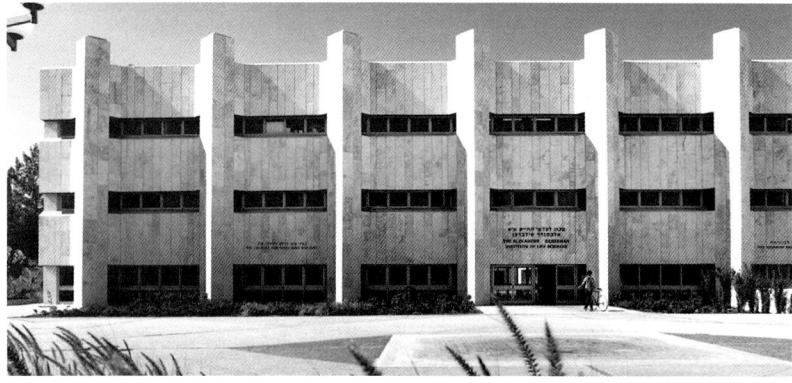

Photo of the main fassade

the remaining functions, Lecture Halls, Library and Administration (b) and Service and Maintenance areas (d), which run from north to south, forming the woof. Part of the ground floor has been freed to allow for garden and landscaping. This type of a pattern provides for great flexibility, with completeness at every stage.

a. Research laboratories
These embrace Biochemistry, Genetics, Physiology, Botany and Zoology. (It is intended to add a first-year teaching wing to these). Each wing has its respective teaching laboratory at ground level for second-year studies onwards.

b. Lecture Halls, Library and Administration
These have been grouped together on both sides of an arcade linking the northern and southern entrances, which lead off to the various wings. The arcade has been visualized as a meeting place for research personnel and students, providing opportunity for cross-fertilization of ideas.

c. Teaching Laboratories
Maximum flexibility has been achieved by locating all the teaching laboratories within one continuous space, to be subdivided as necessary, with direct access to the arcade and the various wings.
d. Service and Maintenance

This is at lower ground level, reached by a service road. This level is directly connected to the different wings by vertical shafts, lifts and staircases.

The Structure
The structure is of reinforced concrete, partly cast in situ and partly in the form of large pre-cast beams, mass produced, and assembled on site. The intersections of the "warp and woof" pattern of the building form structural cores, spanned in the east-west direction by deep beams cast is situ. Large pre-cast beams have provision for housing the slabs that in turn span them, eliminating the need for scaffolding during construction. The north-south sections of the building bridge across between structural cores. This unique structure is flexible, economical and saves construction time, while answering complex functional demands made by a building of this nature.

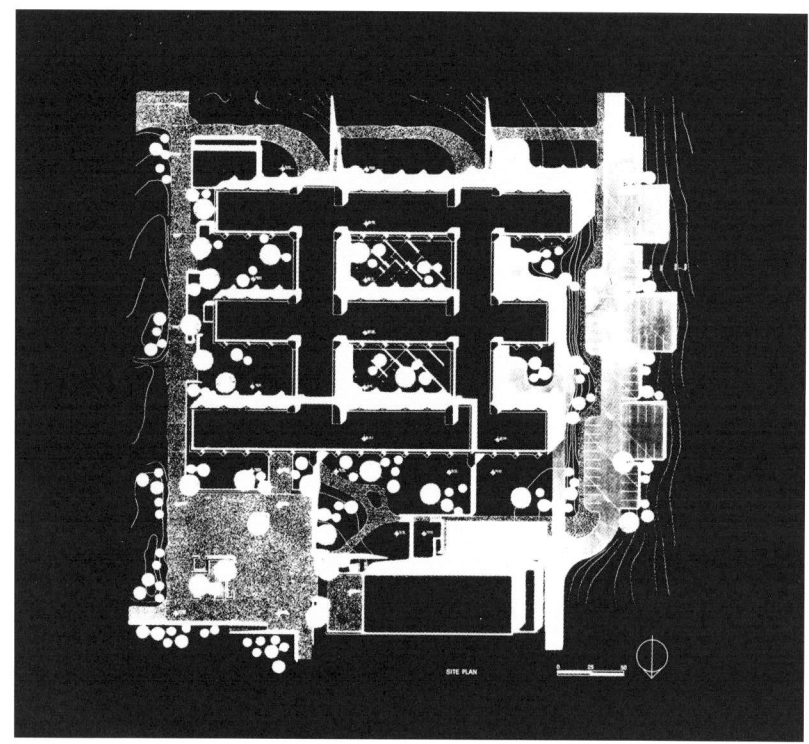

The Electromechanical Systems

The outer walls form the "shell" of the building, which remains constant. The inner spaces that it contains are flexible – adaptable according to different functions and programme requirements. The shell also includes spaces to house the sophisticated electromechanical systems forming an integral part of the building. These are logically conducted from basement plant rooms to the various parts of the building via a basement service tunnel, vertical cores and horizontal ducts to the various parts of the building. The main vertical service cores are located within the structural cores at the inter-sections of the "warp and woof" pattern. They are readily accessible for servicing, and for any future changes that may be called for. Maximum flexibility is provided in that individual circuits can be closed off at will, without affecting the remainder of the building. Vertical stacks, which may not be necessary in all the cores during the first stage, may be added as required, with no inconvenience whatsoever to the building. Main horizontal supply lines branch out of the vertical service cores at each floor level, with

6. Other Projects of Zarhy Architects

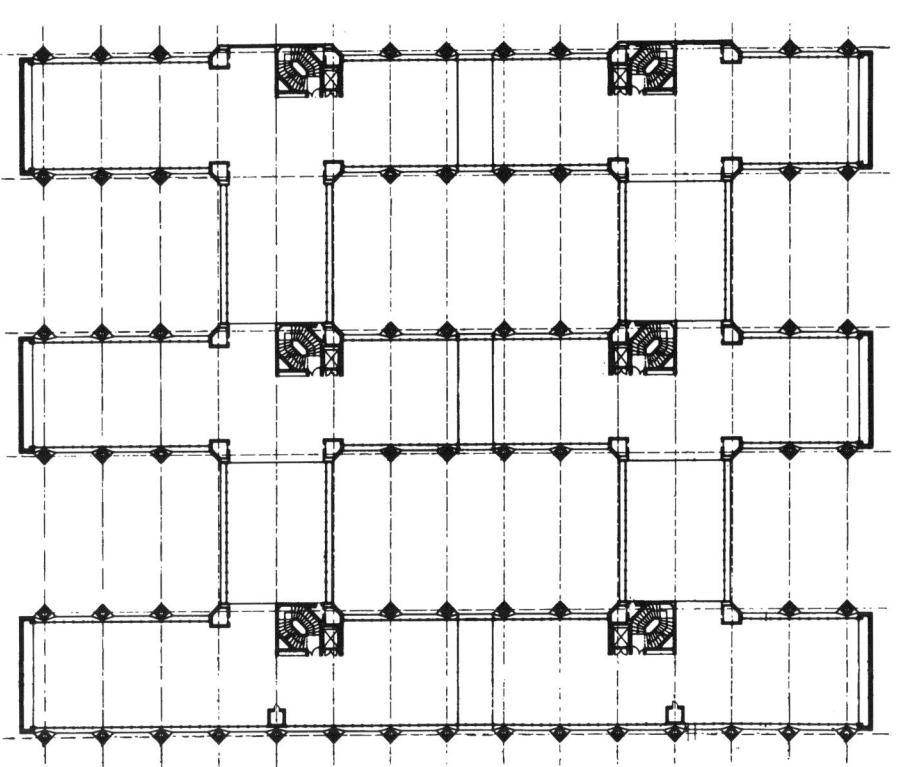

Typical laboratory floor without partitions

pipes for air-conditioning led in fully accessible ducts above the windows, and sanitary installation and other plumbing below the sills. Waste water is conducted via these below-window accessible ducts to separate vertical stacks, which also contain rainwater disposal pipes, all collected below ground level.

A fan and coil air conditioning system was chosen as most suitable for this building because of flexibility of operation, efficiency, and the isolation that it provides between the respective laboratories. Units can be matched to the individual requirements of the respective laboratories which they serve. Placing units on a specially provided ledge above the windows allows maximum flexibility for dividing up the different areas, with minimum disruption of existing functions during execution of new work. The main electricity supply lines will be connected to main-boards and sub-boards at the respective floors during the first stage, when secondary horizontal supply lines will be also installed. Sub-boards for the various rooms and supply lines to stands will be installed as the laboratory equipment is installed.

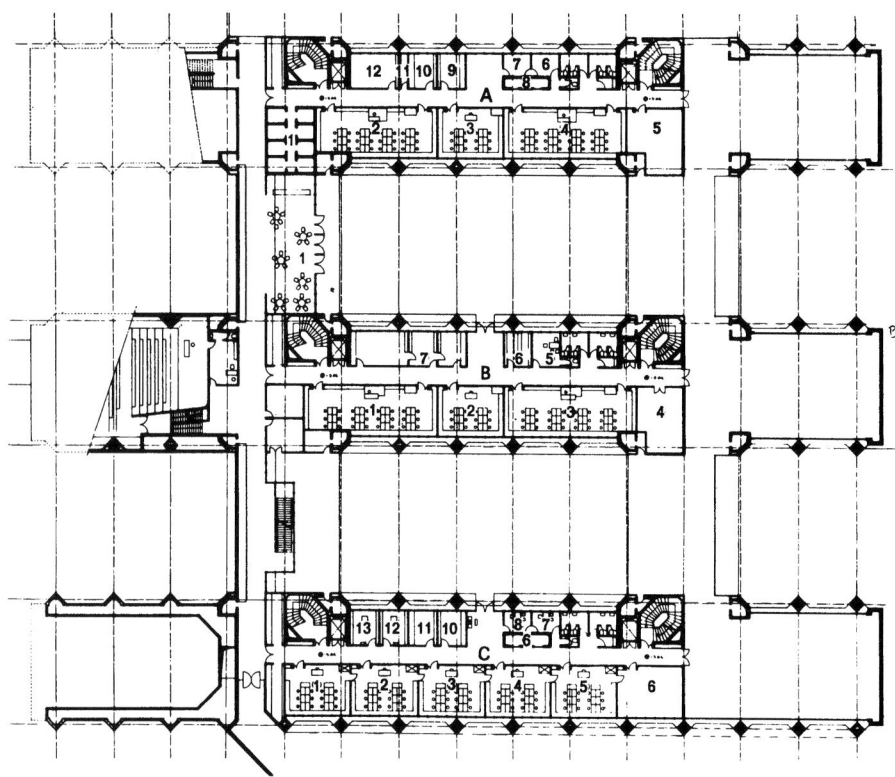

Teaching laboratory floor – level 3

A.   Physiology teaching
1.   8 Constant temperature room
2–4.   Teaching lab
5.   Lab. For teaching equipment
6–7.   Lecturers' rooms
8.   Low temperature room
9–10. Preparatory lab.
11.   Experimental animals room
12.   Teaching store room
1.   Common room and cafeteria
B.   Genetics teaching
1–3.   Teaching labs
4.   Constant temperature room
5.   Lecturers' room
6.   Teaching store
7.   Preparation rooms and kitchen
C.   Biochemistry teaching
1–5.   Teaching laboratories
6.   Lab. For special instruments
7–8.   Lecturers' rooms
10–11. Preparation laboratories
12.   Teaching instruments store
13.   Chemical store

6. Other Projects of Zarhy Architects

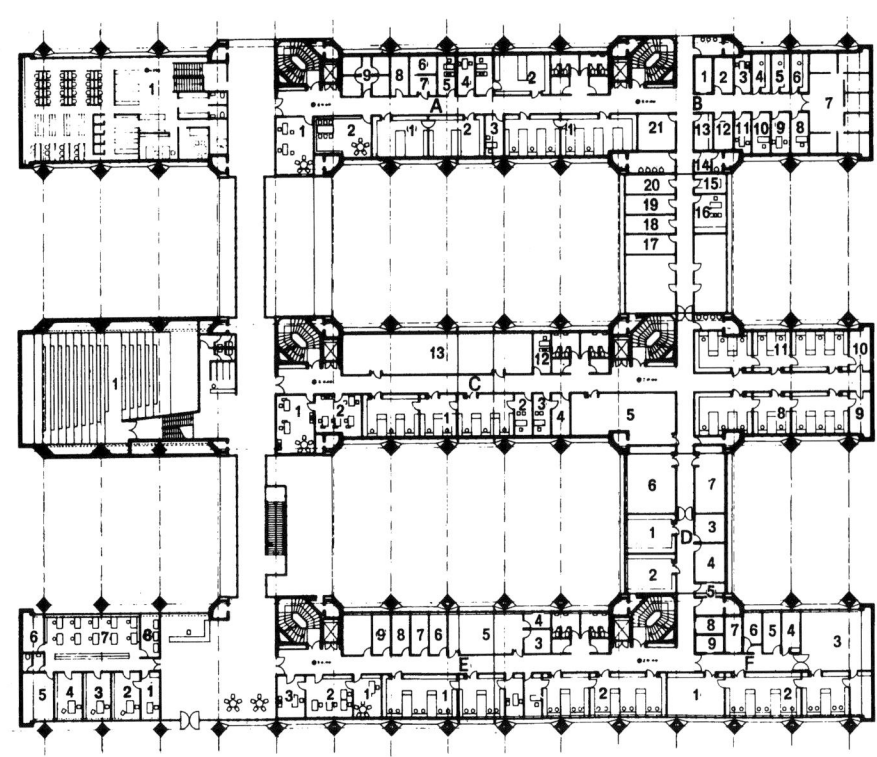

Entrance floor – level 4
1. Library, reading hall

Physiology administration
1. Secretariat
2. Library

A. Environmental animal physiology
1–2. Standard laboratories
3. Room
4–5. Lecturer
6–8. Equipment rooms
9. 4 Rooms
1. Lecture hall

Genetics administration
1. Secretariat
2. Calculating machines

Administration
1. Chairman's secretary room
2. Chairman's room
3. Chairman of teaching committee
4. Administrator's room
5. Archives

6. Duplicating
7. Secretariat
8. Calculating machines room

Biochemistry administration
1. Head of department
2. Secretariat
3. Administrator's room

B. Electroneurophysiology unit
1. Low-temperature room
2. Histology room
3. Lecturer
4–6. Laboratories
7. Center working spaces
8–11. Lecturer
12. Dark room
13. Reptiles
14. Fume hood
15. Store room
16. Electronic engineer's room
17. Workshop
18–20. Mammalians
21. Operation room

1. Additional research lab.
2. Guest lecturer's room

C. Standard research unit group A
1. Formal and developmental genetics
2–4. Offices
5. Lab for special apparatus
6. Constant temperature room
7. Lab. For tissue culture
8. Bacterial and viruses genetics
9–10. Offices
11. Fungal genetics
12. Office
13. Kitchen: cleaning cooking, sterilization and Autoclaves. Kitchen store

D. Bioelectronics
1. Chemical lab.
2. Electronic lab.
3. Electronic instruments room

4. Senior lecturer's room
5. Dark room

E. Biophysics
1–2. Standard labs.
3. Dark room
4. Weighing room
5. Special equipment lab.
6. Optical instruments room
7. Cary o.R.D.
8. Optical instruments room
9. Analytical centrifuge

F. Biotechnology
1. Heavy equipment
2. Standard lab.
3. Fermentation pilot plant
4. Preparation lab.
5. Tools store
6. Sterile room
7. Low temperature room
8–9. Thermostatic room

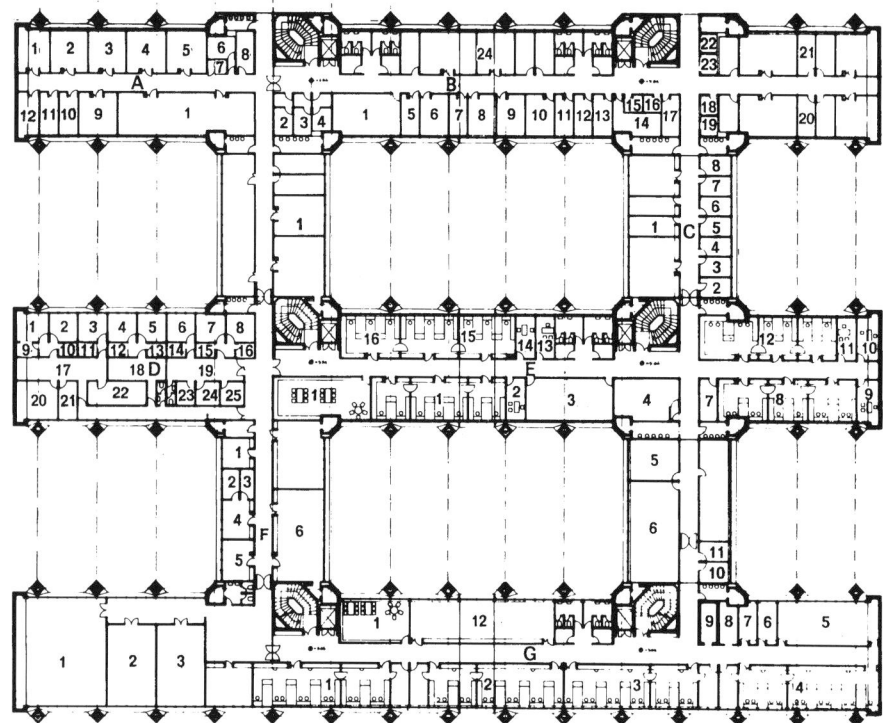

A.	**Plant anatomy unit**	
1.	Equipment room	
2–5.	Research laboratories	
6.	Dark room	
7.	Fume hood	
8.	Tissue growth	
9.	Research laboratory	
10–11.	Lecturer	
12.	Laboratory	
1.	Additional research lab. unit	
1.	Library	

A. Plant anatomy unit
1. Equipment room
2–5. Research laboratories
6. Dark room
7. Fume hood
8. Tissue growth
9. Research laboratory
10–11. Lecturer
12. Laboratory
1. Additional research lab. unit
1. Library

B. Plant physiology units
1. Unit c research laboratory
2–4. Dark rooms
5. Constant temperature room
6. Technician
7. Rough work room
8. Optic instruments
9. Centrifuges
10. General equipment
11. Calculating machines room
12. Secretariat
13. Kitchen and cleaning
14. Counting

15. Fume hoods
16. Weighing room
17. Glassware washing room
18. Chromatography room
19. Constant temperature room
20. Unit a research lab.
21. Unit b research lab.
22–23. Low temperature room
24. Unit d research lab

C. Physiology of membranes
1. Standard research unit
2. Cold room
3. Glassware washing room
4. Sensitive equipment
5. Instruments room
6. Weighing room
7. Growth room
8. Centrifuges

D. Electron microscopy unit
1–8. Electron microscope
9–16. Developing rooms
17–19. Preparatory rooms
20. Photography room
21. Technician
22. Photography room

23. Technician
24–25. Microtom
1. Library

E. Standard research unit group B
1. Cytogenetics
2. Office
3. Special equipment
4. Dark room and photography
5. Constant temperature room
6. Growth room and lab
7. Archives of genetics records
8. Human genetics'
9–11. Offices
12. Biometrics and evolution
13–14. Offices
15. Biology of the cell
16. Cytogenetic service

F. Inter-departmental equipment
1. Office
2. Spare parts
3. Freezers

4. Counters
5. Measuring and optical instruments
6. General equipment

1. Informal discussion room
2. Seminar room
3. Seminar room

G. Standard research unit group A
1. Biochemistry of membranes lab.
2. Enzymatic biochemistry lab.
3. Molecular biochemistry lab.
4. Comparative biochemistry lab.
5. Spectrophotometers
6. Chemical store
7. Dark room
8. Thermostatic chamber
9. Low temperature room
10. Fume hood
11. Weighing room
12. Heavy scientific equipment

6. Other Projects of Zarhy Architects

Research floor – level 6
Standard research units group B
1. Sterile room
2. Physiologic biochemistry lab.
3. Chemistry or the cell lab.
4. Biochemistry of peptides lab.
5. Biochemistry of development lab.
6. Weighing room
7. Fume hoods
8. Heavy equipment
9. Preparation room
10. Hydrogenetic
11. H.V.E.
12. Low temperature room
13. Storage room
14. Chromatography
15. Additional research unit

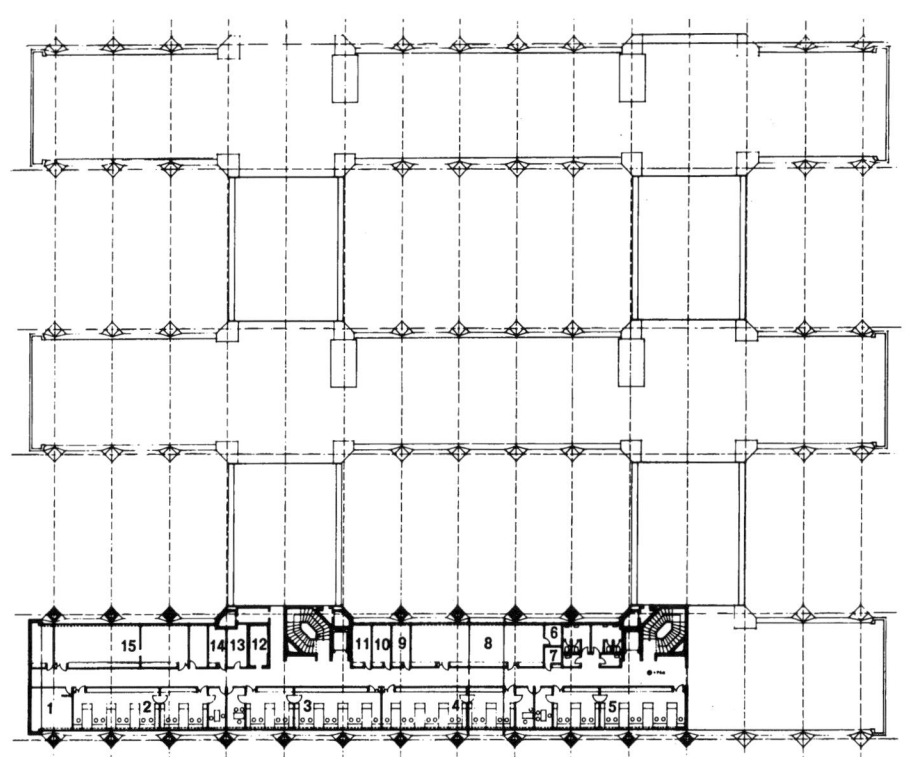

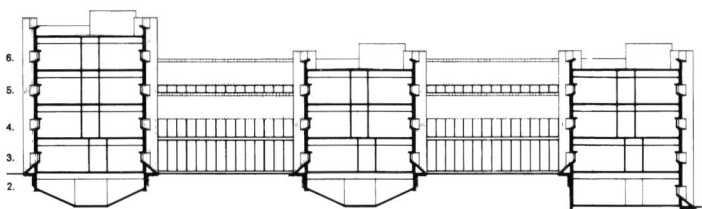

North-south section

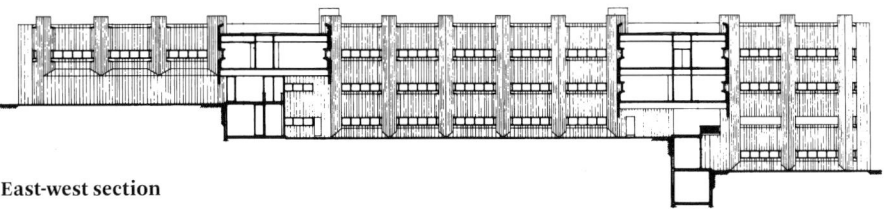

East-west section

Technion – Israel Institute of Technology –
Nuclear Engineering Research Building, Haifa

Haifa, 6,000 sqm, 1978–1985

The building is located at the Technion – Israel Institute of Technology – campus in Haifa. The program called for two distinct elements – workshop areas and offices for researchers. Since the workshop areas have highly specific requirements such as insulation from high radiation and flexibility, the building is divided spatially into two parts. The workshop areas are articulated as large floors extending into the rolling hills of the surrounding site, while the offices create a welcoming façade and friendly workspace for the building's inhabitants, and maintain a direct connection to the adjacent workshop areas.

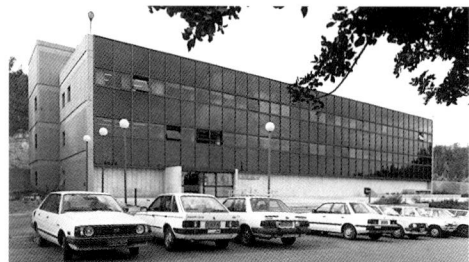

Nuclear Engineering Research Building, Haifa

Jerusalem International Convention Center

Jerusalem, 1961–1971

The International Convention Center (ICC) – Binyanei HaUma has been a byword for excellence for the past 60 years. Its lounges and halls tell the story of a center that has seen it all: receptions of presidents and world leaders, exhibitions by distinguished artists, monumental business conventions and spectacular performances.

In the description of the official website is to be read, that Zeev Rechter was the architect, but he died in 1960 and the project was built between 1961 and 1971. So, Yaakov Rechter and Moshe Zarhy were the architects at that time.

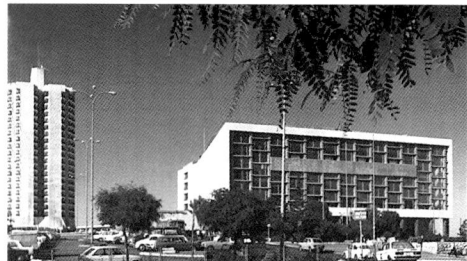

**Jerusalem International Convention Center,
built between 1961 and 1971**

"The largest auditorium in Israel is named after Menahem Ussishkin and designed by the architect Zeev Rechter, who also designed the Convention Center and the "Habima" theater, among others. With its spaciousness, first rate acoustics, state-of-the-art equipment and the finest support services available, the auditorium provides the perfect solution for hosting

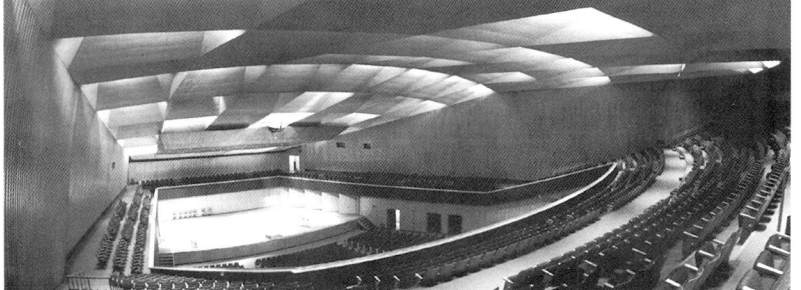

**Ussishkin Auditorium
for a maximum occupancy of 3,000 people**

6. Other Projects of Zarhy Architects

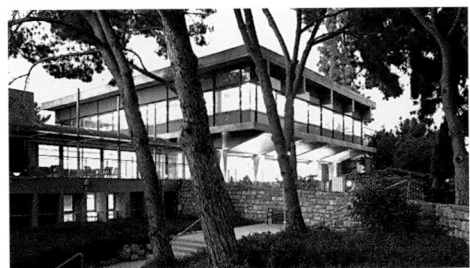

Physics Library, main building

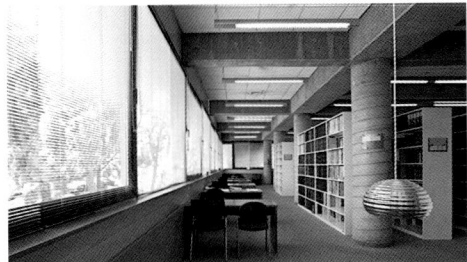

Physics Library, reading zone

large scale conventions, conferences, lectures, spectacular performances, concerts and rock festivals.

· *Maximum occupancy – 3,000 people: orchestra stalls 1,371 seats, mezzanine 1,495 seats, gallery (both sides of the stage and behind it) 134 seats.*
· *Stage Depth 13 meters, width 23 meters, height 11 meters (8 meters effective height)*
· *Entrances – three doors (each 1.48 m wide by 2.05 m high) and one door (2 m wide by 2 m high).*

Special equipment and facilities – 30 monitors (20 electric), one stage, three-phase electric power outlets, three translation cubicles, recording and broadcasting studios for radio, TV stations for live broadcasting."
www.iccjer.co.il

Physics Library, Weizman Institute of Science
Hovering concrete and glass slab as a library
Rehovot, 1,500 sqm, 1994

The library forms an integral part of the Physics Complex in the Weizman Institute of Science. The architectural concept for the building derives from its central location at the main intersection of the complex. It was envisioned as a hovering concrete and glass slab that would serve not only as an extension to the existing physics building, but would also create an accessible vestibule for the complex. With its gracefully elevated design, the library seemingly floats over the ground floor. This leaves the entry level free to serve as an entrance to the existing buildings and generates a covered social space protected from the beating sun. The building is a cubic form constructed of structural elements presented in their most pristine condition. Inside, it is an open space with bookshelves in the center and individual working spaces along the naturally day-light glass facades. In its essence the building is ascetic and pure, achieving harmony between interior and exterior spaces.

Left: Physics Library, detail of the massive concrete construction

Right: Night view of the building

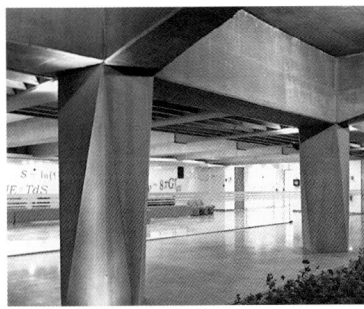

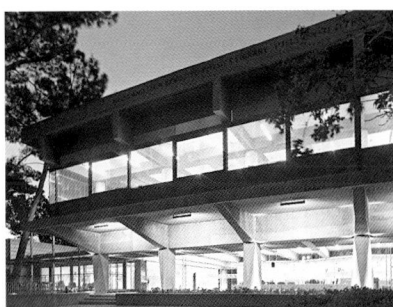

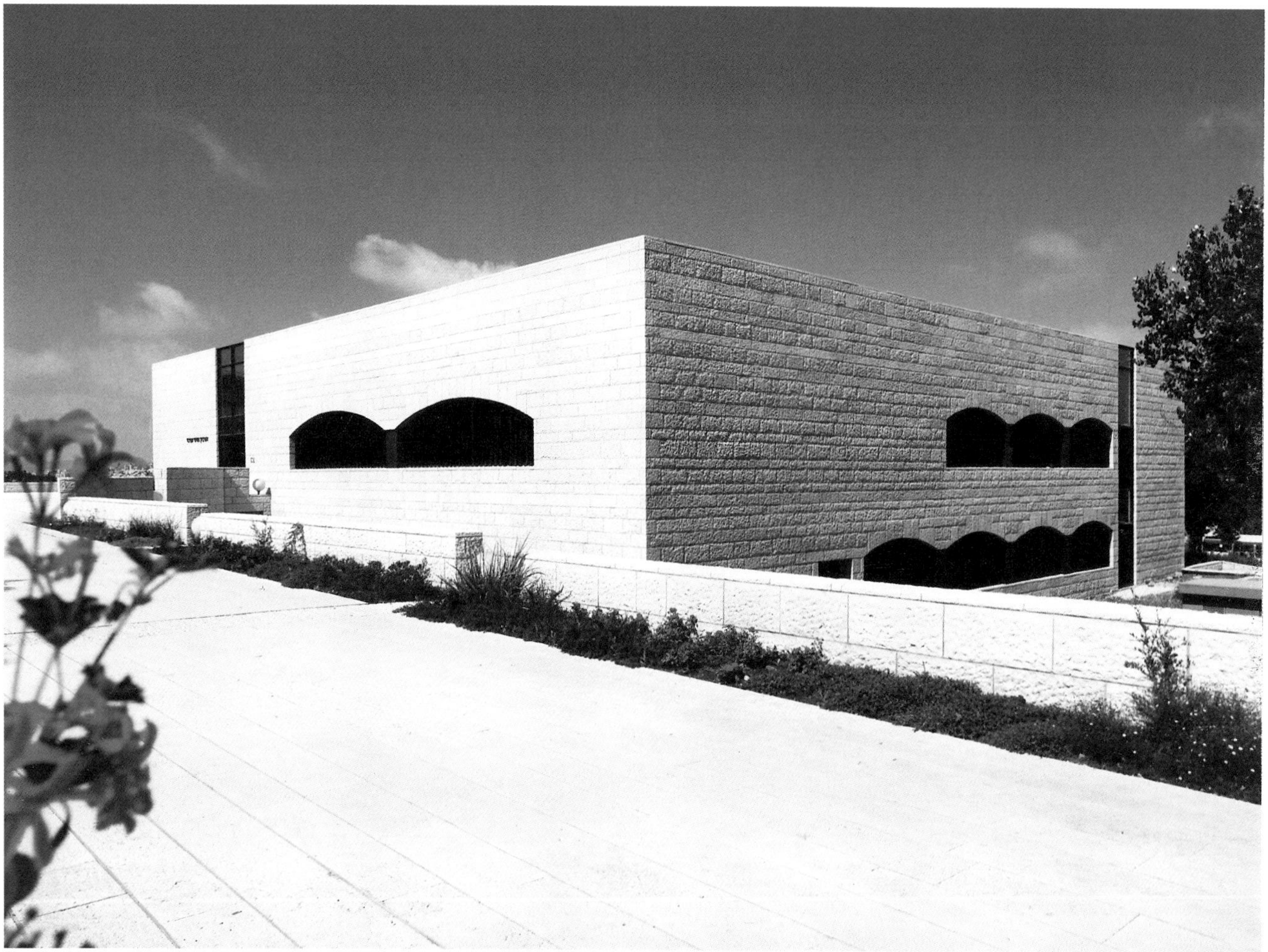

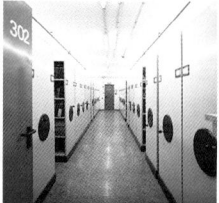

Zionist Archives, Jerusalem

6,000 sqm, Jerusalem, 1980–1987

The building is located at the western entrance to Jerusalem next to "Binyanei HaUma". It functions as the main archive of the historical documents of the Zionist movement. The premises consist of two different programs – the archive itself, which requires special storage conditions and is therefore located underground; and a public library, reading room, and offices which are located above ground. This two story horizontal building, clad in Jerusalem stone, offers a new interpretation of both the modern strip window and the oriental Jerusalem arch.

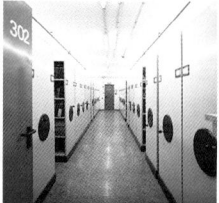
Archive shelves

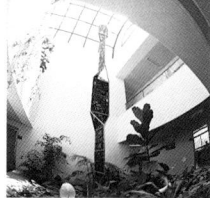
Inner courtyard

Top: overall view

6. Other Projects of Zarhy Architects

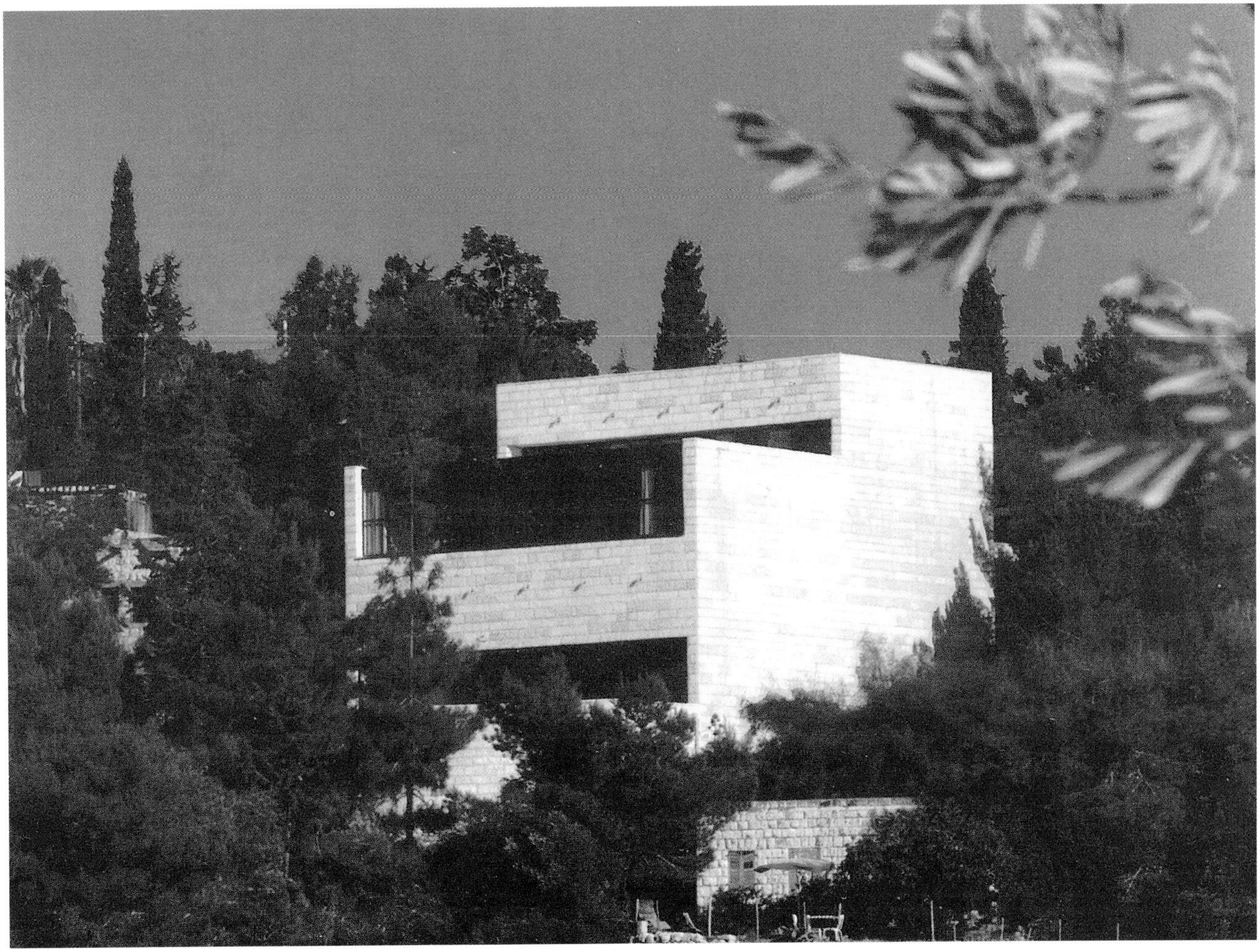

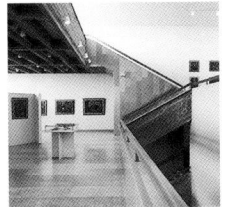

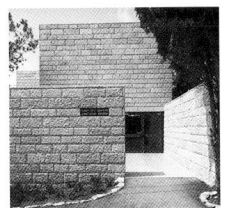

Exhibition hall   **Main entrance**

Top: overall view

Janco Dada Museum – Ein Hod, Haifa

1,600 sqm, Haifa, 1981–1982

Sitting in the hilly terrain of the artist village of Ein Hod, the museum is seamlessly integrated into the landscape. The structure is simple and aspires to be a continuation of the modernist spirit that Janco, one of the founders of the Dada art movement, imbued. At the same time, the building maintains the local architectural vernacular. The visitor accesses the building through a small open courtyard and continues inside. It is perceived as a single story building and evolves into split-level volumes, which make up the main exhibition spaces, continuing into a roof terrace with views out to the surrounding landscape and the sea.

Synagogue and Jewish Memorial, Moscow/Russia

2,000 sqm, 1993–1998

The building is located in the Poklonnaya Hill park in the heart of Moscow. Situated in the midst of an urban park, this symbol was created for the Jewish people of Moscow who fought with the Russians during the Second World War. The architects wished to create an abstract and simple building, yet one that would sustain a presence in the landscape. They refrained from introducing direct symbolism into the design, thereby allowing each visitor to have a different interpretation of the subject memorialized and encouraging a distinctly intimate experience.

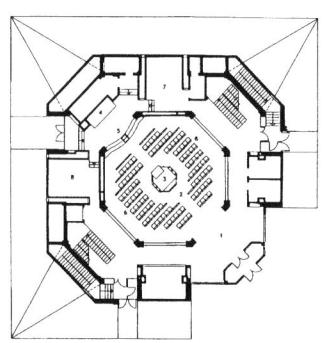

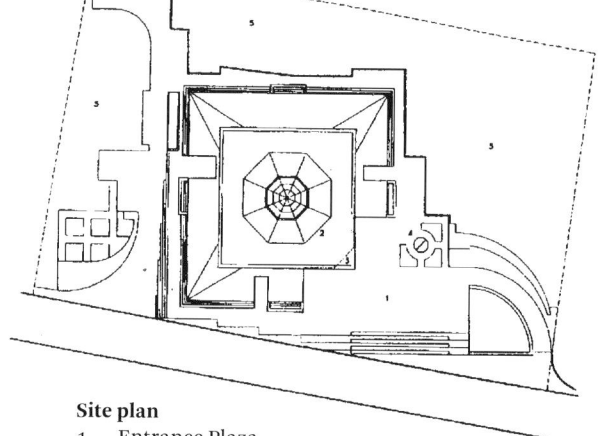

Entrance plan

1. Main Entrance Anteroom
2. Prayer Hall
3. "Bima"
4. Torah Scrolls Ark
5. Cantor's Podium
6. Men's Pews
7. Rabbi's Office
8. Reception Hall

Site plan

1. Entrance Plaza
2. Memorial Synagogue
3. Main Entrance
4. "Menorah"
5. Natural Grove

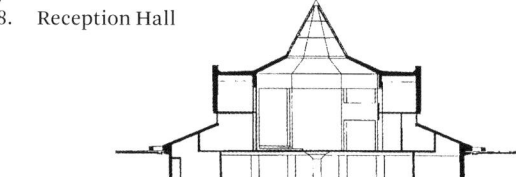

Section

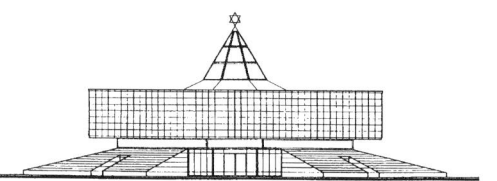

North elevation

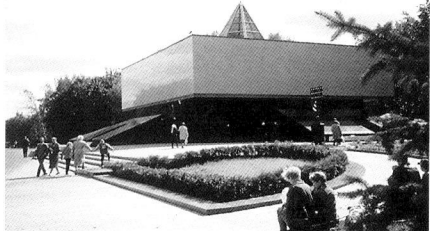

Overall view

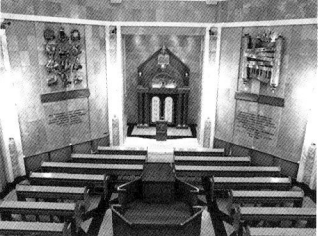

View into the synagogue

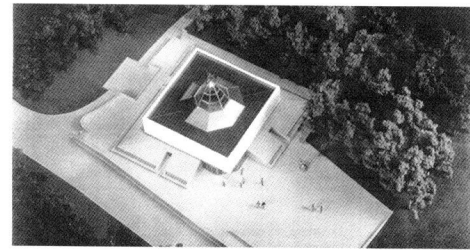

Aerial view

6. Other Projects of Zarhy Architects

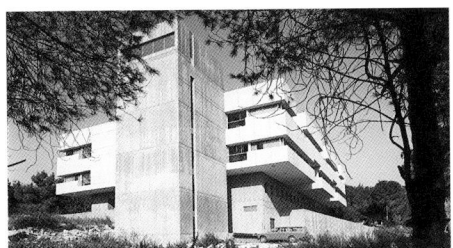

Solid State Physics Building, facade

Solid State Physics Building, Technion, Haifa

4,000 sqm, Haifa, 1970–1973

The building, which houses a workspace for the research of Solid State Physics, is located at the Technion – Israel Institute of Technology – campus in Haifa. We wished to create a flexible laboratory area both in terms of size and infrastructure. By locating a ring of laboratories around a large central shaft, a maximally efficient area was created. Another ring encompasses the laboratory ring, creating additional workspace for researchers. By occasionally cutting into the outer ring, the building's mass was articulated and views between the interior and exterior areas were revealed.

Microelectronics Research Institute, Haifa

Haifa, 3,000 sqm, 1984–1989

The building is located at the Technion – Israel Institute of Technology – campus in Haifa. This building forms an extension both academically and spatially of the Solid State Physics Building. The program called for the most sophisticated laboratory space requiring a high level of clean-rooms and vibration free spaces. These clean-rooms are sandwiched between two technical levels – plumbing utilities underneath and AC above. The façade of the building is articulated by cutting into the main volume by means of the entrance section and fenestration. The materials aesthetically extend the façade of the Solid State Building, built almost 20 years earlier.

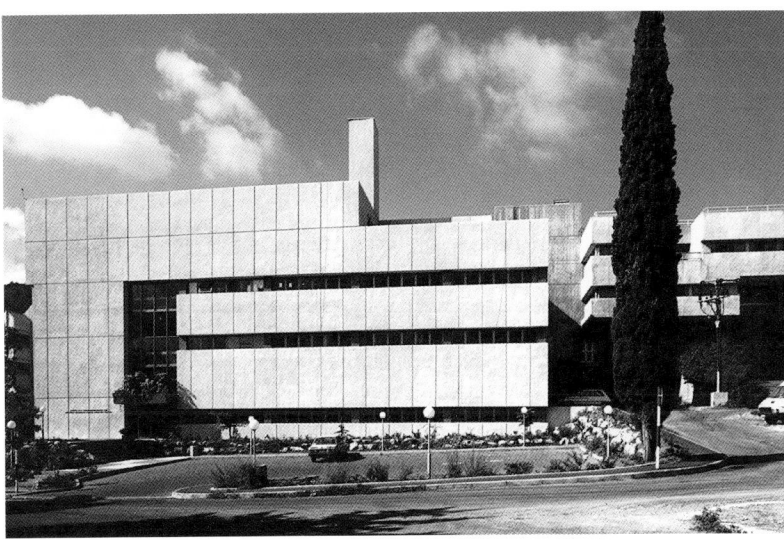

Microelectronics Research Institute,
view from south

Swimming Pool, Technion Haifa

Haifa, 4,000 sqm, 1979–1980

The building is located at the Technion – Israel Institute of Technology – campus in Haifa. The swimming pool is part of a master plan for the sports facilities on campus. The building is composed of two volumes – the covered Olympic swimming pool and the locker room facilities building. Designing an indoor Olympic swimming pool requires bridging large spans. In this case, the structural solution enhanced the architecture – the covering is made of a series of pre-cast concrete elements, each in the form of a three-hinged arch. This solution created an elegant, slender, and fluent structure

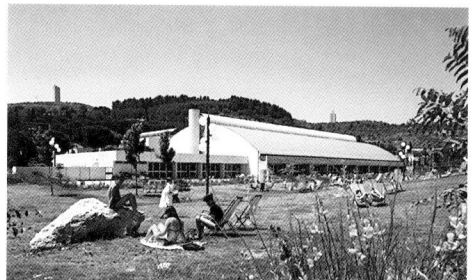

Main view of the covered swimming pool

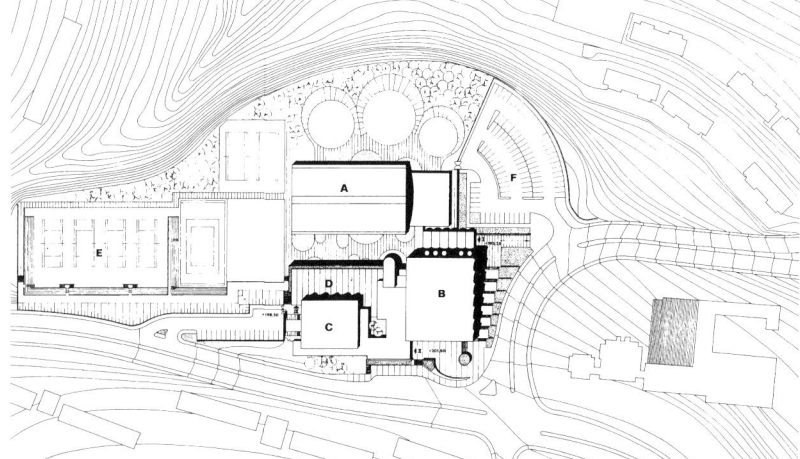

Site plan
A. Covered swimming pool and lockers
B. Central sports hall
C. Secondary sports hall (existing)
D. Various sports halls and miscellaneous
E. Sports grounds
F. Parking (100 cars)
I. Main entrance
II. Audience entrance
III. Secondary entrance and parking

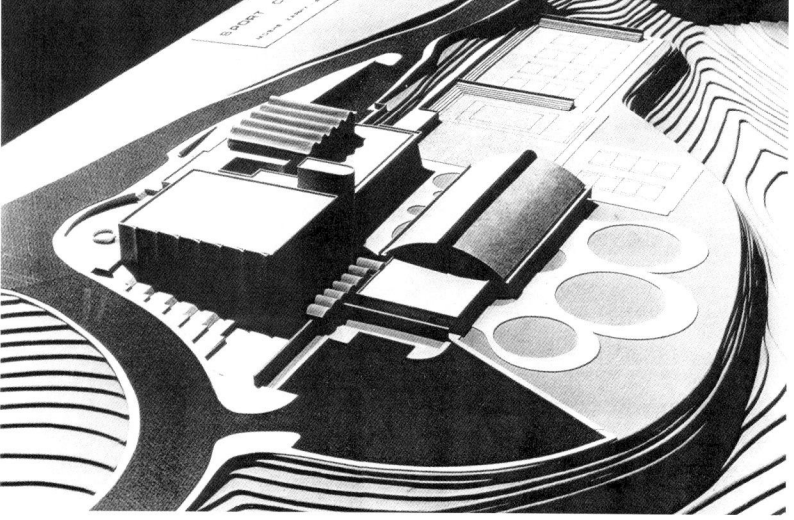

Model of the sports complex

6. Other Projects of Zarhy Architects

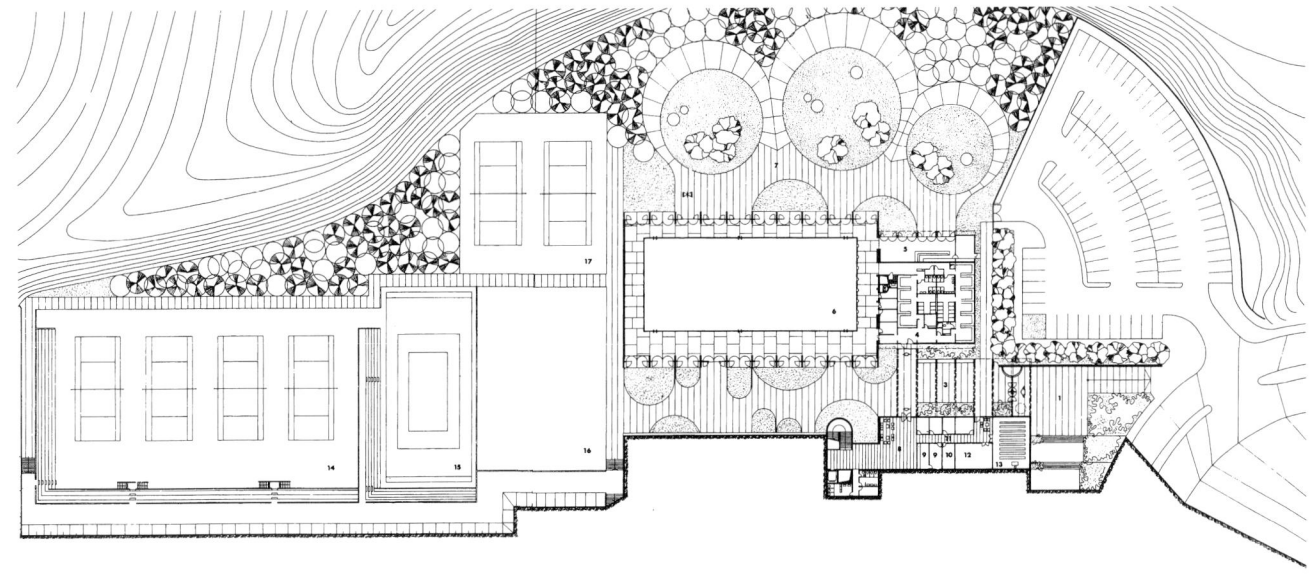

Plan at level +193.25

1. Main entrance
2. Entrance gate and control
3. Covered entrance area
4. Swimming pool, dressing room and utilities
5. Buffet
6. Covered swimming pool
7. Swimming pool open area
8. Entrance hall
9. Buffet and storage
10. First aid
11. Administration offices – head unit, secretariat and sports coordinators' rooms
12. Chess and bridge club
13. Lecture hall
14. Existing tennis courts
15. Existing basketball courts
16. Multi-purpose court
17. Tennis courts

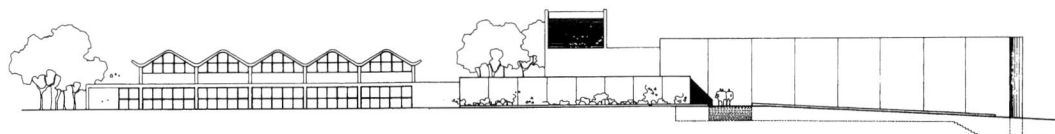

South elevation

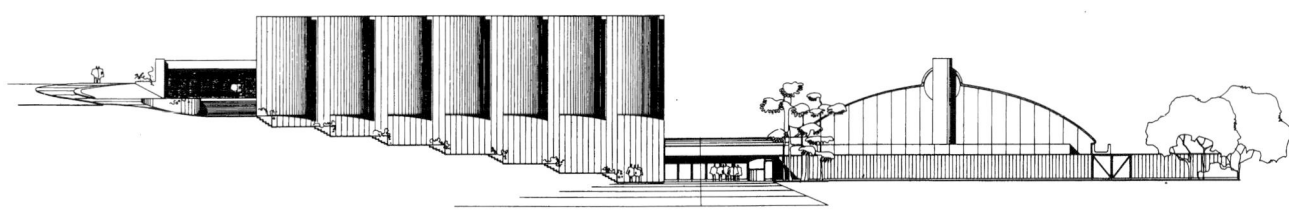

East elevation

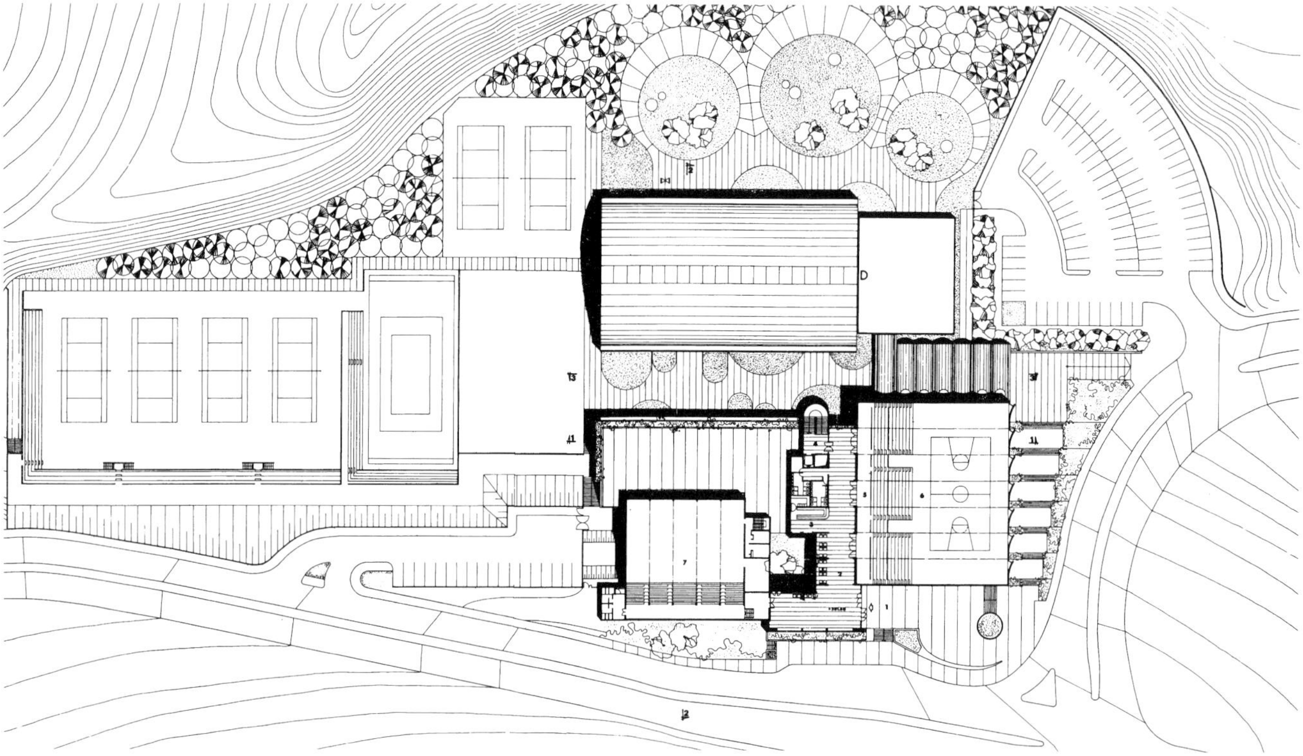

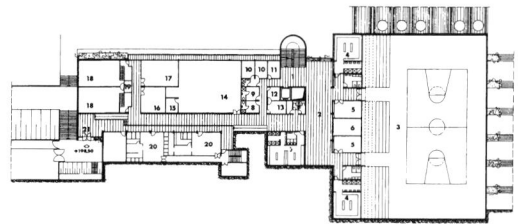

Plan at level +201.50

1. Audience entrance
2. Entrance hall
3. Buffet
4. Stairs and elevator lobby
5. Audience tribunes
6. Central sports hall void
7. Existing secondary sports hall

Plan at level +197.75

1. Stairs and elevator lobby
2. Lobby
3. Central sports hall
4. Lockers
5. Team room
6. Equipment storage
7. Female lockers
8. Instructors' unit
9. Teachers room (female)
10. Teachers' room
11. Seminary room
12. Doctor's room
13. First aid
14. Gym hall
15. Equipment room
16. Weight lifting room
17. Gladiator's room
18. Squash hall
19. Storage
20. Existing lockers
21. Secondary entrance

6. Other Projects of Zarhy Architects

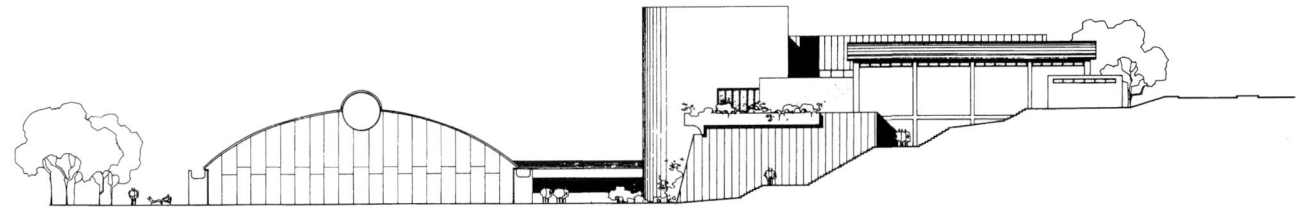

West elevation

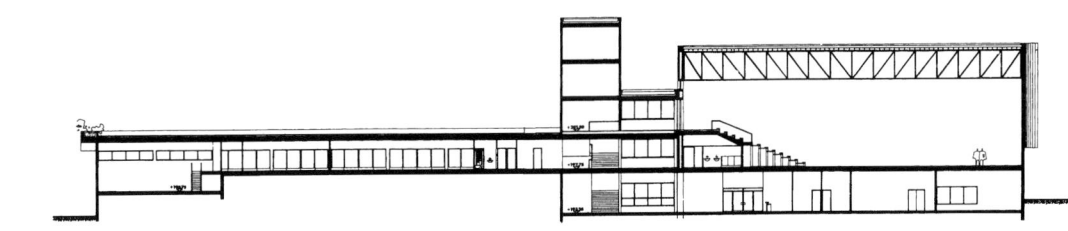

Section 1-1

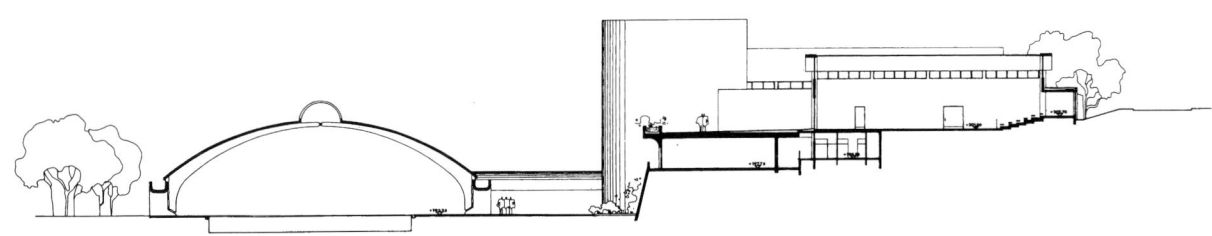

Section 2-2

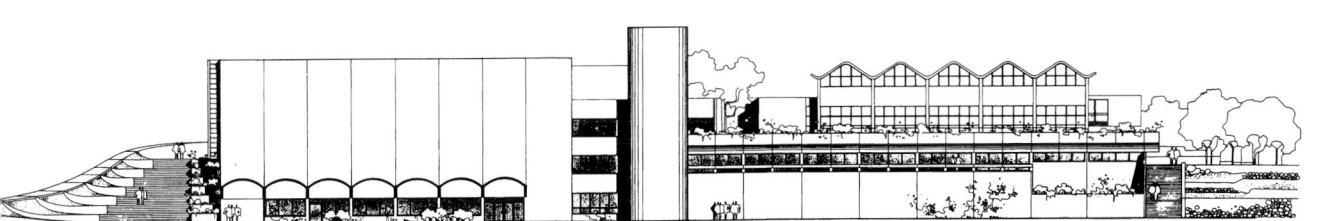

North elevation (Section 3-3)

Hi-Tech and Science Based Industries

Iscar Industries, Upper Galilee

Tefen, Upper Galilee, 90,000 sqm, 1985-2000

Tefen, the site of Iscar's campus, is a mountainous rural area in the Galilee, in northern Israel. The campus is designed as a park with independent structures scattered throughout the landscape. The buildings define an open and central garden with a ring service road surrounding the site and servicing the buildings via a multi-purpose yard. Special attention was paid to landscaping and integrating the buildings into the natural environment. The buildings are articulated as simple, horizontal, rectangular volumes made of pre-cast concrete elements. They function as open systems enhancing flexibility and change, while generating a formal aesthetic language attained from the gestalt effect of the campus' configuration. Data Program: Tool plant, Hard metal plant, and a marketing and training building.

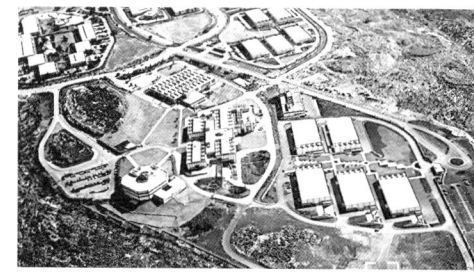

Aerial view

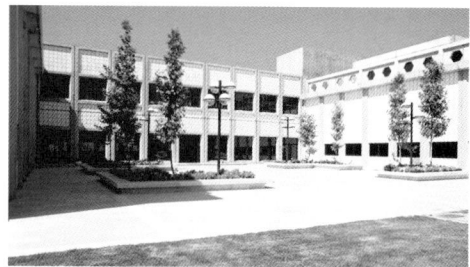

Facade

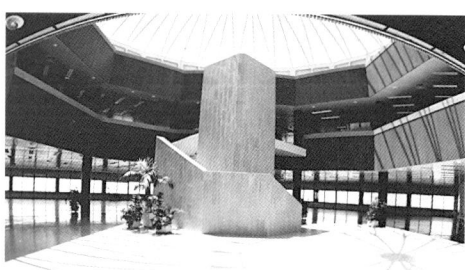

Entrance hall

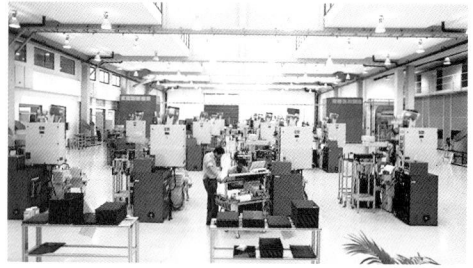

Production zone

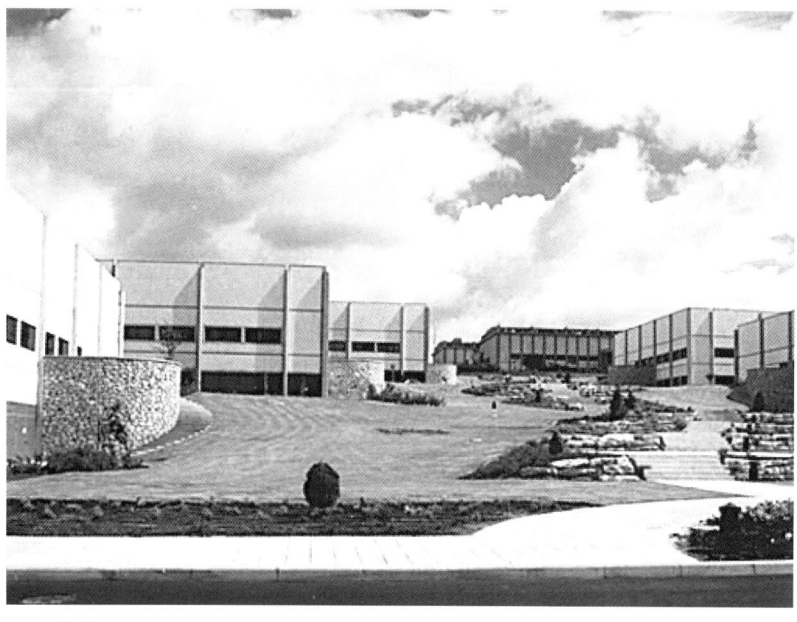

Overall view

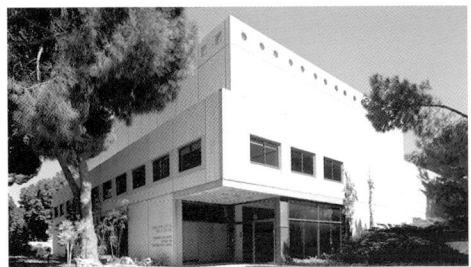
**Weizman Institute of Sciences,
main entrance**

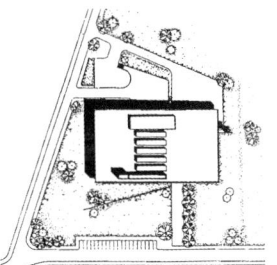
Animal Breeding House, site plan

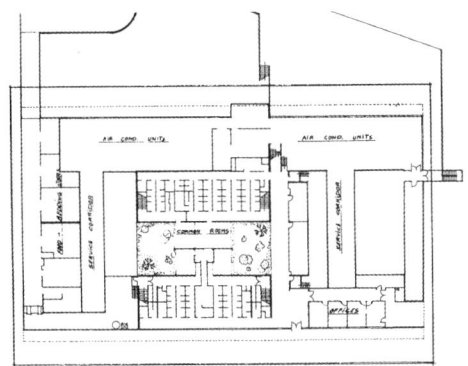
Animal Breeding House, plan of lower floor

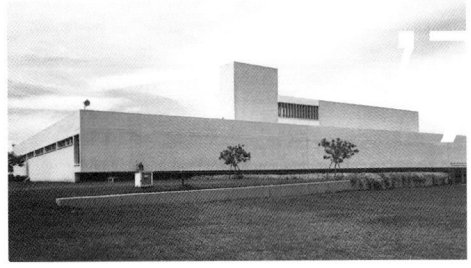
Animal Breeding House, main view

Weizman Institute of Sciences
Rehovot, 5,000 sqm, 1999

The Sub-Micron building is situated in the Physics Complex at the Weizmann Institute. It is designed to house the semi-conductor research facilities. The premises are designed as a box within a box. The research spaces, clean rooms, and laboratories are arranged as an internal structure, disconnected from the external one in order to comply with strict micro-pulsing requirements. The internal box is a three-layered structure: the laboratory level is sandwiched between an upper technical level for AC and HVAC and a lower one for MEP. A perimeter ring of research offices surrounds the box of clean rooms. The building is clad with pre-cast stone and concrete elements, creating a clean and simple appearance.

Animal Breeding House, Rehovot
5,000 sqm, Rehovot, 1967–1969

At the same complex of the Weizman Institute of Science, Zarhy Architects built a huge animal breeding house. It is a very functional building in a cubic modern architecture. The laboratory Animals Breeding Center is situated within the Weizmann Institute complex, on a sloping site bounded by streets on the south and west. The building was conceived as a simple envelope, enclosing four distinct and predefined zones. These are: a small animal wing (for breeding mice, rats and hamsters), a large animal wing (for breeding rabbits, guinea pigs. etc.), a specific Pathogen-Free Unit, and a Diagnostic Laboratory wing. It was necessary to provide for traffic flow between "clean" and "unclean" areas, and moreover, these areas had to be isolated from one another. We were faced with the additional problem of joint use of various services, such as food and bedding supplies, cage washing in the different areas, etc. The building was designed on two levels. Technical areas are located on the lower level, as are staff change rooms, toilet facilities and cafeteria. All productive functions are carried out on the upper level. Each of the four sections of the building; are self-contained with distinct traffic routes. In addition, the small animal wing and the large animal wing are subdivided into "clean" and "unclean" areas, with a one-way traffic system conducting the movement of materials. Air-conditioning, ventilation, plumbing and electricity systems likewise follow the clear-cut separation of functions.

Mixed Uses

ATIDIM, Industrial Park for Science-Based Industries

50,000 sqm above ground and 50,000 sqm below ground,
Tel Aviv, 2000–2011

The complex is comprised of buildings specially designed for high-tech based industries. The building is part of this complex, whose master plan was devised by our office in the 70's. Its design philosophy established a new paradigm for high-tech campuses in an urban environment and has triggered major development in its adjacent areas and created Tel Aviv's main employment quarter, mixing workplaces, leisure and retail. The building's design needed to overcome a major incongruity: How to create vast horizontal floor area in a high-rise building, while maintaining maximum natural light? The solution of Zarhy Architects creates maximal envelope in relation to floor area: The building is conceived of as two intersecting volumes creating a flexible floor plan that allows for either a division into several companies or unification for a single corporation. The building also includes public amenities on ground level, such as indoor retail spaces, that will function as the new heart of the entire campus. Architecturally, the elevations of the two volumes are articulated differently, one horizontally and the other vertically, helping to lighten the building's mass. It was developed a unique technology that treats both the glass and the stone cladding as a curtain wall. This sophisticated system reinvents the use of stone as a cladding material.

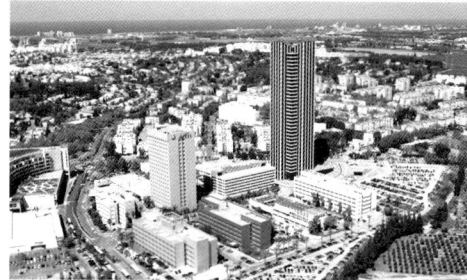

Aerial view of ATIDIM Complex
Photo: Zarhy Architects

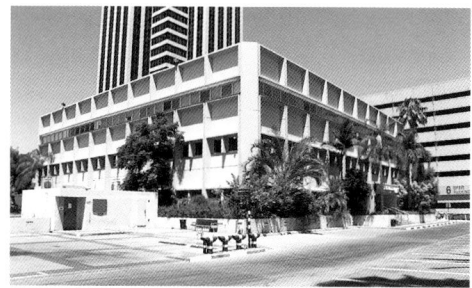

Laboratory: view from south-west

ATIDIM Main Laboratory

4,000 sqm, Tel Aviv, 1973–1980

One of the first projects in this area has been the Hospital Main Laboratory for the whole Tel Aviv Region. It was no longer economic to operate the laboratories in the various hospitals, this building was projected and built by Zarhy Architects between 1973 and 1980.

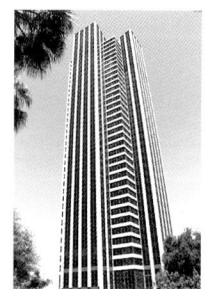

ATIDIM Main Building

The Weizman Multi Use Center, Tel Aviv

140,000 sqm, Tel Aviv, 2007

Weizmann center is a multi-functional complex, in the context of an existing major medical center in the heart of Tel Aviv. In order to accomplish contextual integration, the large constructed area is articulated in three separate buildings connected by a covered commercial street, a galleria, acting as the complex's spine.

A garden is located on top of the commercial center, extending the adjacent "Ahad-Asar" garden. The main entrance from Weizmann Street creates a continuation of the street through an urban plaza and establishes a natural connection to the city and the hospital.

All buildings are clad with stone and glass, however, each one has a unique façade articulation. Thus, architectural coherence is maintained while sustaining each structure's own character. The internal façades of the covered street continue the external façades of the buildings, simulating the feeling of an urban street.

Data 140,000 sqm built above ground. Commercial Center – Contains a commercial area of 3,600 sqm. Retirement Home – Houses apartments for independents, four geriatric wards, and public areas for use by residents. Office Tower – Contains hotel, medical clinics, offices and Retirement Home apartments. Parking lot – can contain 2,300 vehicles, 700 of which exceed the project's demand, for staff and visitors of the medical center.

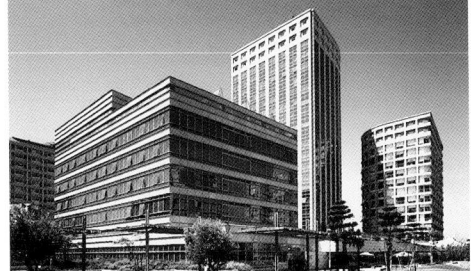

Geriatric building

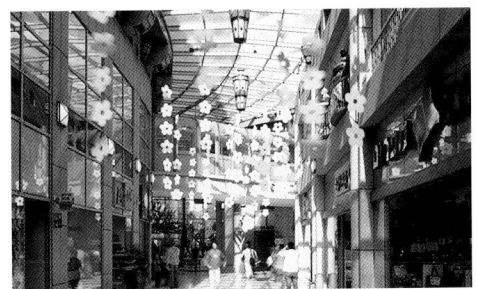

Commercial hall

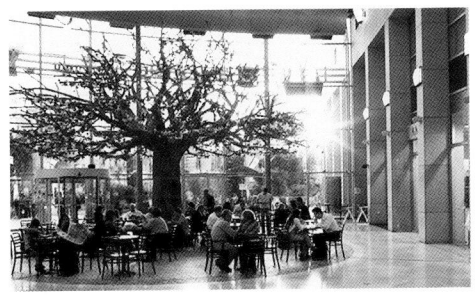

Cafeteria

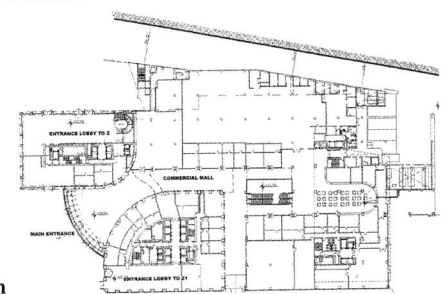

Ground floor plan

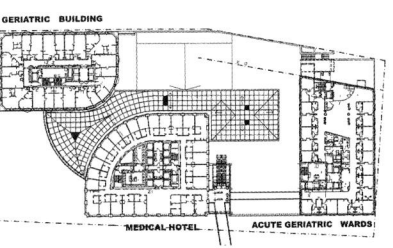

Typical floor plan

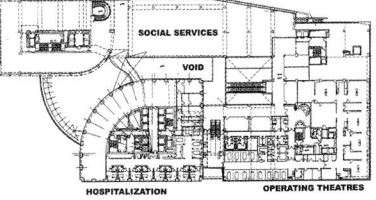

First floor plan

7
Papers

1. The high tech laboratory design architectural considerations

Lecture presented to the I.D.F. Authority in Jerusalem in 1970

Most of the principles of the laboratory design we described in the first part of this paper are applicable to most types of laboratories. (Thinking along the lines of systems rather than using conventional architectural vocabulary). But while the conventional laboratory maintains "normal" environmental conditions for the sake of comfort for the staff (except in certain working places where special conditions are needed) in the high-tech laboratory we have to adhere to very strict functional constraints in order to insure maintenance of certain environmental and infrastructural requirements.

Some of these requirements are listed here:

a. To maintain the desired level of air cleanliness in work places and workrooms.
b. Protection of people from harmful particulate matter discharged by the process and prevents work process being contaminated by particles shedded off work people.
c. Screening-off the facility from outside polluted air and protects the surrounding area from toxic undesirable contaminants discharged from the building.
d. Supply of high-purity liquids and gases needed for research or production process.
e. Eliminate possibilities of cross contamination between adjoining work places.
f. To keep and control a low level of vibration in working rooms, especially in working places.
g. To maintain air pressure, temperature and humidity within close tolerance.
h. Create a very flexible partitioning system in order to enable frequent changes in their configuration and increase their adaptability to hooked-in bulky equipment.

Clean room technology cannot be implemented unless these requirements are strictly fulfilled. Specialists, consultants and companies, supplying clean room components, can guide the architect, designing the facility and give consultation concerning their field of specialization.

It is beyond the scope of this paper to discuss these requirements in great detail.

The architect designer must have a general understanding of these requirements and their meaning in terms of function, operation, cost physical appearance, material and their relationship to other systems in the facility.

This understanding is necessary, because it is the architect's task to relate the systems to each other and create the optimal functional composition in order to get the maximum operational capabilities at a Minimal cost.

The high-tech laboratory building is virtually a machine. It must be a nice good machine. All these constraints, and others, dictate the building's composition. They generate its structure and architecture. The experiments to express the high-tech laboratory and the new trends in laboratory design by symbolic architecture are complete nonsense.

Efficiency of conventional laboratory design can be measured by the ratio of the total length of workbench to total floor areas.

It expresses number of working places per total given built up area which means actually, the best design configuration (net to gross area as some experts think).

Efficiency of unclear research laboratory design can be measured by its decontamination properties (as the facility is concerned) regardless the right location of certain functions according to the work process.

This means arrangement of functions according to the level of contamination hazards.

One must bear in mind that decontamination process can jeopardize or paralyze the work in the laboratory for months (what will one do with the scientists during the decontamination period not to spear of risks of life?).

Designers of high-tech clean room research and production laboratory strive for zero deficiency facility, as clean room technology is concerned. This is their contribution to minimum rejection of the laboratory's product.

Another problem is corrected with cost effectiveness of the facility. Cost of a square meter of utilized are in conventional laboratory in the order of 1,000–1,500 US$. The cost of a square meter of working clean laboratory is in the order of ten folds of that of the conventional laboratory.

On the top of the costly operation there is the risk of creating a "white elephant" in case we don't get the right performance of facility and it will not get its operational certificate. This might happen because of wrong design criterion, design failures or bad workmanship on site.

Our concern in this paper is the best design of a given design criterion. Because of many constraints in clean room technology and because the architect receives, sometimes, contradictory from expects of the various different disciplines of the high-tech clean room laboratory, it is obvious that we deal here with an interdisciplinary problem.

The architect is in the best position to produce the best optimal design due to his training to understand enough in each field of specialization and his experience in manipulation and combine them in best and efficient configuration.

i. Anti-vibration precautions. In choosing the proper location of a clean room facility site special attention must be paid to anti-vibration precautions. Avoidance of proximity to heavy traffic route and other sources of vibration. Soil vibration testing of proposed site must be carried out before a final decision on site choice is taken.

Design of the facility itself must take into account the following considerations:

a. The floor carrying the clean room laboratories (the "table") must be separated from the rest of the structure in order to avoid any transmission of vibration from the other parts the building to the laboratory's floor and hence to the working place. The separation of the "table" from the rest of the building is to be defined clearly to form a vibration free area, or independent structure carrying the free standing partitions of the laboratory area. We get here, actually, a building within a building, a box in a box.

b. The "table" is to be heavy solid block, usually carried out in cast in-situ concrete "Waffle" slab, supported of pillars to leave room for service floor under the "table". Another alternative is to locate the "table" right on the ground, on proper fill. In this case the problem of services void (mainly support and waste disposal piping) is partly solved by provision of trenches and tunnels. This system has the drawback or rather limited possibilities of changes.

c. Another anti-vibration precaution is the avoidance of any rigid connection of pipes, ducts, conduits, elements of construction of other building components between the table and the rest of the structure.

The anti-vibration precautions dictate, as matter of fact, an independent building housed in an "envelop structure" bridging the "table" area.

A. Air cleanliness

The air cleanliness requirement is the decisive factor dictating the conceptual design. A tremendous amount of cubic feet of air has to be circulated per hour in order to achieve the required degree of air cleanliness. The space needed to house the machinery, the air-ducts, and the filters etc. termed" air circulation machine" is very great in proportion to functional laboratory space. The "system" of air cleanliness, based on the Laminar flow phenomenon, comprises the following components:

a. Filtered outside inlet

One must pay attention to its location and relate to considerations of environmental pollutants as well as to the position of the building's air outlet and scrubbers.

b. Air handling units

Because of the huge quantities of air to be circulated the air handling units are very big. Their function is to treat the air and circulate it. On one hand they have to be located not to far from the clean room laboratory area in order to avoid clumsy duct work, but on the other hand they are a source of vibration and noise and should not be located too close to the laboratory area. The decision on the location of the air handling units in the facility is a major decision.

c. The ducts network

The ducts carrying the air from the air handling units to the laboratory's ceiling are voluminous. They occupy almost all the area above the laboratory's ceiling. The height needed to house them is about 5–6 meters. The space consumed by the ducts network is more than twice the space of the clean room laboratory itself. The ducts have to be hanged from the top ceiling, the "bridge" and to have their connection to the Hepa filters, located at the clean room laboratory's ceiling, via flexible connections. These precautions are necessary in order to avoid any transmission of vibration. The Hepa filters, through which the air passes and flows to the clean room laboratory, are cased in metal does open at the bottom. They occupy most of the ceiling area, leaving very little place for "eye-drop" lighting fixtures, smock detectors etc.

d. Air flow in the laboratory

Clean room laboratories are classified according to their "cleanliness class", (100,000, 10,000, 1,000, 100 and 0) measured by maximum permitted dust level or particles per cubic foot of air. The lower the class is the more difficult it is to accomplish it. The right pattern of flow of air in the laboratory is very important factor; one can say that it is a crucial factor in the process of getting the desired degree of cleanliness class. The right pattern of airflow depends a lot on the arrangements of the Hepa filters in the laboratory's ceiling.

e. Return air track

Track of return air starts from continual opening in the laboratory's wall panel, at floor level, or through a perforated floor. It flows to the service chase and exhausted via return air ducts to the air handling units to be retreated and recirculated. In some cases the return ducts system is eliminated and space in used as "Plenum". Return air is pumped from this space right to the air handling units. In this case the architect has to design and specify the envelope's building as a sealed box, a very tough job.

Three more problems have to be mentioned in connection with the air cleanliness "system".

The energy conservation problem. The amount of the treated air consumed by the facility uses a great deal of energy. This is a running cost problem, especially in Israel where cost of energy is high. Possible solutions to this problem are beyond the scope of this paper.

Another problem is the location of energy center of the facility in relationship to the air handling units. The energy center and the units are interconnected by pipes carrying cooled and heated water.

One more problem is the removal system of toxic gasses, mainly from confined working places.

It consists of a closed system of ducts, relatively of small cross-section and scrubbers located usually adjacent to the facility. The air outlet is via a stack. The height of the stack, velocity of discharged treated air and it's composition have to be coordinated with the health authorities.

B. Protection of people

Protection of people and prevention of work process being contaminated by particles emitted – off work people consist of two categories, conduct of people according to instructions and physical means. The two categories are tied together and will be described jointly.

People penetrating the clean room area have to pass change rooms. They have to get off their street clothes and wear "bunny suits" which will cover their body completely. Penetration to the clean room area is through an air shower cabin designed to shed particles off the "bunny suit".

All other conduct instructions concern behavior of people. For example, any abrupt movement of people in the laboratory will disturb, for a time, the cleanliness "balance" in the laboratory. It is the architect's task to design the facility in such a way that lines of movements will be as simple and as clear as possible.

Flexible partitioning system

The philosophy of flexible laboratory design existed for a long time. Certain systems and elements of flexibility were implemented, here and there, long ago, with considerable success.

· The free of columns laboratory space.
· The interstitial service floor.
· The service chases and service basement.
· The flexible industrial partition system.

These elements of design and many other innovations existed before the clean room technology came into being. But they were not an absolute necessity; in many cases one could design the laboratory space otherwise. In the case of clean room technology it became a must. All innovations were put together and a complete philosophy is created.

The clean laboratory area, the "table", is free of columns. Its design consists usually of central clean corridor with a row of working bays on both sides and service chase in between the working bays. A perimeter service corridor is designed on the circumference of the laboratory area. Modules of design have to coincide with modules of the waffle slad. Because services run in the basement service floor and can penetrate only in cases of the waffle slab. Clean room partitions are constructed, on modular grid, or self-separating framing on the waffle slabe. Flexible partition systems became, by now, an industrial product and can be purchased in the open market. We have discussed, briefly, flexibility of the partitions system. We have to bear in mind that flexibility is attained only if all components are flexible. Services and electro-mechanical system included.

Conclusion

The clean room laboratory design is a complex problem. Many trades and specialties are involved in the design. It became an interdisciplinary operation. The pace of progress is very rapid. The success of the operation depends on optimal fulfillment of all requirements of all trades. This can be achieved through design, which takes into account all infrastructure requirements and "melts" them unto balanced integral design. We have mentioned here only some of the requirements of high-tech clean room microelectronic laboratory in order to demonstrate an architect's approach to this complex problem.

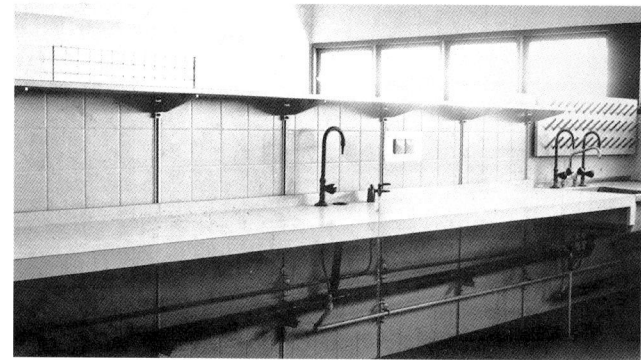

Safed Hospital, typical laboratory

2. The high-tech laboratory – an Israli experience

Abstract of a lecture, presented 1970 to the I.D.F.
Authority in Jerusalem

3. Change of scale in building in Israel

Lecture presented to Ministry of Housing,
1970 in Tel Aviv

The high-tech laboratory is intended to satisfy sophisticate environmental needs of modern research and production in various and diverse spheres. The classical laboratory could no longer provide adequate working conditions for the advanced technology developed in the last two decades. The infrastructural requirements for research and development in the field of microelectronic, electro-optics, biotechnology, genetic engineering, robotics and in many other areas called for a new type of laboratory- the high–tech laboratory. The need to accommodate research activities of these variegated fields created various different types of high-tech laboratories. The present paper deals with architectural aspects of one type of high-tech laboratory. The microelectronic clean room laboratory intended mainly for research and production of microchips. It will, I hope, demonstrate an architect's approach to the complex problem of the design of high-tech laboratories.

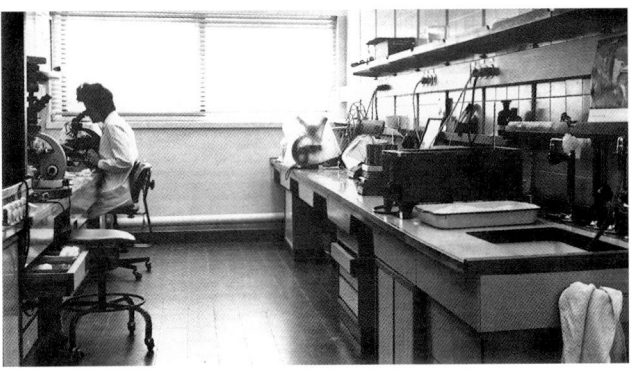

Meir Hospital, typical laboratory

We are presently witnessing a process of change of scale in building in Israel; the urban and general landscape may be said to be undergoing a metamorphosis. High-speed roads, connecting the large town, are being constructed. Here and there are to be seen – in other words: the landscape known, for better or for worse, from the highly – developed countries, a landscape of traffic axes and bridges – is now establishing its presence in Israel. New towns, planned in advance, have risen during the last decade on previously desolate areas, such as the town of Arad, Dimona, Carmiel etc. In these towns there exists, to a considerable extent, a nicely-calculated balance between social infra-structure, employment and transportation development and consequently – construction on an appropriate scale. In the large town we are witnessing, for the first time in Israel, a process or urban renewal. New buildings are taking the place of the old. This is generally accompanied by an alteration in the purpose of the site. Low-standard dwellings make way for hostelries, commerce etc. The three or four storied houses are replaced by multi-storey buildings. The scale is changing. Incertion fortunate areas urban planning covers an entire neighborhood. New districts in the older towns are common phenomenon. New university campuses are moreover being built in Jerusalem, Tel Aviv, Beer Sheva, Haifa etc. New medical centers are being built for purposes of hospitalization, cures, research and instruction. Preplanned industrial towns are also a common phenomenon wherever there are population concentrations.

As the scope of construction had increased, the use of building materials has assumed characteristic patterns. The building component manufacturing industry has grown. As a result of this ramified activity in the field of development and construction it is evident that in the not-too-distant future, different belts of the country will units into continuous built-up areas, like the one along the Mediterranean coastal strip, or the one which will connect Jerusalem with Tel Aviv. In order words we are approaching the well-known, intricate problem of the megalopolis. All this entail the loss of the values of natural landscape and the megalopolis of an environment of human design. The question has more than once been asked: have we not left in until too late to control this gigantic process and are we not creation a robot which will turn against its marker? At the same time the public is developing a landscape-preservation consciousness, which has come to stay. Difference currents and schools of thought are crystallizing, and fighting over the steps to be taken to prevent the cancerous spread of building as a perpetual source of mortification.

In the light of the aforesaid are to be viewed the problems with which the planner and architect in Israel must now hold firmly. At the present time, as district from previous period, it may be said that the tools exists. Will architects meet the challenge and fine modes of expression for creation of dwelling-place for society?

a. Characterization of the plants

The plants mentioned in sub-paragraphs 1, 2, 3 of the previous paragraph cab be classified:

1. Plants that completed the development of their basic product / products and are in full production and are continuing in research and development of additional products (or that will include the existing products).
2. Plants that did not complete the development and production of their Basic product / products and have

not reached yet industrial take-off. Their emphasis is on research and development and semi industrial production.

b. The plant's requirements

The plants that are in industrial production phase will require large production areas for their facilities and the auxiliary services – this in addition to the laboratory and office areas. These plants will want to assure themselves expansion possibilities. Their location will be suited to their size and character – or in specific building suited to their needs or in multi-purpose structures with the production halls the dominant element. The plants that are in early development phase will require mostly laboratories and semi-industrial production (comparatively small areas). Success in product development will cause the need for fast expansion. That many even justify moving from structures of a certain character to structures in which the production halls are the dominant element. These plants will need strong communication with the university at the development phase. They will also require the services of the suburb. These plants will strive for minimal investments (in order to lesson the "risk") and will avoid long-term leases. Their natural location will be at first in multi-purpose structures with the laboratories as the dominant element. Various service plans – their location in multi-purpose structures (dominant element-laboratories and offices). The above said does not prevent the possibility that plants in full production will not locate in multi-storey, multi-purpose structures, but points out the "reasonability of the needs".

c. The size of plants

It is hard to determine the usual size of the science industry. We can divide the plants into three categories:

1. Small plants – 5 to 20 employees, especially "infant plants", from research institutes and laboratories, service plants.

2. Medium size plants – 20 to 100 employees.
3. Large plants – over 100 employees.

Area of industry: An acceptable thought is that the required area per employee in the small and medium plants (excluding service industries) is 20 sqm. These industries can be found usually in multi-purpose structures.

The area required in the large plants depends on the automation in the production phases. Here also we can assure a key area of 20 sqm. per employee of research and development, but it is difficult to determine a key for the production employees.

A survey of science industries in Israel shows that excluding large plants, the average area is between 500 to 1,000 sqm.

d. Designation of areas within the plants

From local surveys, present experience and literature – we get the following picture regarding the area designation:

Production	Research plants	Plants in 1st devel. Stages	Plants in full
Offices	20–25%	30–60%	20–30%
Laboratories	65–75%		
Production / semi industrial production		30–60%	50–70%
Auxiliary areas and warehouses	5–20%	approx. 10%	approx. 10%

e. Manpower composition in plants

One of the significant points of the industry is the high rate of academics amongst its employees. This rate changes with the character on the plant, but even in large plants dealing in high volume of production this rate will not be lower than 10%. The usual is about 20–30% academics of all employees.

f. Plant's production

According to data published by the national committee for research and development- science industries- S. Danieli (May 1970), the production in 1969, in 39 science industries surveyed was about IL 47,000 per employee. It is self-understood that the production in industries rich in capital and science was higher than in plants in which the capital input was relatively lower.

h. Investment

The investment per employee according to the same source varied so much from plant to plant that it was difficult to come to conclusions. Included in the survey are plants that are in rented structures and plants that have invested considerably also in the structures. "Scattering" of investment per employee in the mentioned plants was between IL 3,500 to IL 50,000.

The Economic Designaturion of the Suburb

Assuming that on an area of about 86 dunam it is possible to erect approx. 50,000–60,000 sqm. of industrial structures. The following is a comprehensive picture of the suburb:

a. The plant's area   50,000–60,000 sqm
b. The no. of employees in the plants

         2,500–3,000 employee
     calculated according to 20 sqm / employed
c. Total investment in the plants   75–100 million
d. Anticipated yearly production of
all the suburb industries   120–150 million
e. Area of centers (incl. Parking)   Approx. 4,400 sqm
f. No. of employees in the services   50–75
g. Investment in the services   Up to 10IL million

Basic Assumption

a. The possibility to expand and develop in characteristic of all the suburb plants. We have learned from experience that it is the nature of science industries to constantly change and renew their products and procedures, and are expanding in a fast rate. The growth rate of "infant plants" mentioned above is so fast sometimes (after the development of the "basic product") that they are fully justified to move to a new site. Plants that have finished the development of "the basic product" expand during their first years of existence at an average rate of 25%. But some reach even a higher rate of growth especially between the first and second year of production. The development of the suburb and population policy must assure the expansion possibilities without splitting the plant into its various units. It is necessary to enable this growth to be executed in several stages.

b. The uncertainty as to the plants to occupy the suburb on the one hand, and the renewed character of the plants on the other hand is necessitating great flexibility in use of the structures. Accordingly, the planning must be based on modular structures that can be joined one to the other and to divide the interior areas to suit the arising and changing needs.

c. Planning emphasis was put on economy in building expenses. The structure that must give efficient operation must not burden the tenant with purchasing/leasing expenses that would cancel the advantages stemming out of the incentives given to science industries.

d. An atmosphere of an "academic industrial community" must be created that must be different from ordinary industrial areas. This atmosphere can be achieved by high service standard, convenient parking facilities, and keeping the aesthetic character and prestige of suburb.

e. The small area and the high cost obligate its full usage. It should be emphasized that the suburb's area of 86 dunam is not enough and will make wise population difficult. There is reserve land close by (agricultural). The planning must organically include this area or part of it within the suburb.

f. The plant's demand is that is the research and developments will not be cut-off from the production departments. This demand must guide the planning.

g. There must be convenient communication to assure the attachment between the suburb and the university, which will also enable the use of the computer center by the plants.

h. The supply of power and auxiliary services to the plants by the service center seems desirable when the suburb's population will justify it. Accordingly, the erection of several service centers, power and auxiliary sevice ecnter and refrigeration were considered.

Chapter B – Planning Guide

1. Area Data

a. Site location (see plan no.2)

The suburb of science industries in Tel Aviv will be erected on an area designated for it, close to the northeast boundary of Tel Aviv(with the Tel Aviv jurisdiction), on blocks:6338-the following plots:

Old	New
3	3
5	13
6	24
7	15
10(road)	10(road)
9(")	20(")

Total 86–87.8 dunam

On the north – west side of the area – Eser Tahanot St.
On the south – Dvora Hanevia St.
On the east – the area borders with agricultural land.

b. Size of the area

The area now at the disposal of the science industries is about 85,000 sqm. From this – the area allocated for the plants is not more than 52,000 sqm. This area will not justify development of the services that should be developed, and is much smaller than the area of subsidiary companies in Jerusalem, Haifa and Rehovot, and does not assure the required flexibility in its population. The plants must be able to expand – and this requires land reserve attached to the original site. The size of the area today does not answer these demands and stops the vital process of the expansion.

c. Reference to existing urban planning
1. The area was including in the script of the contour plan no. 738 that was approved on 12.1.1967. In this plan the area was designated for industry.
2. Urban planning scheme No. 721 is referring to the above area, and includes script for a detailed plan 721, which is part of the general contour plan 738, that was approved for deposition on 27.4.1971.
3. Because of parking needs, and our recommendation for building of not more than four storeys, it is not possible to utilize all the building percentage mentioned according to the regulation (200%) but 100%.

d. Existing objects in the area
1. Objects belonging to the science industries:
   Soccer field.
   Paved basketball court, including a shack (7 x 12 sqm).
   A Shack near the soccer field (7 x 3 sqm).
   A Shack used as a synagogue (7 x 10 sqm).
   High (low) tension line (4 posts); high tension line (2 posts).
   Electrical posts (5)
2. Objects that are on the access road to the since industries:
   Soccer field.
   Paved basketball field, including a shack.
   A Mikveh (ritual bath); a synagogue.

e. Topographical structure
A 1% land slope from west to east – downwards
A 2.5% land slope from north to south – downwards.

f. Soil quality
The soil in the area is red loan containing red soil – in depth the red loam becomes sandy and sand. Deep water is found is the soil at the depth of more than 10m.

2. Access Roads and Communication
a. Access roads to the suburb (see plan no. 1)
The area has to access roads from the west side, connecting it with greater Tel Aviv and the university:
1. Esser Tahanot St. – Rokeh Brvd. And connection to the university from the south.
2. Dvorah Haneviah St. – Rishpon Rd. and connection to the university from the north.

Today there is no connecting road to the east, to the Petah Tikvah, Kfar Saba area etc. The continuation of Esser Tahanot St. or Dvorach Haneviah St. up to Geha Rd. would connect the suburb with the Industrial and residential area east of the area. There is a need to affirm that this access road will indeed be executed. Connection to greater Ramat Gan will be A. H. Silver St.

b. Communication
It is necessary to ascertain that the Communication Ministry will allocate.

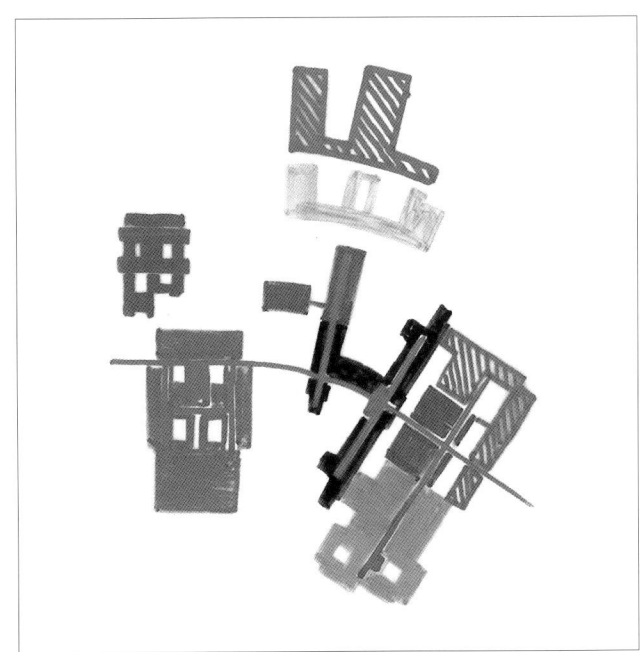

Meir Medical Center – Sapir Medical Center
Phases of construction 1956–2006

4. Science industries

Presented 1970 to Tel Aviv Municipality and Tel Aviv University

The purpose of this document is to represent the basic data for the planning of a suburb for science industries to be erected in the industrial area in the north-eastern section of Tel Aviv. The document consists of a "general" chapter, giving general background to the program and another chapter giving planning guidance. The document does not deal with the populization policy, condition of handing over areas to the tenants, management of the suburb, sale of services etc.

Essential Points

1. The program is based on definitions of the company's aims as established by it temporary Board of Directions.
2. As one of the means for achieving its aims the company intends to erect and develop a suburb for science industries. The company now owns an area of about 85 dunam in the north-east section of Tel Aviv – Jaffa.
3. As far as access roads to the area, topography and soil quality – the area is convenient to develop, but a substantial investment is required in sub-structural work.
4. A stipulation for the development of the area is the clearing of various objects such as electrical lines, and various structures. Likewise, the area must be cleared to enable paving municipal access roads to the area.
5. Since the area is quite small, it will be difficult as far as populization policy and probably will not justify development of all services that ought to be included in a suburb of science industries. Efforts should be made to acquire additional area that will be used as land reserve for the suburb.
6. The populization policy and the guiding lines will be:
   - The suburb is planned as a homogeneous unit that enables the creation of an industrial community both from the atmospherically viewpoint and the services developed there.
   - Each industry in the suburb will have its privacy. This privacy will be assured also if there will be more than one plant in a building.
   - The area and the structures will be planned so as to assure their flexibility, both in the manner of its use and the possibility of expansion of the area set aside for the plants.
   - The populization policy will be to centralize as many industries of similar character in close areas to the suburb, while keeping reserve areas for their expansion.
   - The company will strive to always have a stock of unrented area. The stock of unrented area will be decided from time to time, but the feasible minimum seems to be about 3,000 sqm.
   - The structures will be built economically, but will include all the required elements for science industries.
   - A communication system with the Tel Aviv University must be assured.
7. According to a master plan there will be about 52,000 sqm. of industrial buildings and additional 4,500 sqm. of service structures.
8. There will be 3 types of industrial structures:
   Multi-purpose structures – multi storey
   Multi-purpose structures – single storey
   Specific structures.
   A multi-purpose structure – multi storey will be between 4,000–5,000 sqm.
   - 3 or 4 storeys, the structure will have piping for power supply, cold and heat, water and a disposal system.

- A multi-purpose structure – single or double story will be mostly a structure of production halls, on an area of about 1,500–3,000 sqm.
- The specific structures will be built to suit the initiators while keeping the uniformity of the suburb.

9. Service structures will be developed to suit the suburb's development. These structures should provide all the services required by an industrial community, such as: central supply services, auxiliary services (workshop), hand administrative services (post office, bank, restaurants, etc.).

10. The suburb will develop in stages. It is proposed that stage 1 will include municipal sub-structure development (chapter 2, para. 9–1), sub-structure development by the company and the erection of 2 multi-purpose structures. The direct investment of the company at this stage based on summer 1971 prices (before evaluation) and not including evacuation expenses, management, taxes etc. will be approx. IL 7 million. The estimated investment of the municipality have not been coordinated yet with the parties involved. A time table for execution will be set after approval of the plan, but execution of stage 1 should not last more than 18 months.

11. According to estimates there will be about 2,500–3,000 employees in the final stage of the suburb, and their production value should reach approx. IL 120 –150 million a year.

Definitions

The municipality .... Tel Aviv Jaffa Municipality
The university .... Tel Aviv University
Suburb .... Suburb of science industries
A plant .... A scientific industrial plant in the suburb
Typical plant .... A plant in need of production and research area of Laboratory type, office or production halls.
Specific plant .... A plant in need or production area with a structure and character specific to it.

Initiator .... A future plant in the suburb
Structure .... A structure in the subarea including a plant or Plants
Supply services .... Those services that the suburb intends to centrally supply to all plants.
Central services .... Those administrative and community services that will be available to all the initiators within the suburb
Auxiliary services .... Plants and workshops that will supply various services that are not within the limits of their designation

List Of Plants

1. Access roads
2. Site location
3. Soil usage and road system
4. Key plan for laboratory structure
5. Key plan for typical plant structure
6. Key plan for production hall structure
7. Plan showing laboratory and production structure
8. Placement of services in the suburb
9. Service center and multi-purpose structure
10. Present day situation

Chapter A – General
1. Background
a. Aims and functions of the company for science industries
- Initiation, encouragement and construction of science industries.
- Initiation and encouragement of communication between the above plants and the Tel Aviv University, in the field of research and development, scientific consultation, and the use of the University's research facilities.
- Planning and erection of centers of science industries.
- The erection of structures for the purpose of renting, leasing or selling to science industries and / or providing areas within the center for the initiators

for the erection of structures according to the master plan.

- The construction of service for the supply of services to the plants, their operation and maintenance, or passing on the operation to sub-contractions.
- The existence and maintenance of the centers.
- Obtaining incentives from the government, the municipality and other bodies and their allotment for the development of the centers and the plants.

b. The suburb in north-east Tel Aviv

As one of the means of achieving the aims of the company and fulfilling her duties, the company will construct and develop a suburb for science industries block 6338 covering about 86 dunam in north east Tel Aviv – Jaffa (see map no. 1).

c. The criterions for examining science industries

The financial proportion between research and development and the yearly turnover.

- The numerical perdition between the scientific technological employees and the rest of the employees.
- The financial relation between the cost of material and the cost of product, while considering the added value stemming out of the plant's activities.
- Research ties, consultation and utilization of university know-how, research centers etc.
- Utilization of advanced technological know-how, while giving preference to know-how developed in the country and especially at the Tel Aviv University.
- A plant that is aiming the development of know-how and research, the supply of services and products for the purpose of research for various scientific institutions, including research laboratories and services.
- A plant that requires the research facilities of the university for part of its activity and / or academic personnel of the university.

2. A Suburb for Science Industries

The suburb for science industries will include three basic elements:

a. Plant structure
b. Service centers
c. Roads and public areas.

a. Plant Structures

Will be made up of three types of structural:

1. Multi-purpose structures – their dominant element will be the area designed for research and development, short production lines or semi-industrial and offices.
2. Multi-purpose structures – their dominant element is in the Production field.
3. Specific industrial structures – planned to meet the demands of the plants by prior arrangement with the company.

b. Service centers

Will be compounded as following:

1. Supply services.
2. Central services.
3. Auxiliary services.

The designer can recommend the erection of services in separate structures or centralized ones. A detailed program as far as the center's essence, their scope, details and their contents will he prepared by the designer.

In chapter B paragraph 7 – more details for service centers.

c. Roads and Public Areas

A high standard of communication services and convenient access to the suburb must be assured. Special attention should be given to the parking problem, A parking area of 0,5 – 0,6 per employee will be allotted.

d. Stages of the Suburb Development

The functions of the company arc to assure the initiator a construction area which he can occupy immediately, with services supplied without having to invest large sums of money. Accordingly – the development stages of the suburb will be:

Stage A

· Physical development of the sub-structure and imparting a character of a prestige suburb.
· Erection of multi-purpose structure that will be a „reserve" area for initiators (size of the proposed „reserve" – 3,000 to 5,000 sqm.
· The erection for structures according to commitments with initiators.
· Development of supply and power centers etc. (for example cold and heat center). Its side and scope will depended on commitments to populate the suburb.

Stage B

· Strictly keeping a "reserve" area as mentioned above and additional structures as needed.
· Erection of structures according to commitments.
· Erection of general services, expansion of power services, and erection of a core for auxiliary services.

3. The Plants

a. The main types of industries considered for the suburb

Industries, laboratories and research institutes active in the area:

1. Electronics, physics and optometry –
   including combinations of these areas.
2. Chemistry and its various branches.
3. Biology, microbiology, pharmaceutics etc.
4. Various services such as – environmental examinations, programming etc.

It is different to foresee which plants will be admitted to the suburb, but the master plan must consider that all the above mentioned plants may be included in the suburb.

5. Comments on Israel architecture and housing

Presented 1972 to the TAC (Technological Advisory Committee) in Jerusalem

Foreword

Members of the Technological Advisory Committee of the Ministry, of Housing and the Jewish Agency Committee on Housing, were provided with technical data and statistics concerning the present state of building activity and housing in Israel. This activity consumes about 10,000,000 sqm. of land annually, has a decisive influence on the environment and consequently on the people's state of mind. Among different problems of building the housing problem is probably the most important one, from the point of view of effecting the living environment. Housing projects comprise most of the building space in the country. They cover huge areas and they actually determine the urban environment in which we live.

The influence of the architect, or any other individual for that matter, on the forms and character of housing projects is limited. Government offices, local authorities, town planning solutions, development and construction companies, economic interested of building industries, transportation problems and last but not least, public opinion and social conceptions – all these have decisive influence on the nature of housing.

Therefore, all or most residential areas in Israel have – more or less – the same character. That does not mean that it cannot be changed, but it seems to me that this change, which is a must in itself, cannot happen suddenly. It is a gradual process, it should be directed and the different factors should have their right proportions. The committee will miss its target if it does not take into account, while making its recommendations, aspects of the housing problem, other than how to build quicker and cheaper. It will be helpful if we try to view the problem in retrospect.

A Period in Retrospect

The struggle for Israeli architecture began at the end of the nineteenth century with a succession of romantic searching and imitations of oriental styles, which were highly fashionable at the time. The early pioneers took this as a way of identifying themselves with the environment. Later, the third and fourth waves of European immigrants tried to recreate the forms they had known in their native countries. Next came the stage of attempting to imitate the big international trends and Israeli architecture was seen to strike cut, among other things, along the path of functional rationalism.

The newcomers, from different countries and civilizations, confronted the architects with new criteria based on experience gained within the framework of their new home. Such confrontation has been going on since the beginning of the first "Aliya" and is not characteristic of the last generation only. The basic problem was lack of common way of life. New forms of life had to be created out of nothing and in essence the struggle involved much more than actual architecture. It involved the new ways of life. The different experiments that marked these unceasing searches were in most cases by-passed by the requirements of reality and the many frictions have in the meantime been abated by the emergency of new ways of thought; some barriers between different civilizations have fallen. Heterogeneous ways of life found a common denominator, which had to be given a form of expression. Attempts were made to express this synthesis formally. It had to have an appropriate style. Awareness of new values on the part of the people, the leaders, the architects, has enabled certain building and residential areas programs to be worked out. The strenuous efforts of the architects achieved a genuine level of merit when they began to draw inspiration from the creative force of collective enthusiasm. The proclamation of the State in 1948 marked the outset of an entirely new epoch, previously, building programs and had been initiated by various non-governmental organizations. Since the creation of the State, the programs have been made up either by the Government or by other public organization. The major part of the building drive was concentrated on housing for new immigrants and on the creation of new urban and rural centers. The programs for these different centers were started, more or less. According to the master plan for the country's physical development, drawn up soon after the creation of the state by the National Planning Office. The master plan, that initially provided for a population of two millions, became very soon out of date and a new plan was worked out for population distribution at a national level, providing for a population of 3,250,0000. This plan is now outdated as well. Present development does not adhere strictly to the master plan, although it is within the framework of the overall policy of decentralization, that is – dispersal toward thinly inhabited areas. It is worth stressing that one of the essential reasons that make such planning possible is that most land in Israel is state property, thus the Government can make decisions without raising problems of the ownership and can ensure the development of new centers.

New towns have raised during the last decade on previously desolate areas, such as the towns of Arad, Demona, Carmiel etc. In these towns a calculated balance between social infrastructure, employment and transportation development and consequently construction on an appropriate scale, has been reached to a considerable extent. In the large we are witnessing, for the first time in Israel, a process of urban renewal. New buildings are taking the place of the old. This is generally accompanied by an alteration in zoning. Low-standard dwelling make way for hotels, commercial building etc. The three of four stories houses are replaced by high rise buildings. In certain fortunate areas urban planning covers an entire neighborhood. New suburbs in the older towns are a common phenomenon. We are presently witnessing a process of change of scale in building in Israel; the urban and general landscape may be said to be undergoing a metamorphosis. High-speed roads connecting the large towns are being constructed. Here and there interchanges are to be seen, in other words – the landscape known in the highly developed countries, a landscape of traffic axes and bridges, is now establishing its presence in Israel. It is the end of an initial period and the beginning of a new era. It is a turning point in Israeli architecture and housing.

The Challenge

As a result of this diverse activity in the field of development and construction it is evident that in the not-too-distant future, different regions of the country will unite into continuous built-up areas, like the one along the Mediterranean coastal strip, or the one which will connect Jerusalem with Tel Aviv. In other words – we are approaching the well-known, intricate problem of the megalopolis. All this wiII result with the loss of the values of natural landscape and the emergence of man-made environment. The question has more than once been asked: what are the steps to be taken to prevent the cancerous spread of building as a perpetual source of unsolved problem? Have we not left in until too late to control this gigantic process and are we not creation a robot which will turn against its maker?

This is the background of the problem that we have now to confront. At the present time, as district from previous period, it may be said that the tools exists, the opportunities are available and a spiritual climate prevails. It is now our job to grasp the new scale of the country, to fuse the new values, painstakingly acquired, to regroup dispersed efforts and adapt them firmly and faithfully to architecture and housing in Israel. The necessary elements certainly seem to be available.

Shall we meet the challenge and find modes of expression for the creation of LIVING PLACE FOR OUR SOCIETY?

6. Professional education in view of expected social and economic developments

Presented 1974 to the TAC (Technological Advisory Committee) in Jerusalem

Subject No. 1

It is a well-known fact that the only established school of architecture and engineering in Israel is the Hebrew Technion in Haifa. I am prepared to take the risk and say that the school of architecture in the Technion still continues to a certain extent, its professional education along the lines that prevailed during the Bauhaus period. No effort has been put into adjusting the professional training to new demands of our country. The same refers to the training of technicians, draftsmen etc. This situation caused the sporadic formation of many evening schools, some of which are a far cry from any reasonable standard. I think that we reached the point where a second school of architecture is a must. I also think that this new school of architecture (which could be a part of the University of Tel Aviv) has to be oriented more towards town planning and the study of human needs rather than towards technology. We all know that technology is an integral part of the building, but integration of technology in architecture cases to be purpose in itself. Another thing which is an urgent is a foundation of schools for building technicians of high standard. These technicians should fill the gap between the architect and the man on the site. Undoubtedly, our colleagues abroad could be of help to us in achieving this target. But, as much as we need help in this field, we can still share our experience with developing countries

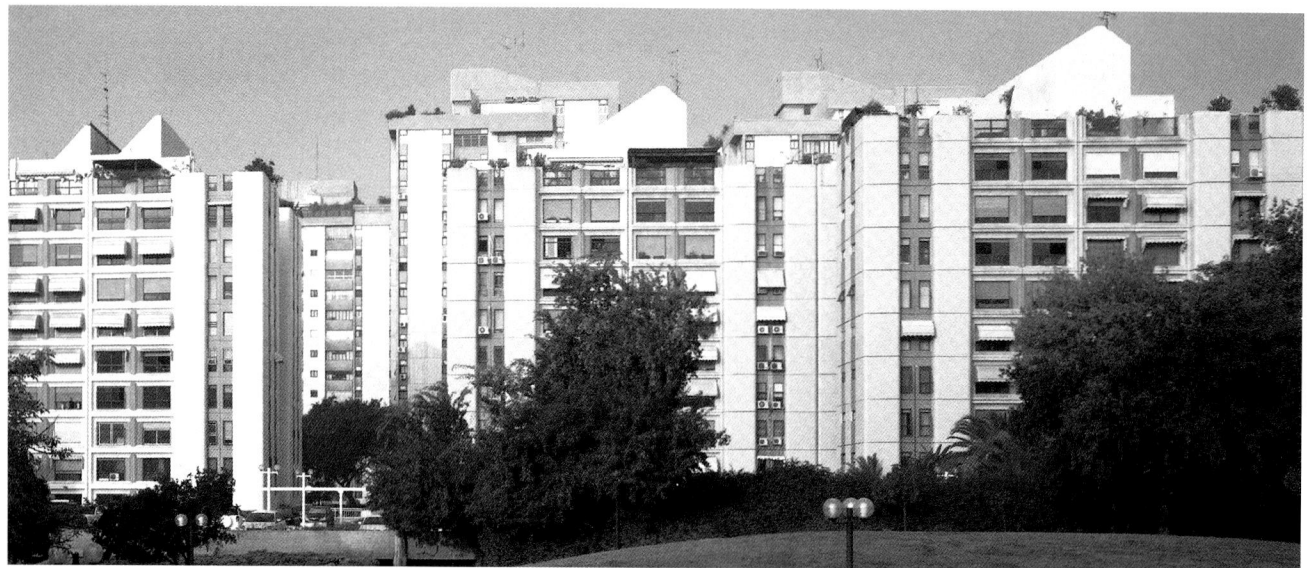

Residential Blocks in Ramat Aviv, 1991

and help them lay the foundations for their professional education, I can tell you from my own experience that when I prepared a report on urbanization for the state of Chad in Central Africa, I could not find a single local person who could help me in my work. The situation was not much different in other African countries where I also did some work for the local governments.

Only the means have changed during the different periods. What are the new means at our disposal? These means are actually, as we mentioned before new way of thinking, How can we combine these powerful means and master the industry without overlooking human needs, landscape and nature, without spoiling the most precious thing we have – space. The problem becomes even more complicated if we take into account that industry takes over the construction field and industry's first necessity is production in series. So it looks as if the only way to solve this problem is to look at it as one intricate project in a scale of our country, at least, (when it applies to organization and components of building) in such a way, that will enable the architect to design the particular site with the freedom necessary to integrate it with the landscape and its occupants. When such time comes we'll surrounded by harmony rather than ugliness. If a new thesis bases on the above mentioned lines will be created, we shall probably abandon old conventions and find ourselves in a new era.

Subject No. 3: Large Extension Towns

The phenomenon, which is well known all over, the wold begins to appear here in Israel. It is especially apparent along the coast strip. Let us be aware of the problem of the human being in this micro-megalopolis, Let us study similar cases abroad and draw the necessary conclusions, before it is too late. Before we are strangled by loops of roads, before we are drowned in sewage, before we are suffocated by polluted air and before the sight of a tree during an hours' ride to work becomes a wonder. I don't know if this forecast for Israel is optimism or pessimism but one thing I know for sure; the situation has not reached this point as yet. This gives us hope and possibilities to avoid this catastrophe. So, let us face it and plan a great city, not only in dimension but also in spirit. Let us think in terms of the beginning of third millennium.

7. Residential development in Israel

Presented 1974 in Jerusalem

I would not merge myself into a detailed description of the planning process of a residential development and into all the difficulties involved in getting the required permits, room the due agencies, in order to make its implementation a feasible one. This subject matter has received the due attention of numerous committees and symposium.

There are several written descriptions of the procedural sequence in getting plans approved and building permits issued. Recently much attention has been devoted to that problem in Israel as well.

The professional Association of Architects and Engineers established a committee, of which I was privileged to be Chairman. The Task force was designated the roll of investigating means by which the length of the period of construction could be shortened, as well as, suggesting channels by which they could be implemented. The Technological Advisory Committee (TAC), after a long examination of the diverse aspects of the legislative procedures and their impact on the final implementation phase, could not avoid joining the general dissatisfaction from the existing process and mechanism. The investigation analyzed past experiences, filtered through the relevant ideas and generated some new ones of its own. All aspects were well defined, correlated and edited as a coherent unit. This report will be available, shortly, for those who are interested in the specifics of the subject.

This is neither the time nor the place to devote any further attention to the causes leading to the present frustration of those involved in the planning process. Let me use this rare opportunity speaking to this distinguished audience to suggest a different planning process and approval mechanism which could be applied to specific residential development. It does not attempt to solve the general problem or to improve the existing procedures but rather to outline a legislative framework upon which the planning process could be built.

Before describing the Proposal itself let me give some relevant words. In many cases a new idea is not a new one and that's the way that things occurred forever. It will suffice to mention by past proposal for community design responsibility to which I kept referring at previous meeting of TAC. I suggested the establishment of a structure in the planning process of the residential environment, in the ambient of which the total responsibility of the community design will be accorded to qualified architect-planner.

Such circumstances did exit in several cases in the past, but was seldom applied up to and missed the required status for good management. The fact that such a process, has been used, in the past, with due successes gives me vigor and strength to continue my burden. I would like to state with satisfaction that after the last meeting of TAC, the Ministry of Housing formed a committee to consider the proposal. After investigating it in depth recommendations were made and some new procedures are already implemented in the course of the design of residential development.

I hope that the results will justify the expectation.

As we can see, a proposal which initially was rejected by the Ministry, of Housing on the podium of this very forum has been proven as an operative one. Hence, a new proposal, a proposal which in essence is not a new one but attempts to legitimize processes which will to now take place as matter of fact. This will apply to development which can be considered as comprehensive planning units and as such with due dimensions. I would like to avoid calibrating a dimension which will vary from one development to another but in all cases will not be smaller than several hundred units. In the planning process of such development many design aspects have to be considered simultaneously, such as: the design of the new urban environment and its compatibility with the existing one, the design of the vehicular and pedestrian movement systems, the designs of the buildings and the dwelling units, the landscaping etc.

All of those have to occur at the same time with the application for the due permits. Over designing any of the above will result in neglecting one of the other aspects and thus lengthening the process. Hence, we should seek for those projects a privileged status well anchored in the legislative framework which will foresee for the comprehensiveness of the design and for a coherent implementation mechanism.

We have to create the notion of "a privileged Planning Development" (PPD). Let is make it clear; we don't seek any special laws but rather suggest that the responsibility of implementing the existing ones could be delegated to the architect. Hence, there will be no need any more to follow the traditional procedures of getting the required licenses and permits. We could create a legislative framework which limits the developer by building codes and restrictions but frees the planning process from the bureaucratic constraints. We suggest that under the special status given to the designer of the PPD the responsibility will be given the architect to ensure and reinforce existing codes as well as to provide all the bureaucratic services required to reach the implementation phase.

This will guarantee not only the continuity and comprehensiveness of the planning process but will secure their very own shortening. I hope that the ministry of Interior will not object a framework according to which "PPO" avoids the very own agencies. Let's face reality, the existing licensing mechanism was built from horizontal layers, which were places one on top of the other, rooted in the Ottoman period, the Mandat era and bearing more recent additions since the foundation of the State of Israel. This machinery was built and addressed to a reality of parcels, properties, and neighboring relationships which could reflect a scenario which relevant. There are too many built-in breaking points within this system, legal time periods, legal objections, etc. The conditions in the new settlements are entirely different. For those we have to create a new procedural and legislative situation which will enable us to accelerate the planning process without harming its very own perfection, a perfection which emerged from a spirit of collaboration of teamwork for the benefit of future residents. Let's face rarity again. Construction has been started on many sites with no permits whatsoever and with a knowledge and approval of all those involved. Are those exceptions or necessities?

Should we adapt the law to reality or bend our backs under outdated procedures? As I already mentioned special procedures were already adapted in the past to meet the needs of specific developments. Let's mention the planning procedures for Developing Settlements. My proposal builds upon past experiences and existing situations which cause a dictated reality, as well as on the analysis of the new conditions which offer entirely different practical opportunities.

The designing of a new residential development is a task which requires an in depth research phase, data collection, the establishment of a structure which permits team work as well as coordination between the consultants. All planning efforts are pushed by a creative idea which assumes its momentum as the design proceeds. One should be able to identify, in the final product comprehensiveness and continuity which will generate the required elements for a well-coordinated implementation.

8. Competition for the design of a residential development summary

Published in December 1974 in the "Engineers and Architects newspaper" Tel Aviv

The Association of Engineers and Architects and the International Technical Cooperation Center sponsored an open conceptual competition for the design of a residential development.

The framework for residential construction evolved through the years, and was modeled by concepts accepted by the public. Most of the construction presently executed, by the Ministry of Housing, the private and public construction companies; it dictated by those establishes schemes. If construction will go on like today, a disaster will occur to the quality of life.

The central problems in designing the residential developments should be seen in the light of the general development of the country. We should find the ways to face future's challenges.

The residential construction, forecasted for the next decade, will change natural landscapes into man-made environment. It will have long range impact on the environment we live in and even on future life patterns. Many architects feel, that they have too little say in the designing of the residential environment, and that too effort was devoted to advance the basic thought of designing it. The competition aims to help advancing the design of residential development and to let the architect express his say. The competition focused on general concepts.

The planner had to face foreseen future challenges, identify the cardinal problems and propose proper solutions. Designing a residential development is a complex problem anywhere in the world. We have, here in Israel, additional problems to solve: demographic, heterogenic population, geographic, political, and the uncertainty about future immigration.

38 architects participated in the competition. 28 of them in the full-scale and 10 in the limited version open to students and architects having up to three years of experience. Efforts were devoted to face today's problems and those of the foreseen future. The proposals emphasized a variety of aspects. They accentuated the problem's dimension and its complexity.

After reviewing the proposals and after long deliberations the jury decided to award four equal prizes, three acquisitions and one honorable mention. In the limited version competition only second prize was awarded. Regarding this competition – the disappointment was great. The association and the school of architecture at the Technion should inquire why, this central problem in Israel, did not capture the young architect's imagination. Each of the four winning proposals dealt with a diverse aspect of designing the residential environment.

We hope that such a competition for the design of the residential environment will not be an isolated event, without follow-up. We should examine, periodically, if the way that the residential areas are built is the right one. We should allocate energy and forces to advance the basic thought in the field of designing residential developments.

We hope that The Ministry of Housing will join the Association of Architects and Engineers and the International Center of Technical Cooperation in a common effort that will turn ideas emerging from the competition into reality.

Project No.7 designed by architects Rachmimov, Havutan in collaboration with A. Avrami, S. Dor, S. Grinshtein. T. Ben Tovim, N. Belson, built a comprehensive framework which could be implemented on various construction sites. The designers learned from local past experience, collected advance thought here and elsewhere, building a coherent conceptual framework, which could contribute to the shaping of residential developments in Israel.

The designers foresee a hierarchical system which has six levels: the flat as the private domain, to which the proposal devoted special attention, the group of flats, the sub-neighborhood, the neighborhood, the quarter and the residential zone. The conceptual framework locates each level in relation to the movement system, designed as a grid connected to major arteries. Options are left open for the development of more avant-garde movement systems as the standard of living increases. The proposed urban unit could be self-sufficient integrated into an existing urban continuity or part of a large urban development plan. Unfortunately, the designers did not reach a convincing urban design when applying their diverse construction prototypes to the urban structure.

Project No, 9, designed by arch, R. – R. Megido, in collaboration with A. Meller, propose a brave but feasible solution for the design of urban spaces. The designers propose high density of construction, the integration of residential units and services and development of urban space within the residential building. Their proposal devotes the dwelling unit to the role of fulfilling the private needs of the inhabitants whereas concentrating the social activity in the urban environment. The structural solution of the high-rise construction is innovative but plausible as well.

The designers focused their efforts and managed to offer a physical expression to an urban quality by shaping the central urban space. The designers foresee a movement network which merges into the urban core, where the main interchange node is located, as well as a ring type artery, around the residential development, along which parking silos and exchanging stations between the express and local system are situated. Their statement that some of the dwelling units' functions will be transferred to urban spaces, is not a convincing one. It also seems hard to implement the proposed movement systems in the foreseen future.

Project No. 16. designed by arch. K. Frank P. Bogod, Y. Luterman, A. Niv-Krandel, proposed an alternative to the existing residential development in dense urban areas, and emphasizes the need to restoring its human dimension. The designers envision the possibility of developing relatively small residential units, on mountain slopes, by inexpensive construction means, and connecting those residential units to the metropolitan core by public transportation modes. This development policy aims to stop the growth of existing cities along the coast, and channel new developments, of moderate scale to mountain slopes, strengthening existing development settlements. The designers' proposal is a departure point in the basic thought on the location and character of future residential areas in Israel, and could be implemented in many places in Israel. This proposal, when implemented, will contribute to a better distribution of the built areas and to the creation of right mutual relation between the individual and the environment we live in.

Proposal No. 23, by arch. AI Mansfeld, D. Gatt, Urbanists, in collaboration with P. Koifman, G. Goor, H. Kehat, proposed a controlled urban development along transportation lines. Directing such urban developments will limit the un-restrained sprawl of built areas. The designers foresee chains of urban units, having a dimension in which the individual and communal needs could be integrated. The growth channels, of the urban units, are composes of residential zones along the transportation lines and confined by open spaces. Such urban unit will allow for good inter-connection and their integration into the metropolitan network. The urban unit builds upon a hierarchy of movement axis, squares, etc. which allow for local pedestrian and vehicular movement. The structure of the proposed residential site builds upon elements that will offer a rich and varied urban landscaping. In the implementation of the design principles, on a residential site, the designers created a good layout around small spaces, creating an impressive urban landscape.

No.1 (acquisition) proposed by arch. Salo Hershman
The focus is on the structure of the residential unit and on the clear movement system, which allows for direct access to each dwelling unit. The assembly of residential units creates an interesting urban entity, which build upon a right hierarchy of spaces.

No.5 (acquisition) proposed by Arch. M. Burman, Y. Goor, in collaboration with B. Frum. The designers emphasize the rapid decrease in free access to natural resource – the beach. The proposal deals with a layout, on a typical longitudinal site designed by the shore and an expressway. Open spaces are left between the built area and the sea. The dwelling units are grouped in three building prototypes: hi-rise linear construction, hi-rise tower and low-rise sprawl. The organization of the building prototypes creates good urban space, with complete grade separation among the vehicular and pedestrian movement systems. Although the hierarchy of movement paths, activity centers etc. is a nice one, the assemble is not a convincing one.

No. 17 (acquisition), by Arch. Robert and Rebecca Oxman from Prof. Idelman's Office. The designer envisions an urban entity of 5,000 dwelling unit. In the core an urban center which connects a number of quarters. Each quarter has its own center with the needed services. Internal roads that cross at the lower grade connect the quarters among themselves and to major arteries. The quarter itself builds from neighboring units that include the public facilities. The basic social interaction occurs at the level of the primary unit, 100 dwelling units each.

No. 24 (honorable mention) by Arch. Nava Rozenfeld, Edna Ishai, Aliza Oko. The essence of the Proposal is a protest against the disconnection between the special requisites of a specific site and the designed residential environment. Even though the competition focused on general principles, without being relevant to a specific site, it is impossible to ignore its character when they are to be implemented on it.

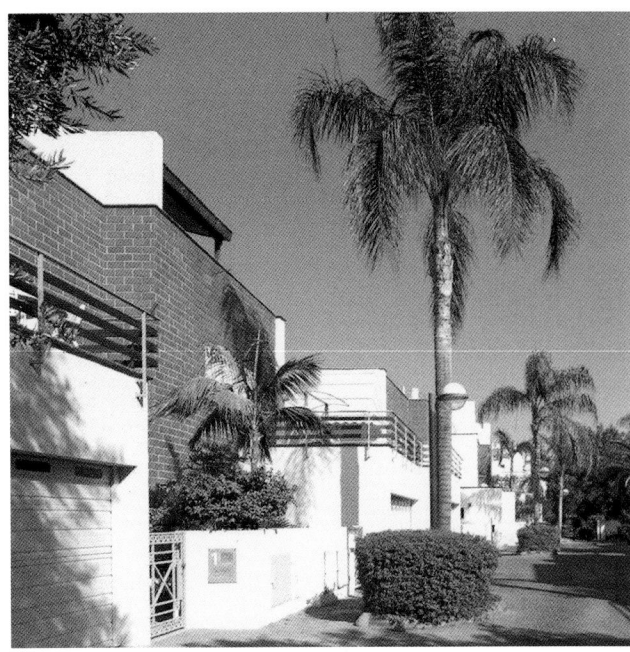

Ramat HaSharon
A residential neighborhood of semi-detached single-family houses between 2 and 3 stories high. The layout is modeled on the Dutch town of "Woonerf". While holding true to the Mediterranean tradition, the houses, in the form of simple cubic volumes, are of modern design. Red brick cladding was used for the façade to establish a local identity.

9. Module beton Israel housing schemes

Presented 1975 to the Ministry of Housing in Jerusalem

The Ministry of Housing in Israel provides housing for various population groups which the government decides to help (new immigrants, young couples, needy families etc.). Some of these housing schemes are carried out by Modul Beton of Israel, mostly in the northern region of Israel. Module Beton of Israel has been operating for the Ministry of Housing for about seven years. During these years Module Beton has built several thousand dwelling units per site. An average housing scheme comprises two to three hundred dwelling units. In most cases the Ministry of Housing prepared the town planning scheme and the site layout, and determines the program for flat type as well as the number of types for the various sites. This is the outcome of the yearly government budget program.

The main concern with the first projects was mastering the new techniques, adapting the Jespersen System to the plans, working out new developments to satisfy Israeli needs and providing the opportunity for teams in the factory and on site to learn the new methods of construction. For these first projects very simple designs were produced. Any complications that may have occurred in more sophisticated designs were avoided. These designs were based on standard deck and wall elements, one type of staircase, limited types of facades and simple arrangements of utilities. These were usually four story row buildings, two flats on cache floor served by one staircase. Then came the second phase (at that time the company was bought out by "Clal" and had undergone many changes and reorganization). In this phase a

variety of new types of flats were designed. Buildings of up to 8 stories – four flats per floor served by a new type of staircase, new façades etc. During this phase studies were focused on the design of the different types of flats. The designs were improved to make maximum use of the restricted given area of the flat for the benefit of the dweller. It was tried to provide plants that would enable families of different backgrounds to lead their life according to their ethnic habits and ways of life.

Now comes the third phase – the developing of a new project based on the acquired experience and on the idea that despite all the above mentioned constraints a system must be provided that will enable planners to create harmonious living environments. This project has been conceived so that certain basic designs may be used in a great number of combinations, resulting in varieties of buildings and their groupings. This overcomes the monotony which is usually inevitable in free-standing buildings. The program dictated by the ministry of Housing requires five types of flats (2 to rooms), and calls for a strictly predetermined area of each type of flat. Therefore the basic designs are five types of flats and two types of vertical transportation cores (staircases and lifts). The common denominator of the flats is that any chosen two, three or four flats can be arranged around either of the two types of vertical cores, and that all flats can be arranged to form continuous buildings. The possible building shapes are determined by the number of floor combinations. This project aims to create the greatest variety of spaces using the smallest number of elements. This system has been experimented with for the past few month and new possibilities are being discovered. The great number of feasible combinations results in a built-in flexibility which enable the planner to design each site according to its specific features. This design system allows complete freedom for the creative mind and the opportunity to create a great variety of spaces. It provides the planner with the necessary tools for achieving his ultimate goal – the erection of a living environment that can be happy with.

10. Community design responsibility

Prepared 1974 for the Second Symposium of the Joint Technology Advisory Committee of the Ministry of Housing and the Jewish Agency Committee on Housing

The object of this provocative introduction is to open discussion on a key problem concurring the physical planning of residential areas.

The influence of the architect, or any other individual for that matter, on the form and character of housing project in Israel is limited. In most cases there is no architect in charge of the design of the project, coordinating it from beginning to end. There are too many people involved. Every planner is responsible for a certain phase of the design.

Let us briefly describe the present situation for our overseas members, and follow the typical design procedure of a residential area in Israel.

After a decision has been taken by the Ministry of Housing, or any other developer, to create a new community, a Town Planning Scheme is prepared by the Ministry of Housing or by an architect and town planner. Today, it is a document that arbitrarily defines zones, density, public spaces, sites for public buildings, etc., along with a so-called "buildings layout plan". This plan is a part of the Town Planning Scheme but sometimes it is entrusted to another architect who has to follow the approver Town Planning Scheme in order to avoid new negotiations with the Regional Town Planning Committee. "The building layout plan" defines the shapes of the various buildings, their dimensions and their heights. Now an architect is commissioned to plan the buildings if "typical plans" are not used. This architect is responsible for the design of the buildings, and his plans are used as contract documents between the developer

and the contractor. In some cases the architect works directly for the contracting firm. The public buildings in the community are usually designed by other architects. Very often "typical plans" are used without giving much thought as to whether they fit the particular site or not. Public open spaces are designed by landscape architects, pedestrian networks and roads by road engineers. Their plans are based on information supplied by the various architects concerned. One can define the as horizontally split responsibility.

Among these various architects, coordinators are hard put to coordinate the different designs. This puzzle or mosaic of plans is in the best cases mechanically fitted designs. It can never be an architectural entity, a result of a creative mind.

There are too many designers and no one is really responsible for the overall design of the community in question. This procedure brought into being many residential areas. Most of these communities remind me the story of Shalom Aleichem which starts like this: "I came to a 'Shtatel' where all buildings 'shteit in droisen' (stand outside). This compounding of phases of design, searching each other to make an overall community design, resulted in de-humanization and anonymity, leaving its mark on the end product.

I have described a typical procedure, under control of the Ministry of housing. In other areas under control of local authorities of private developers the situation is even worse. An area is parceled up and different architects are commissioned to design the buildings, each responsible for his own particular site. One can see the outcome all over the country. These are lost cases. Buildings are clustered to form defense masses of built-up areas. The arbitrary shapeless spaces in-between buildings are "left-overs". Nobody pays attention to the organization of the spaces forming the streets. How can we, in the Seventies repeat this kind of failure and reproduce such unsightly residential areas?

The first move towards a better design procedure would be to commission one architect planner to design the

11. Proposal for the 1975/78 triennial activities of the U.I.A

Proposed by the Israeli Section

community to be planned. Let him be solely responsible for the design from the beginning to the end. In every architectural job there is a responsible architect, why can't this be the case here too? He would be in a position to study the demands of his client, the specific features of the site, its landscape, topography, its character, climate and existing facts. He would be able to study and master the technology of the building system to be used on this site. He would be able to consider all these factors, weigh up their importance and assign them their right priorities in determining the design.

When submitting his Town panning Scheme he will have certain ideas at the back of his mind, and the legal documents will cover these. Thus the procedure would see reversed. The Town Planning Scheme is finalized after the project has been conceiver.

Before concluding I wish to raise one more point. Good community design can be based on any building technology. It is my belief, and I hope that this committee will back me that there is no contradiction between the need to build quicker, using disciplined industrialized sophisticated systems and the aspiration to build better houses, functionally and aesthetically. The architect responsible for the project will have the option to express the beauty of these modern systems.

To achieve this goal we have to take the first by recommending that total responsibility of the community design be accorded to a qualified architect planner.

I have described a rather grim picture. There are exceptions, of course – examples of good planning. However, I have intentionally emphasized this aspect in order to bring about a fruitful discussion.

Planning with Scarce Resources

Mr. Chairman! Fellow Colleagues,

As part of the next triennial activities we propose to focus on the topic of planning with scarce resources.

Our era is characterized by the dynamic changes that occur all over the globe in the well-being and welfare of human kind. The past years could be characterized by the speed that those changes occurred and by the recognition that resources on earth are of limited nature.

The emergency of a diversity of life styles, in the last decades, originated quite a variety of urbanization patterns, each of which dependent, at a different extent, on a wide range of services. To provide those services, great amount of energy under multiple forms are required. Presently, when resources became, scarce new and more efficient ways of propelling our cities are to be found and urban areas have to be designed accordingly. The architect's creative mind should team with the engineer's technical know-how to design buildings, which make use of clean and available resources of energy, which are abundant of unlimited nature and free for the use of all.

We propose that the UIA working groups in the discussion of their specific topic would devote much attention and care to the use of human and natural resources. The reports should provide us with guidelines for planning with scarce resources.

12. On modernization of hospitals in urban areas

The I.H.F., Tokyo Congress, U.I.A. – Public Health Group –
May 1977

Meir Hospital Case, Israel

The basic problem in rationalizing the layout of the medical services is to convince the client that one has to bring the suitable medical personal to the patient, in the right medical service, and not to scatter the patients in different wings which are often built as a result of pressure by a noted medical personality.

Doctors, department heads, administrators and head nurses have great influence, very often, on the size of the department and on its location within the hospital. These influencing factors are changeable. When there are new medical developments in supply and service methods, or when there are staff changes bringing different outlooks on operating methods, the planned hospital structure faces such strong pressures that there is hardly any administrative power that can prevent changes and adjustments in the building. This process refers especially to the medical and supply services. These services comprise about two thirds of the building's area. From the moment that this process begins there exists a danger of general deterioration up to a loss of the building's image. Rooms and departments have a different function than originally designated. Each corner or space is being "occupied" for different needs, by those adjoining these spaces. Changes are made. These changes are usually done unprofessionally. Many disruptions are created in the traffic routes. Valuable property deteriorated and facilities are not functioning properly. Danger of contamination increases. Suffering of the patients increases, and so does the tension of the medical staff. This process also damages the medical work, costs a fortune and causes anguish to all those involved. Every effort must be made to prevent such a process. There is no simple answer to the question of how we can prevent it. There is no doubt that the problem is connected with administrative problems, with the programmatic structure of the medical institutions, and with many other problems that should not be discussed here.

We shale only deal with the projection of his problem on the planning of the medical institution, or rather what is the impact of the fast changing requirements and the phenomenon described above on the thinking of modernization of an existing hospital.

The "life span" of the building is much longer than a reasonable service period of department heads and greater than a time period of a certain working system. Therefore changes in the building cannot be avoided when the time comes.

The mind must be directed to this problem while conceiving the preliminary planning of the medical institution. The basic structure of the plan should form the "skeleton" and foundation of the traffic routes, passages, main supply system, etc. The basic plan must allow for growth and enlargement. The basic structure must have dimensions that are acceptable now and in the foreseeable future. The layout of the department of the medical institution must allow additions without harming the main idea of the institution's concept.

While conceiving rationalization and reorganization of an existing hospital and while thinking of modernization of its structure, one has to replan the institute and reestablish a new route system. In other words, one

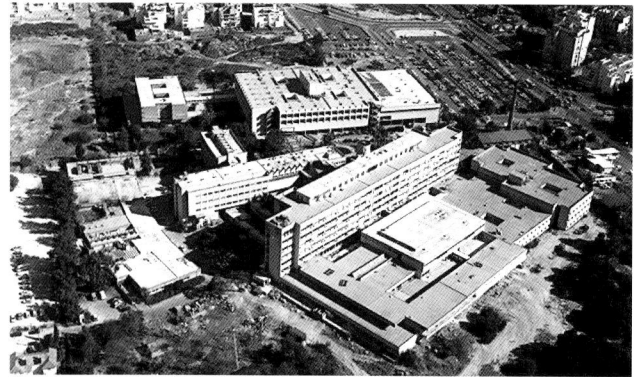

Meir Medical Center, general view

has to reconceive a comprehensive master plan based on far-sighted requirements. It seems that the general guidelines in planning a hospital include two directives opposing one another. The first directive says – plan each department specifically to suit its function; plan it for specific jobs – as described by expert, but plan it in a manner so that it will be able to function properly even with a change in working methods. We have to mention here that different medical expert very seldom agree with one another. Therefore, a ward of medical service should not be planned to suit one personality. All medical and supply departments should be planned in such a way, that future options of various ways of operation are left open. The other directive says – plan as universally as possible, so that you will not be "stuck" after a short period (sometimes before the building has been completed). Or in other words, plan the wards and the departments with a common denominator dictated by the general concept of the building so that in each department, changes and extensions can be made independently of the other departments. Creating a common denominator means: planning based on preferred modules, planning modules, functional modules, structural modules, mechanical modules, etc.; repeated use of facades and openings; "open-end" planning of departments that can expand, etc., and site-plan layout that allows for future growth, based on the pre-set principles. Planning principles impose no limitations on

design freedom. They bring order and discipline – they are a good tool. They serve as guidelines upon which design can be based and from which architectural creation can emerge.

We have to emphasize here the importance of the master plan. This plan forms the outline upon which the hospital plan is built. With the passing of time different wards and wings change their interior divisions or even their designation, while the main traffic axes exist, usually, for the lifetime of the institution. This traffic axes system grows and branches during the years, yet it is very difficult to change the location of the vertical and horizontal traffic axes. In other words, it is difficult to change the concept and the principles of planning after they have been set. Hence the master plan is decisive importance. The master plan of the hospital defines the main traffic routes, the location of the various buildings or wings, the connections between them and the direction of the institution's expansion in its various stages. To simplify the problem, there are five main categories of functions to be considered:

1. Hospitalization services.
2. Medical services.
3. Administrative services and miscellaneous.
4. Supply services.
5. Outpatient department.

It is understandable that in reality there are many exceptions to this division and it is presented hare only to enable discussions of the desirable connections between these categories of the various wings.

As already stated, the least changing of the hospital wings is the inpatient department. The demands for alterations in this wing are small in comparison with that of medical and supply services, where the changes and expansions are more frequent. However, in hospitalization services, the inpatient department repeats itself several times. This fact enables the planner to locate the inpatient departments on top of each other without special complications. The result is a building block of several stories. Vertical traffic cores connect the floors. In the medical services there is an advantage in having horizontal connections because of the attachment of various services to one another, and the attachment of certain medical services to the casualty department (in emergency cases). As mentioned above, changes and additions in the medical and supply services are frequent, and therefore the advantage of having them to the ground floor is great.

It is necessary that the visitor's passage from the main entrance to the hospitalization services will not cross the route system of the medical services. It is desirable that food and medical supplies will reach the various departments without having to cross too many of the traffic axes of the medical services. It is necessary to create a scheme, an infrastructure flexible and universal, that will be good and usable and will withstand the changes occurring in the working systems in the various services.

The horizontal system pattern chosen for the main traffic axes in the medical services floor depends upon the specific conditions of the case, the geometry and topography of the site, the specific program, etc. In any case, simplicity and clarity of the scheme must be achieved. We can compare this problem to a town-planning problem on a small scale. The traffic flows in the traffic routes, while the traffic to the various departments branches as into "cul-de-sac". It seems that there are two systems of traffic axes – the vertical one of the inpatient services, and the horizontal one of the medical and supplies services.

The relationship of these systems to one another creates, actually, the "skeleton" of the master plan. The horizontal system can be a main "road" and "side-road" perpendicular to it, or, a system of two parallel main roads and perpendicular "side-roads". These are examples of "linear" solutions that enable us to start construction in the first phase on a small scale, and then expand and enlarge the complex according to a pre-set principle.

13. Aspects of the modernization and existing health and hospital-care facilities in Israel

Warsaw 1981

Background

The collective effort began at the turn of the century, when doctors, architects and others dealing with medical administration were few, performing their job pioneering spirit, as did other pioneers at the time. They worked in those days under very stringent conditions, and only their inner strength enable them to carry on. Over the years the tools have improved and the few became many. Organization was established. Many medical institutions were built. Some of them had developed, but usually their development was not anticipated by their founders. Reality was the strongest factor.

Serious planning and construction of health services and hospitals only really commenced towards the end of the first decade of the existence of the State of Israel. At present, after three decades of planning medical institutions, being in constant contact with medical, administrative, and technical staff, following-up life in hospitals, and comparing facts that have materialized against preliminary planning of these institutions – all these have led me to the thought, that Modernization of exiting Health and Hospital Care facilities, creating or rather recreating the proper physical environment and preserving the values that prevailed in the past will be our main concern in the near future.

Some of the problems we face are of international nature, common to all countries. Other groups of problems which manifest themselves in hospital design in Israel are specific to the country.

These include actual dispersal of population and anticipation of population increase, limited budgets, coordination with local authorities, political pressure such as may be exerted by local inhabitants, problems of national security, particularly with regard to border settlements, national characters customs and population attitudes, all play their part in coloring the overall picture.

What is the core of the problem? We face now in some of our existing institutions the Danger of Physical Deterioration. The "modus operandi" of the medical services is based on acceptable methods and is influenced by the outlook of the client or operator of the hospital. When there are new advances in methods of supply and medical services changes in the planned hospital structure become inevitable.

These changes usually affect the building's physical image. From the moment that this process begins, there exists a danger of general deterioration up to a complete loss of the building's appearance. Rooms and department take on functions other than those originally designated.

The areas being altered, tent to take on a temporary and disorderly appearance. Traffic routes are disrupted. The attitude of the staff, patients and visitors to the building becomes one of disregard.

Valuable property deteriorates and facilities do not function properly. Danger of contamination increases as does the suffering of the patients and the tension of the medical staff. The end result is the relocation of division, so that the shape of the built-up area is altered until it is impossible to recognize the original plan. This process also impairs the medical work, is extremely costly and causes anguish to all those involved.

A follow-up of these developments in various hospital and medical facilities indicates that not enough was done to prevent this deterioration. There is no doubt that the problem is connected with administrative difficulties. The programmatic structure of the medical institutions and with other problems is not discussed here.

We shall deal only with three main aspects of this problem:
1. Allowance for changes and additions.
2. The "joint services" concept.
3. The master plan of the health and hospital care facility.

Allowance for changes and additions
The "life span" of the building is much longer than the reasonable service period of a departmental head and then the duration of a certain working system. Therefore changes in the building cannot be avoided as advances in methods of medical and supply services occur.

Attention must be given to his problem during the preliminary planning of the medical institution. The basic plan must allow for growth and enlargement. The structure must have dimensions that are acceptable both at the time of the plan's inception and in the foreseeable future.

14. Living environment based on a comprehensive pre-cast concrete building system

Warsaw, may 1981

In existing hospitals we must face the challenge of contemporary needs and allow for changes and additions without harming the main design concept of the institution.

The "joint services" concept

Hospital equipment is often technologically sophisticated and also extremely expensive. Finding suitable staff to operate such equipment is a perpetual they have been set. Hence the master plan is of decisive importance to the physical appearance and environment of the hospital. In existing plants we have to resist any pressure put on us and keeps the main features of the institute's master plan unharmed. At the same time we have not only to modernize the hospital but also strive for its humanization.

Conclusion

Hospital design is both: complex and intricate, demanding a mature approach to a problem that is both technical and cultural. The essence of culture is the relationship between man and his fellow man and between man and his environment. The architect is creating an environment in which the patient often undergoes a critical period in his / her live. The patient may be greatly influenced by this environment, which, if it is a positive one, can contribute to the patient's recovery, or at least prevent unnecessary suffering.

Thus, along with mastery of complex functional problems, a principal challenge for the architect is to create an optimum relationship between the physical environment and the patient.

This paper describes a living environment project based on a comprehensive pre-cast concrete building system. The dwelling units are geared to recognized behavioral patterns of new immigrant and middle-income Israelis, the envisioned dwellers in this environment. Identity, privacy and individuality will be achieved through a unique design developed specifically for the building site.

The components of the building system will be produced in large series and assembled according to a rigid set of rules whose special rhythm and language are based on production constraints and erection patterns. Apartments are assembled around a standard staircase core, within a changing multi-story structure, thus creating a continuous environment and offering a variety of living spaces. Harmony will emerge from a design in which the proposed system is adapted to the inherent characteristics of the site and where the future dweller will find his own identity expressed.

The project has been conceived so that certain basic designs may be used in a great number of combinations, resulting in varieties of buildings and their groupings. This overcomes the monotony, which is usually inevitable in free-standing "block" buildings.

The basic designs comprise 5 types of flats (X1, X2, X3, X4, X5) and 2 types of vertical transportation cores.

The common denominator of the flats is that any chosen two, three or four flats can be arranged around either of the two types of vertical cores, and that all flats can be arranged to form continuous buildings. The possible building shapes are determined by the number of floor combinations.

Our aim in this project is to create the greatest variety of spaces using the smallest number of elements.

As a demonstration, let us examine how many arrangements of these 5 types of flats can be found in a typical floor of an H-shaped building, based on the assumption that we take into account the feasible arrangements, and that for this purpose, mirror-imaged flats are of the same type.

1. If the floor is made up of one type of flat we have:

X1 X1 X2   X2 .... X5
X1 X1 X2   X2 .... X5

5 possible floor arrangements

2. If the floor is made up of 2 types of flats we have:
In the case of 2 flats of each type

X1 X1   X1 X2   X1 X2
X2 X2   X1 X2   X2 X1

3 arrangements

In case of 1 flat of X1 and 3 flats of X2

X1 X2
X2 X2

1 arrangement

In the case of 1 flat of X2 and 3 flats of X1

X2 X1
X1 X1

1 arrangement

Thus for 2 chosen types we have 5 possible floor arrangements.
Number of possibilities to choose 2 out of 5 is:

$$\frac{5}{2} = \frac{5}{2!.\,3!} = \frac{5 \cdot 4}{2} = 10$$

i. e. Altogether we have 5 X 10 = 50 possible floor arrangements

3. If the floor is made up of 3 different types of flats we have:

In the case of 2 of X1, 1 of X2 of X3

X1 X1   X1 X2   X1 X2
X2 X3   X1 X3   X3 X1

3 arrangements

In the case of 2 of X2, 1 of X1, 1 of X3

3 arrangements

In the case of 2 of X3, 1 of X1, 1 of X2

3 arrangements

For 3 chosen types we have 9 possible arrangements.

Number of possibilities to choose 3 out of 5 is:

$$\frac{5}{3} = \frac{5!}{3!\,.\,2!} \quad \frac{5 \cdot 4}{2} = 10 \text{ possible arrangements}$$

i. e. Altogether we have 9 X 10 = 90 possible arrangements

4. If the floor is made up of 4 different types of flats we have:

X1 X2
X3 X4

4 arrangements

Number of possibilities to choose 4 out of 5 is:

$$\frac{5}{4} = \frac{5!}{4!\,.\,1!}$$

i.e. Altogether we have 5 x 4 = 20 possible floor arrangements

The total number of possible floor arrangements is:
5 + 50 + 90 + 20 = 165

This was an analysis of only one case – a typical floor of an H-shaped building.

We have been experimenting with this system for the past few years and keep discovering new possibilities. The great number of feasible combinations results in a built-in flexibility, which enable the planner to design each site according to its specific features. This design system allows complete freedom for the creative mind and the opportunity to create a great variety of spaces. It provides the planner with the necessary tools for achieving his ultimate goal – the creation of all environment in which people can enjoy living.

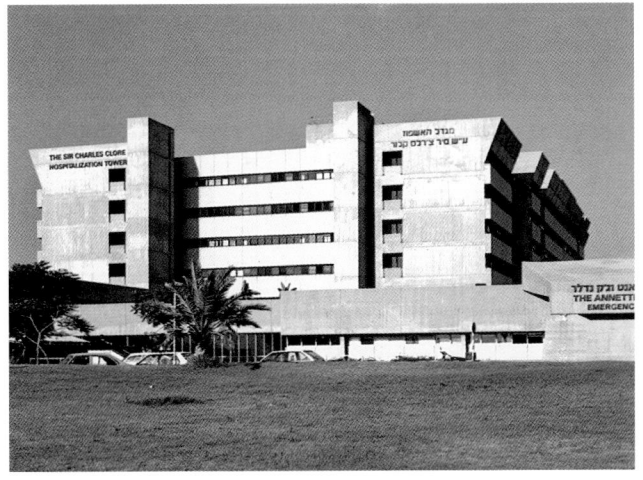

Clinical and Research Laboratories

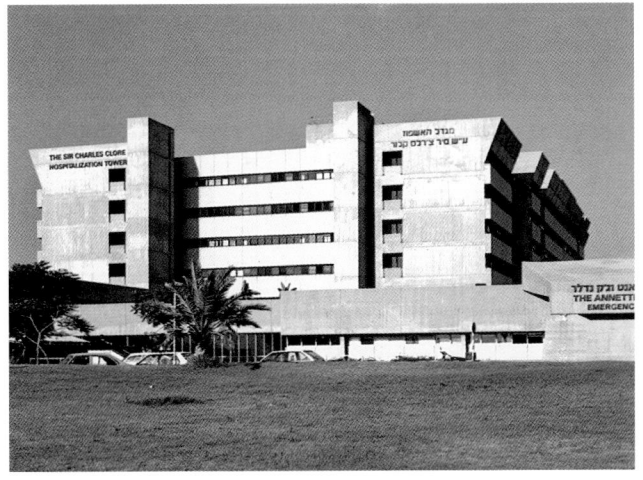

Sheba Medical Center

15. Planning, building and organization of medical research facilities – Three developments in Israel

In: World Hospitals, Vol. XVII, No.2, May 1981

1. New Laboratory wing. Chaim Sheba Medical Center (Tel Hashomer), Ramat Gan

The Chaim Sheba Medical Center (Tel Hashomer) is the Israeli Government's largest center hospital. It has been functioning since Statehood in 1948, in the military barracks which served as a hospital during World War II. Recently, the construction of a new hospital, which is Part of the Chaim Sheba Medical Center, was begun. In the first stage it will house all the medical services. The complex is being erected on a site adjoining one, and is planned for approximately 1,000 beds. The general composition of the hospital buildings is arranged around a main east-west axis (the spine) which is also the axis for the wards, with secondary axes (the ribs) housing the health and maintenance services. The scheme permits the complex to be planned so that each wing can be enlarged independently if necessary. A new laboratory wing has been designed based on the following philosophy. In most hospitals in Israel, routine work on samples taken from patient and research work, lire carried on side by side. For the planner, there is no difference between the shape of routine and research laboratories. The area required for routine laboratory work depends mainly on the volume of work, which is a function of the number of beds and outpatient clinics in the hospital. The research laboratory area depends entirely on the extent of the research carried out at the hospital. In recent years the relative size of the laboratory department within the overall area of the hospital has increased.

Our experience shows that it would be a mistake to plan a laboratory department without allowing for its increase. The laboratory department must be able to be enlarged without reference to other hospital departments. In addition to the routine and research laboratories, some hospital contains a sub-department for radio-active isotopes and radiation services for therapeutic purposes. Also, an animal house is sometimes attached to the laboratory department, for tests and experimental surgery. Taking into consideration the need for constant updating of working methods and instrumentation, and the rapid development of scientific working methods, as well as changes in composition of staff and the subjects of work and research, a plan was devised which permits internal changes to be made by the maintenance staff, without requiring basis changes in the structure of the building, The design which has been proven effective is based on uniform, modular, two-stage planning of the entire area of the laboratory department.

According to this philosophy, the entire area of the laboratory should be planned uniformly, without regard to purpose. The exception to the rule is specific areas for radio-active isotopes, glassware washing and other services common to all the laboratories. The planning is bases on a fixed, standardized laboratories module. First-stage planning includes the construction and main supply systems, without reference to divisions according to purpose. In this stage, the entire invariant planning components are laid down. These components include the structural system of the building, the system of external openings and sometimes the passages and main internal opening. Also, the first stage includes the main supply and waste disposal systems.

The actual building work can be carried out according to the plans prepared in this stage. The first planning stage should be undertaken without the cooperation of scientists. In the second stage, the purposes and details of the area, the furnishings or the laboratories and the functional supplies to the laboratories are planned. This planning can only be effected with the full cooperation of the scientists. Generally the second stage of the planning proceeds while the building operations of the first planning stage are being carried out, according to the rule: "design as you build".

Planning the laboratory department according to this philosophy requires considerable experience, since the first stage must be designed in such a manner that the second stage can be completed without running into complications. The first-stage planning must take into account most of the data on uses of the area, and the type of supply and waste disposal systems to be used. The decisions taken in this stage will determine the options of the second-stage planning.

The uniform planning of the laboratory areas are, as we have seen, based on a fixed module. This module is determined according to an analysis of the operations to be carried out in the laboratory unit. In our experience, the axial width obtained from the job analysis concerned is 3.20–3.60 m. This is confined by actual working conditions. The "depth" of the modular laboratory is given by the conditions prescribed by the division or the area and by reasonable proportions relating to the movements or the workers in the laboratory unit. Experience shows, that in dividing the laboratory areas according to purposes, it is often necessary to provide for areas smaller than the modular units. These areas are assigned for the "laboratory office" or for small special-purpose laboratories.

In large laboratory departments, there is a tendency for section heads to concentrate the equipment, needed for their work, in their departments. This trend is particularly marked in research laboratories. Such equipment can generally be used by several sections or even the entire laboratory department. The concentration and installation of such equipment in a manner enabling it to serve all the sections which need it, results in a working system and a distribution of areas according to purpose based on the "joint services" principle.

The joint service may be of a pure service nature, like washing and sterilizing of glassware, or of such a sophisticated nature as electron microscopy. The planning of the department's work according to this principle occasionally meets with resistance on the part of the scientists. The designer of the department must take the possibility of centralized services into account, even if the scientists do not agree to it to begin with. Scientific equipment is becoming more expensive and complicated by the year. Work in a laboratory department which is not based on centralized serviced results in duplication of equipment and inadequate use of the equipment acquired. Without any doubt the day will come when it will be practically impossible to supply expensive laboratory equipment to each separate section. Moreover, there is the question of specialization in the use and maintenance of such equipment. Centralization of equipment makes it possible to make better use of this equipment. Planning the work of the laboratory department according to the "joint services" principle permits each scientist to make the maximum use of the equipment available to the department; experience shows that this is not the case in departments where the expensive equipment is located by the different sections and the section heads in charge of it.

Decision on the system of supplies and waste removal are extremely important. To all practical intents, they determine most of the data characterizing the laboratory department as to possibilities of dividing the area according to purposes. One may say that these initial decisions lay down the "rules of the game" for planning the laboratory area. There are several possible solutions for the provision of supply systems; each has its own advantages and disadvantages. The choice of a given solution depends on different aspects of the project concerned.

From the preceding discussions it seems that the general guideline in planning a hospital laboratory department includes two contradictory directives. One says – plan to suit its function; plan it for specific jobs – as described by experts. (We should mention here that experts seldom agree with one another). The other directive says – plan as universally as possible, so that you will not be "stuck" after a short period (sometimes before the building has been completed). Or in other words, plan the laboratory department with a common denominator dictated by the general concept of the building. To eliminate the seeming contradiction, it should he pointed out that the specific case (planning to suit function) is only one case among many other possibilities. Creating a common denominator means: planning based on preferred modules; planning modules, functional modules, structural modules, mechanical modules, etc. Planning principles impose no limitations on design freedom. They bring order and discipline – they are a good tool. They serve as guidelines upon which design can be based and from which architectural creation call emerge.

Construction of the laboratory wing of the Chaim Sheba Medical Center, according to the philosophy and principles outlined above, is now underway and several departments are already functioning. We hope that the building will be completed within the next year, when the results of this philosophy can then be judged.

2. Institute of life Science, Hebrew University, Jerusalem

The Institute of Life Science is located in the Givat Ram campus of the Hebrew University in Jerusalem. The building was commissioned with the intention of consolidating five biology departments, which previously had been scattered throughout Jerusalem. These include: Biochemistry, Genetics, Physiology, etc. The building comprises an area of about 23,000 square meters with provision for future expansion, such as the development of new departments, as well as the physical expansion of the existing departments.

The master plan was conceived as a complex of interconnected wings woven together according to their respective functions. A "warp and woof" pattern allows for continuous spaces and variation in size of the areas allotted 10 the different disciplines. This type of pattern provides for great flexibility, with completeness at every stage. The use of the entire area falls into four categories: Research

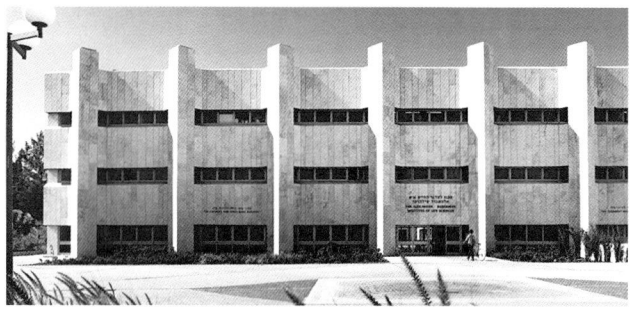
Institute of life Science, Hebrew University, Jerusalem
Main fassade

Laboratories; lecture Halls, Library and administration; Teaching Laboratories; and Services and Maintenance. Each wing of the Research Laboratories has its respective teaching laboratory at ground level for second-year studies on wards. Lecture Hall Library and Administration have been grouped together on both sides of an arcade linking the northern and southern entrances which lead off to the various wings. The arched has been visualized as a meeting place for research personnel and students, providing opportunity for exchange of ideas. Maximum flexibility has been achieved in the Research Laboratories by locating them in a continuous space, to be subdivided as necessary, with direct access to the arcade and the various wings. The Service and Maintenance areas are located on the lower ground level and are reached by a service road. This level is directly connected to the different wings by vertical shafts, lifts and staircases. The structure is of reinforced concrete, part which was cast in suit, and part of which was pre-cast in the form of large beams, mass produces, and assembled on site. The intersections of the "warp and woof" pattern of the building form structure cores, spanned in the east-west direction by deep beams cast in situ. Large pre-cast beams have provision for housing the slabs that in turn span them, eliminating the need for scaffolding during construction.

The outer walls form the "shell" of the building, which remains constant. The inner spaces that it contains are flexible-adaptable according to different functions and programme requirements. The shell also includes spaces to house the sophisticated electromechanical systems forming an integral part of the building. These are logically conducted from basement plant room to the various parts of the building via a basement service tunnel, vertical cores and horizontal ducts. This unique type of structure is flexible, economical and saves construction time, while answering complex functional demands made by a building of this nature. The Institute of Life Sciences was recently completed and is now in use.

3. Laboratory Animal Breeding Center, Weizmann Institute of Science, Rehovot

The laboratory Animals Breeding Center is situated within the Weizmann Institute complex, on a sloping site bounded by streets on the south and west. The building was conceived as a simple envelope, enclosing four distinct and predefined zones. These are: a small animal wing (for breeding mice, rats and hamsters), a large animal wing (for breeding rabbits, guinea pigs. etc.), a specific Pathogen-Free Unit, and a Diagnostic Laboratory wing. It was necessary to provide for traffic flow between "clean" and "unclean" areas, and moreover, these areas had to be isolated from one another. We were faced with the additional problem of joint use of various services, such as food and bedding supplies, cage washing in the different areas, etc.

The building was designed on two levels. Technical areas are located on the lower level, as are staff change rooms, toilet facilities and cafeteria. All productive functions are carried out on the upper level. Each of the four sections of the building; are self-contained with distinct traffic routes. In addition, the small animal wing and the large animal wing are sub-divided into "clean" and " unclean" areas, with a one-way traffic system conducting the movement of materials. Air-conditioning, ventilation, plumbing and electricity systems likewise follow the clear-cut separation of functions.

The building has been used successfully for several years now.

16. The precast concrete industry and the environment

10th International Congress of the Precast Industry
Bibm, Jerusalem, september 1981

Ladies and Gentlemen,
dear Friends,
I am going to talk about living environment project, based on a comprehensive precast concrete building system.

As architects and town planners, our ultimate goal is to design and carryout living environments. These usually consist of a neighborhood, a living zone, living quarters – or whichever name you want to use. The character of the environment in which people live has a strong effect on their life.

Here in Jerusalem, from the time of the British Mandate, a city by-law dictates a stone-faced building. It gives a feeling of permanence, as if to say: it will stay forever.

There is a saying that Tel Aviv has been built temporarily, until we have the time to build it. A certain story by Shalom Aleichem starts with the words:
"I came to small town, where all the houses are standing outside" (Alle Häuser stehen draussen).

In these 3 examples I meant to expose certain characters of living environment in concise foam, like permanence as against temporary.

A living environment is created by out-door spaces, landscaping, bridling materials, repetition of details, colors, and something which is very difficult to define but has to do with the basic feeling of the human being. The shape of the neighborhood is an outcome of a town-planning scheme, nearby network of roads, city zoning, climatic conditions, etc. For each neighborhood a list of requirements is dictated by the client – in most cases the Ministry of Housing, in other cases major building companies of promoters. We call this list of requirements – a Program.

What we understand in the word "Program" for given neighborhood is the total number flats types of flats and in certain cases instructions for arrangements of flats in buildings. Type of flats are decided in the Ministry of Housing, according to immigration forecast, urban renewal programs, national budget allocation for this project, political pressure, local authorities pressure and so on.

We architects and town planners don't have a say in this matter. Our task is urban planning and design of the building of the given neighborhood. We have to give the proper answer to this site. Our work is carried out team-work, in which take part community workers, statuary official planning committees, engineers, road and traffic engineers, landscape architects and other consultants in specify fields like foundations or energy conservation.

Let me start with a few words about the building material

We are dealing here with precuts concrete elements. It is a very good building material, if properly insulated to avoid cold bridges, if properly assembled and connected, and properly face-treated.

From the rather shod period of about 20 years of experience with precast elements, we have confidence that deterioration will not occur. It is much better than plastered buildings. Perhaps they don't age as gracefully stone-faces building, but they keep their performance for a long period of time.

Our system can be carried out only with this kind of cast in moulds building material in the shape of elements, and call be achieved only in technologically developed countries, highly mechanized and administratively sophisticated. This system has the properties of being easily computerized for design purposes and on-site execution.

Now back to the neighborhood.

To create a living environment is a complex problem.

I am going to concentrate only on the problems connected with precuts concrete industry, and the living environment.

From the living environment designer's point of view, we strive for variety of shape, specific design per neighborhood, maximum fulfillment of given conditions of the given site, which are: Geographic location, sloping or flat land, direction of nice views, special character of the zone, the given program for this site, avoidance of anonymity, and so on. During the designing period the dweller is anonymous. He is actually represented by the designer. The wish of the individual dweller is to have a certain corner of his own. So his slogan will be: individuality and privacy, but yet belonging to a community. This community must have a self-identity of its own.

From the viewpoint of the producer of precast elements, identity of elements-large series of production of the same elements – is required for efficiency, cost cutting and confinement of budget. So we have 2 opposing view-points: variety of the end products on one hand, and identity of dements to be produced on the other hand. Our air in this project was to satisfy the 2 goals, without sacrificing one for the other.

Specific urban planning for a given site must he the outcome of the specific conditions of this site. Our project is geared to flexibility in urban planning and building design, based on a limited number of precast concrete elements.

Just for the sake of being clear, let's arrange the urban design components in this hierarchy:
· The neighborhood,
· The cluster,
· The building,
· and the flat.

The Neighborhood in Israel usually consists of a few hundred of flats, with public garden, playground for children, parking lots, public building like kinder-garden, synagogue and some shops or a shopping center.

The Cluster is comprised of a number of buildings arranged to form a sub-neighborhood, a group of buildings.

The Building is a number of flats arranged around a transportation core. It is usually a legal unit, registered in the Land Registry Bureau as a condominium. The dwellers share the same vertical transportation core, and have to take care of their building.

The Flat is the home of the dweller, – in most cases owned by him.

To achieve flexibility in urban planning, we used the well- known mathematical phenomenon that with a limited number of components, a large of combinations is possible.

In my abstract I demonstrated that in the basic designs composed of 5 types of flats and 2 types of vertical transportation cores – there are 165 possible arrangements of flats in a building. For the on-looker, actually there are unlimited possible arrangements, as far as the view appearance is concerned.

While for the plant, for the producer, there are only 5 types of flats and 2 types of transportation cores, the number of elements to be produced for these 5 flats is limited to 62.

A large number of arraignments is possible, because the design is such that any fall can be served in any position of layout by the same vertical transportation core, and any type of flat has the fixed depth, so the result that any arrangement of flats around a stair-case can form a building, and any building can match other buildings to form a cluster.

The end result is, that unlimited configuration possibilities of building arrangements is feasible. We have to choose the appropriate one for the given site, according to the specific site conditions and the specific program for the given site.

So the right urban layout is achieved with a limited number of precast elements. The great number of feasible combinations results in built-in flexibility, which enables the planner to design each site according to its specific features.

This design system allows complete freedom for the creative mind, and the opportunity to create a great variety of spaces. It provides the planner with the necessary tools for achieving his ultimate goal in the erection of a living environment, in which people can enjoy living.

But precondition is: long-range plants, so that enough time is given to study the optimum production plan, in order to cut the cost and raise the quality. In this respect of a long-range production plan, we depend totally on government authorities. We must understand that modern sophisticated industry has a lot of possibilities, but it must match with proper administrative understanding.

I want to use this opportunity and call upon responsible Israeli Government Authorities, to study our building industry possibilities and use its potential for the benefit of the people, by making administrative decisions based on long-range plans.

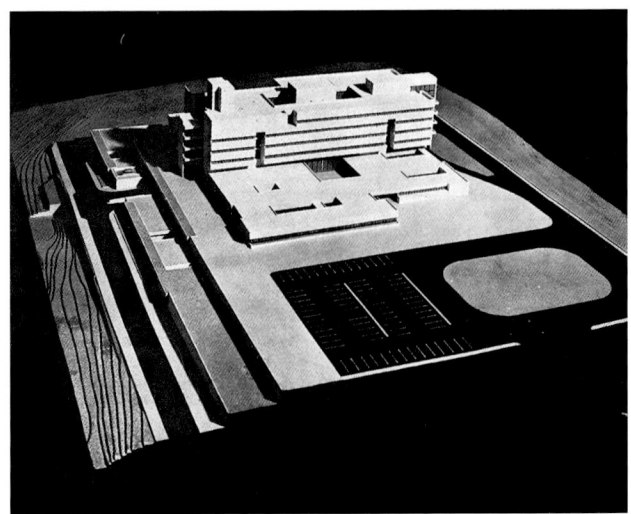

The Safed Government Hospital –
The Rebecca Sieff Government Hospital
View from North-east, model

17. The balanced hospital concept

23rd international hospital congress, Lausanne 1983

Design for Efficiency, Economiy and Humanity

This title refers to hospitals designed to operate, be developed and extended on balance. Three examples of operating hospitals, a regional, a metropolitan and a central hospital, in various stages of their realization, are described:

Rebecca Ziv Hospital – Safed, is a regional general hospital, built to provide medical services to the Upper Galilee. First phase realized, comprising the entire infrastructure, 250 beds with their relevant services, is operating efficiently. The second phase, extension of certain department, is under construction.

Sapir Medical Center – Kfar-Saba, a metropolitan general hospital, is built to provide medical services to the population of the Sharon Valley. For the last two decades, extensions and developments are realized in phases, each one designed according to the balanced hospital concept.

Chaim Sheba Medical Center – Ramat-Gan, is conceived as the largest governmental medical Center in Israel.

The master plan of this new vast center is designed to be realized in definite stages. First stage, the infra-structure and the medical, subdivided into specific departments, are realized and operated one by one. They serve the wards houses in existing barracks. First hospitalization block, containing about 700 beds, is under construction. The balanced hospital concept is a practical method, implemented in the design of hospitals of considerable size under constant pressure of development and extensions. It is based on quantitative break-down of economic constraints and efficiency directives and organizes the carrying out of the project in definite phases. The method results in striking a balance in finding the middle-course among the various factors and leads to harmony of design and proportion.

18. Future hospital design

International Public Health Seminar, Budapest, 1985

Introduction

The design of hospitals in the future in different parts of the world can be discussed only in general terms, due to the great variations in conditions from continent to continent, from region to region. There are, however, a multitude of factors influencing design that are common to all countries. Studying data available to us today can provide a basis on which to consider, and, one hopes even to predict, the shape of future hospital design. Thus, instead of looking into a crystal ball and trying to decipher plans of the hospitals of tomorrow, we must identify and examine today's parameters that may serve as indicators of future developments in hospital design under different conditions.

Representing the Community

Let us begin with a basic assumption: hospitals are a creation of the society they serve. We, architects, hospital designers, should play a major role in hospitals construction by serving as representatives of the community. It is our responsibility to identify trends and foresee developments in society; to contribute to their final outcome as much as possible.

The actual features of hospitals design in the future will reflect the myriad of factors impacting on the development of a particular society. We can, by identifying trends, assist in the process of shaping the hospital of the future. We can have an impact on the policy makers and planners. As the Hebrew proverb states: all is foreseen and choice is given. Thus, the two crucial questions are:

1. What are these trends or factors; and
2. Where do we want to direct or lead future hospital design?

Let us examine some major factors that affect all societies and thereby their future hospital designs; namely, cultural heritage, international and national health planning for the future, the revolution of hospital technologies, social tasks and the futuristic approach.

Cultural Heritage

Hospitals have served their communities ever since they came into being. In past centuries, hospital filled a multitude of functions: asylum, orphanage, foundling home, poorhouse, and, of course, a place where sick people were treated. In the course of time, like religious building and town halls, they became national monuments.

In the service of their community, hospitals in every ear have reflected the social, cultural, economic, political, psychological and spiritual milieu. They have done so in the past and will do so in the future.

The evolution of the hospital building pattern reflects the changes that have taken place in the societies thy served. A brief glimpse at the morphology of the hospital in the western world in this millennium will reveal an uninterrupted evolution of physical environment and related building patterns.

In the early centuries of his millennium, the hospital was an integral part of a religious edifice. It must be understood, within the context, that "medical treatment was inadequate and communications with God was more urgent than with doctors". Here are some examples: the Aisle Hall and Aisles Chapel, the cruciform shape, the radial pattern of more than four spokes, the pavilion Hospital, the Wing-Building, the "Superstructure" and lower floors composition.

These are steps in the evolution demonstrating the relationship between the building pattern and the characteristic of the epoch in which it was erected. The last pattern became possible only with developments in technology, including air conditioning.

Each country has its own cultural heritage. The hospital designer must recognize the importance of the influence of his country's cultural heritage on the evolution of hospitals in the future.

Future International Health Planning

Future hospital design must be considered in the light of the international health planning for the future. The most widely recognized plan of this type is the well known "health for all by the year 2000" – a goal set by the WHO. About 160 governments and many other non-governmental organizations are engaged in implementing this goal. It received recognition in the declaration of Alma-Ata. Most of the resolutions of the plan are related to the prevention of disease by improvements in sanitary conditions and other means, and to the development of primary care systems and follow-up procedures.

The fundamental policies for health for all, in concise form, are as follows:

1. Health is a basic human right.
2. Distribution of resources and accessibility to all people.
3. Participation of people in planning.
4. Governmental responsibility for implementation.
5. National self-reliance and international solidarity and help for execution.
6. Cooperation and coordination of all social and economic sectors.
7. Complete use of international resources.

Let us look at some indicators concerning this plan. World population stands at today at around 4.5 billion. It will be about 6 billion in year 2000. The main increase will be in the developing countries.

Health and related socioeconomic indicators are – infant mortality, life expectancy, birth weight, coverage by safe water supply, adult literacy rate, GNP per capita, public expenditure on health per capita – they are all health and related socioeconomic indicators. Each one of us can examine where his country "stands" in regard to these and estimate their impact on his country's future hospital design.

Health manpower is related directly to total area in square of health care facilities. If health for all is to be realized (and we hope it will) one can calculate the increase of health care facilities coverage needed.

Age structure and urban and rural balance of population are starting points for estimating characteristics of the health care facilities needed.

Primary health care systems are cornerstones of the "health for all" plan. This is especially so in developing countries, but, according to the Bordeaux Conference, their importance has also been recognized for industrialized countries.

Dr. H. Mahler, Director General of WHO in his lecture in Lausanne in 1983 defined the role of hospitals in the overall "Health for all by the year 2000" movement. He examined the problem in and its principles. We must be up-to-date in our thinking, or we shall be caught unprepared.

Revolutionary Developments in Hospital Technology

Other important factors are the revolutionary developments that have taken place in medicine; the evolution of new diagnostic and therapeutic methods; new medical instrumentation and technology; advances in methods of organization; innovations in micro-electronic data processing and communication; new medical supply services; electro-mechanical systems and energy conservation.

We must not only foresee and estimate future progress in terms of time; we must study the nature of the coming changes and be aware of their possible shifts in direction. In general, we can say that developments in technologies related to hospital equipment, industrialization and the commercialization of functions have been very rapid in the last two decades and will gain momentum in the next two becoming independent industries. Such industries supply ready-to-use material-disposable or reprocessed. One must also take into account the tremendous rise in costs associated with these rapid developments.

Social Tasks

Recent changes in hospital developments may require hospitals to fill new tasks and functions in the community, in accordance with national and international health plans. The rising costs of health services, and the consequent closing of hospital doors to the less fortunate economic sectors, may create public opinion that will direct hospitals to new social missions responsive to the needs and demands of the coming generation. Dr. H. Mahler defined the social missions of the hospital. He said, among other things, that these will include: „Developing and protecting health in the community through education and other ways; promoting those factors in people and their environment that protect their health; controlling those factors that damage it; integration or close coordination with the overall health services". How will these social missions affect hospital design?

The new social functions of education, the training of staff for community health programmes, the constant contact with the regional primary health care system, medical research oriented to solve immediate problems of health in the community and other social tasks will have their influence on the hospital's list of requirements and consequently on the hospital's design.

There is another social task that we must consider – that of the architect, the designer, to express the needs of the society for health care; to give architectural expression to the spirit of the new era. This is our social task.

Futuristic Approach

A futuristic approach – imagination and innovation are not contradictory to all that has been said here. They are an integral part of evolution. They put progress in motion. They hinder passivity and stagnation. We architects are expected to seek novelties. We sometimes become the "enfant terrible" of the design team. Risks and prospects are well known, as are the bitter feeling of failure and the joy of the highly praised success.

Recent developments in life sciences, in genetic and bio-engineering, in the science of conception, in sterile and clean room techniques, in micro-electronics, communications, data-processing and data storing, in managerial and organizational methods and in environmental psychology-all these and other new technologies will be harnessed to fill clinical and research requirements. They will certainly have their impact on future hospital design. I can see the hospital of tomorrow. It will fulfill the practical and expressive requirements of the people of the era. People in need of medical aid will cross the threshold of a laboratory-like building. They will be semi-conscious. They will be examined by neo-invasive diagnostic equipment. Results will be registered and patients directed to pass through healing apparatus, from which they will emerge conscious and healthy. If necessary, a medical team will perform a painless organ transplant or replace worn out limbs. Science fiction? Some of these procedures are already on their way. Perhaps the hospital of tomorrow will have a decidedly more human-oriented feeling to it. This, by the way, is much harder to achieve than the "science-fiction" type of scenario I have just described. Perhaps tomorrow's hospital will be designed with people in mind. A patient whose sickness cannot be prevented will penetrate this new healing edifice. Pre-treatment, performed by psychological or bioengineering techniques will ensure his curative state of mind. He will be in a place that conforms to his everyday life, his habits, his cultural background. He will feel at home.

It is up to the creative mind of the designer to draw architectural conclusions. It is up to him to integrate all components into a balanced harmonious complex. It is up to him to utilize all the ingredients to create a physical environment.

19. Hospital design in the computer era

The 10th International Public Health Seminar (Ihps), (1984)
Tel Aviv, 1986

Conclusion

Future hospital design must be looked at in the right context. Is the context that of the "Health for All by the Year 2000" plan formulated by WHO? Or is the context that of the "present and future missions of the architect" in the hospital building team? We must draw our conclusions taking into account some clear trends. These are:

The general consensus that it is a basic human right to receive a satisfactory level of health care; the conviction that we are approaching a "Health for All" era; the implementation of Health for All plans on international, national, regional and local equipment installed in new modern facilities will solve the health problems of the rapidly growing population of the world.

We, architects, hospital designers, must make a thorough study of international, national and local future health plans, and strategies for their implementation. We must draw conclusions concerning the design of health care facilities.

I am aware that my paper raises more questions than it answers. But, if each of us will ask the right questions to the project on his drawing board, a project of any character or magnitude – be it a primary care center, remodeling or extending an exquisite building, adding a new wing or constructing a brand new hospital – he will be able to examine the problem in its proper context.

He will have the opportunity to shape future planning and create a physical environment suitable to the requirements of time and place, and he will have the opportunity to contribute with his creativity. He will be able to express the spirit and state of mind that brought about his solutions and creation.

The Ninth International Public Health Seminar which took place in Budapest about two years ago traced the long history of hospital architecture. We have seen outstanding examples of hospital architecture created during great eras of human history. They reflected the practical and expensive needs of their time.

The typical cross form hospital of the late Middle Ages and the Renaissance, like Santa Cruz hospital in Toledo, built at the turn of the fifteenth century, expressed the belief in God more than in medicine. All beds face the altar and patients hoped for celestial intervention for their healing.

The growing trust in human wisdom and human ability was clearly and openly stated in the Secular large scale Baroque architecture, at the Greenwich Hospital created at the beginning of the 17th century by Christopher Wren and others.

Change of values during the industrial revolution in the 19th century and the fast development of science and technology in the 20th century were all reflected and expressed in hospital architecture of the relevant era.

The need for hospital beds after the Second World War, the scientific and medical development, the new technical possibility and the inexpensive energy brought about the huge compact hospital blocks of the fifties and the sixties. Some call them the atrocities of the sixties, where the patient has the feeling of being a very small cog in a large machine. Antiestablishment movement and public feelings of disappointment in this kind of architecture called for "human scale" in hospital architecture.

The lesson of the past is very clear: Health and hospital care facilities, being the creation of the society they serve, reflect the needs and the spirits of their eras. The question is whether the fast-paces technological movement in modern biology, microelectronics, computers, robotics, automation, sophisticated information and telecommunication systems is just a mechanical improvement or will it bring with it change of values?

We have to ask ourselves whether use of computers and informatics in working places, agriculture, industry, administration, air traffic, tourism, medicine, health and hospital care facilities is just an evolutionary step in the process of development or a revolutionary pace towards different ways of life and a change of human state of mind.

Nowadays, food can be produced by a fraction of the population. More and more people are travelling by air and surface means of transportation. Working hours are shortened. This progress could be achieved only through revolutionary inventions of the human mind. Research, industry, production, management, administration and other related fields connected with these new developments are undergoing revolutionary changes.

New building forms are development, so as to withstand and cope with the new technologies. These types of buildings are designed to ensure not only accommodation of today's technology but to be adaptable enough to cope with future developments. Cost involved in creating this type of intelligent or "smart-buildings" are justified by the possibility or matching the premises for present needs and unforeseen methods with new technical system, thus, building life-span is longer.

In these buildings intelligent environment is created with almost no building constraints on functional lay out. They are easy to service and maintain. Office buildings, too, are undergoing great changes. Information and telecommunication technology radically alters the way working spaces and their organizational patterns are used.

We can even visualize a scenario where administrative work, done today in office building, will in the coming generation, be carried out by individuals at home. With the existence of advanced information and communication systems what is the necessity to move people, create traffic jams, build buildings, and consume energy? Thus, the need for a building to work in is eliminated. Some will say: How can work be performed without human contact? Who knows? Time will tell.

What is the impact of these innovations on future hospital architecture? What is the relevance of introducing comprehensive integrated communication network in health and hospital care facility to its design? New techniques in diagnostic methods and medical treatment will change the layout of most medical services.

Computerizing functions of supply services will dictate their planning. Implementation of computerized new equipment in the laboratory wing will transform the conventional laboratory modules into a plant-like space. Design of the imaging division will have to cope with the new "smart" equipment. The swelling storage for patient' files will disappear altogether. The medical record department will be paper free.

Almost all hospital departments will change their design criteria. Computerization also changed many parameters of programming, design and construction processes. Computerized hospitalization database made health care facility programming and calculating number of beds required, much more reliable.

Introduction of computer aided design, in architectural and engineering offices, changed conventional planning procedures, shortened time needs for production of drawing, enabled storage of huge amount of design information in few tapes or disks.

Preparation of bid-packages, comprised of building specification, bill of quantities and cost estimates became a neat and much faster operation in the computer era. Implementation of computer aided design made the building more efficient and opened new possibilities. In the field of electro-mechanical systems in hospitals and energy conservation, use of computers became very instrumental. As we have seen, computerization had its impact on the design and operation of almost every hospital department.

Let us have a closer look at a key problem: The impact of modern integrated information and communication network on the hospital Master plan. Flow of hospital information in hospital is demonstrated by J. Simpson in his article "Brave New Tools" in simple diagrams. Flow of information among different units is complex.

In order to create an overall database scheme, or a "fully Automated Hospital Information System" (AHIS), certain procedures treating components of information must be standardized.

Discussing different aspects of comprehensive hospital information network, including transmission of voice, data and video is beyond the scope of this paper "Health and Hospital care facilities are information oriented and dependant on communication among the different operational units."

There is no doubt that implementation of up-to-date hospital information and communication system will change design criteria and Master Plan considerations. It will have its impact on the hospital organizational pattern and consequently on the well-known "functional-free" dictating the main lines of the hospital's Master Plan. The Master plan, or as it is called sometimes: The development control plan, defines the main traffic routes, the location of the various buildings or wings, the connection between them and the direction of the institution's expansion in its various stages. This plan forms the outline upon which the hospital plan is built. With the passing of time, different wards change their interior divisions or even their designation, while the main traffic axes exist, usually, for the lifetime of the institution.

Considerations and decisions on the hospital's Master Plan are dependant on the desired proximity of the various departments, on patient's and personnel routes, on supply and refuse methods, on the organizational and managerial methods and mainly on the available information system. With the changing of these considerations, decision on the Master Plan will be different.

Impact of computerization and implementation of up-to-date information network on departmental plan is mentioned. Virtually every department is affected by these innovations. Impact of this new development on the Master Plan of the Health and Hospital care facility is discussed. We can expect, this time, a mutation rather than evaluation in hospital planning and operation. We believe that we, architects, have to keep pace with these new developments.

The goal of this development is to provide every human being with health services in an environment where his individuality is preserved and human digital prevails. This goal is neither the religious belief of the Renaissance nor the Sense of drama and monumentality of the Baroque. But it is the spirit of our era and as such it should be expressed in a new concept of hospital architecture.

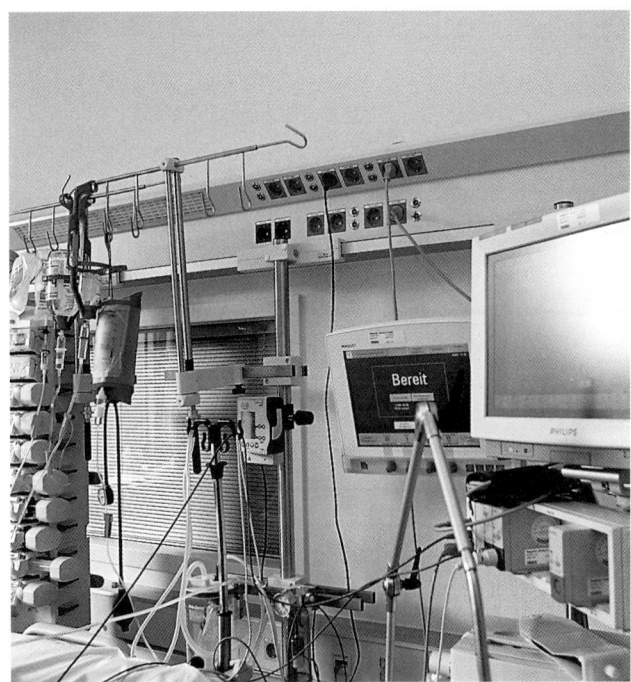

Completely digitalized ICU bedplace

20. Israel – In view of the W.H.O. strategy "Health for all by the Year 2000"

U.I.A P.H.G. XI. International Public Health Seminar, September 1988, Moscow

Preamble

This paper aims to briefly describe Israel's system of hospital and health care facilities relevant to the W.H.O. indicators. It begins with data about the country; its geography, climate, flora and fauna, followed by socio-demographic data, cultural heritage, and information on Israel's economy. Health expenditure data shows some figures connected with the prevailing health system in view of the W.H.O. strategy, "Health for All by the Year 2000". It concludes with some notions on the design of health care facilities and suggestions for further development in designing and maintaining hospital and health care facilities in Israel. The data about the country is cited from official statistics and publications.

Geography

Israel is located on the eastern sea-border of the Mediterranean Sea. Its fertile maritime plain runs parallel to the shore, skirting the Carmel range, extending along the verdant Sharon Valley, and then continuing to the lowlands – merging into the Northern Negev. Parallel to the coast, a range of hills descents from 4,000 feet above sea level in Upper Gallilee through the highlands to the mountains of Hebron.

The Great Rift, which is an extraordinary split in the earth's crust, begins beyond the sources of the River Jordan, extends south-ward through the Sea of Galilee and the Jordan Valley and continues to the Dead Sea – the lowest point on earth, approximately 1,300 feet below sea level. The rift runs south into the Red Sea and Africa. Israel has a land area of 20,500 sq.km.

Climate

For so small a country, Israel displays drastic variations of climate. The coastal plain and inland mountains surrounding Jerusalem enjoy a climate of hot, dry summers and mild, humid winters. The mountains are wetter and colder than the plain, and sometimes have snowfalls. The steeps to the south have a drier climate giving way to semi-desert in the northern Negev. The most southern sector is extreme desert, a rocky and inhospitable region where temperatures can reach a high of 45 degrees C. It is difficult to state the average annual rainfall for there are great variations. While northern Israel enjoys over: 12 inches of rain each year, the amount decreases as one travels south, until in Eilat it is barely I inch.

Flora

The geographic position of the Land of Israel, the variegated structure of its soil, its changing climate, its proximity to the sea, on the one hand, and to the desert on the other – have all contributed to the vegetation rich in genera and species. The land of Israel boasts more than 2,000 species of plants, some of them endemic, others typical to the Mediterranean region, and still others to be found in places as distant as Iran, the heart of Asia, the Sahara Desert and Sudan in Africa. Israel exports a great variety of cultivated agricultural products such as oranges, tropical fruits, flowers and other types of agricultural goods. The limiting factors are water and the irrigation network. Israeli research and development in agriculture fields is very advanced.

Fauna

Each region in the Land of Israel has its characteristic wild life. The deer are to be found in some areas;

in fact "Land of the Deer" is a name which has often been used to denote the land of Israel. The mountain goat lives in the wilderness of Judea and in the bare, rocky mountains around Eilat. Fox and jackal roam the country in large numbers. The habitat of the wild boar is in the swampy regions, and, as these are drained, their number dwindles. There are also many snakes, lizards, mice and other rodents harmful to crops. Birds around particularly when they pass over in northward and southward migrations. Domesticated animals named in the Bible, such as donkeys, camels and sheep can still he found. Livestock, kept on farm using up to date technology, consists mainly of cattle, sheep and poultry. Fish are farmed in artificial ponds.

The People

Variety reigns in Israel not only in the natural conditions but also in terms of the heterogeneous population. Of Israel's just over 4 million inhabitants, the majorities are Jews, with a considerable Muslim minority and smaller Christian and Druze populations. The Jewish population itself consists of people of diverse origins: 60% are Israeli born – nicknamed "Sabra", after the sweet, prickly fruit of the common cactus; the remainder having emigrated from Europe, Africa, Asia, the Americas and Australia. In a country with such a diverse population it is not surprising to find a rich cultural heritage, which plays an important part in the local context, having an impact on health care facilities' design pattern. Primary education between the ages of 6 and 15 is free and compulsory, explaining the considerable drop in illiteracy rates. Secondary and higher education meets international standards. In the cultural scene there is flourishing activity in music, performing arts, literature and the visual arts.

Cultural Heritage

The land of Israel is the cradle of the three great monotheistic religions. Israel is the well spring of the Bible.

Five thousand years of constant habitation, together with its biblical association, have made Jerusalem a unique and special city. It has always been an important junction – a meeting place not only of roads, but also of cultures from north, south, east and west. In Jerusalem one can find the main holy sites of the three religions in close proximity: The Basilica of the Holy Sepulchre; The Western Wall; and The Dome of the Rock. On the slope of The Mount of Olives is the Russian Church of St. Mary Magdalene. All cultures throughout history have maintained some form of water system. The two Roman aqueducts of Caesarea were built in the time of Herod, while the National Water Carrier, constructed by the State of Israel, today pumps water from the sea of Galilee in the north to the arid Negev in the south.

Economy

At the turn of the century, the era of immigration to Israel of the first settlers, newcomers worked mainly in farming, drying swamps, improving the soil and developing agriculture. At present Israel is self-sufficient in terms of food and even exports agricultural products to other countries. However, the economy in Israel is based mainly on industry, advancing towards sophisticated industrial products. Tourism is also an important part of the Israeli economy. The Gross Domestic Product in 1986 was 35 billion dollars, $ 8,750 per capita. This data classified Israel not as a developing country but as a developed country.

Expenditure on Health

The national expenditure on health as a percent of the Gross Domestic Product continues to grow.
The data specific here compares the health expenditure in I952 with that of 1986. The amount divided between hospitals at 43.3% and primary care centers at 32.0% is financed by the public, the government, sick fund and other non-profit organizations. Only a small part is financed directly by private bodies.

The Health System (relevant to W.H.O indicators)

In order to describe the infrastructure of the health system, some background data on population density is required. One should take into account the increase of density in the recent decades. Shown here is the density in 1920 and in 1970. The average housing density has increased while the percentage of families living in density of 3 or more persons per room has decreased. The data concerning life expectancy of male and female compares 1949 to 1985 clearly indicates the improvement in the condition of life. The statistics of the survivors at specified ages out of 1,000 persons born alive, gives a more specific comparison. The improvement of health condition is clearly reflected in the statistics concerning the infant mortality (per 1,000 birth), in born Muslim and Jewish populations, which compares 1955 to 1986. Another detail of statistic providing essential data the system of health care facilities consists of a "net-work" of primary care centers, provincial hospitals, metropolitan hospitals and central hospitals. Medical research takes place in most of the central and metropolitan hospitals. The basic research occurs mostly in universities and at the Weizmann Institute.

Throughout the years, there has been a considerable increase in the total number of hospital beds. This total is divided mainly into general beds and those for mental and chronic diseases. The ownership of hospitals is divided principally between the government, sick funds and other non-profit organization. Only a small number of beds belong to private owners. The data indicates clearly that the majority of hospitals are owned by the public number of beds per 1,000 persons has grown considerable from 1948 to 1986.

The major tendency concerning duration of stay is to shorten the duration and transfer as many patients as possible to an ambulatory treatment in clinics and specialized institute. This tendency has a significant impact on hospital design. The average duration, which has gone down from 1960 to 1986, is still considered too high and should be brought down.

The common calculation in the past had been that a third of the built-up urea in " given hospital was allocated for hospitalization, a third for medical services and the remaining third for supply services and other functions. In the hospitals the space allocation has changed. Some of the space previously used for hospitalization and supply services has been given over to medical services, out-patient departments and institutes.

The Design of Health Care Facilities

In Israel, as elsewhere, design of health care facilities is a collective creation of those who take an active part in the design process and the population at large. Many factors in influence the outcome of the design effort; local conditions such as geography, climate, eating habits, socio-demographic data, economy, cultural heritage, experience gained in operating the existing health care facilities and many other factors which will not be enumerated here. The creation of an Israeli concept of at the turn of the century when doctors and others dealing with medical administration worked under stringent conditions, as did other pioneers of that era. Over the years the tolls have been improved and the few in number have become many. Medical institutions have been built, with each successive generation an improvement over the fast. A general design concept of an Israeli health care facility was created, based on actual multilateral realities. The figures and statistics mentioned here briefly describe some facts connected with the health system in Israel. We architects and hospital designers have to be particularly sensitive to the human aspects of hospital design.

We have to find design solutions suited to the individual human being in a country with a heterogeneous population, a crossroad of cultures, constant political turbulence, economic constrains and an everlasting confrontation of ideologies.

Conclusion and suggestions

Statistics provided in this paper and the Israeli data

relevant to the W.H.O. indicators appear to be satisfactory. Throughout the short history of Israel there has been a consistent improvement in the state of health. This is, however, no reason to become complacent. In a country of contradictions such as Israel, the statistics cannot reflect the disadvantage groups of the population which still need improvement in their state of health. One should have in mind that the Suffering of a single human being couldn't be helped by a satisfactory data of statistics. One should worry especially since public medicine, which has always been dominant in Israel, is at present under turbulence, while private medicine is developing and gnawing at the public medicine, which aims to provide for the disadvantaged. On the other hand, the whole system of health care facilities, which was established in the last three decades, has reached the stage in which strengthening and maintenance have become the dominant problems. This is a problem the authorities still haven't learned to overcome. In a country with so many needs and problems there always seen to be more urgent matters. The system which was established through the hard work of three or four generations of health planners, architects and the sweat and tears of the public is threatened by the danger of erosion. If matters will not he treated in time, the situation in the future will not improve but rather deteriorate. We architects of health care facilities, who took such great part in establishing the infrastructure, have to be especially aware of this subject. We should act as much as possible in order to influence the local authorities to protect the existing infrastructure, renew it and keep it up to date with development and progress in technology and science. Keeping in pace is possible mainly through interactions, meetings and conferences like the one being held here today, which brought us all together. This seminar, it is suggested, should give its recognition to the view that hospitals and health care facilities are of national public interest and should be preserved maintained, and protected by law for the benefit of the people they serve.

THE 12 INDICATORS Adopted by W.H.O. – 34th assembly 1981 – Section VII par 6	
W.H.O. INDICATORS	ISRAEL RELEVANT DATA
1. The lawful right for health for every human being.	Population is covered by insurance organization.
2. People's involvement in National Health Policy.	Through the mechanism of democracy.
3. Minimum of 5 % of G.N.P. for health expenditure.	7.9 %
4. A reasonable percentage of health expenditure for local use.	Needs improvement.
5. Even dispersion of resources.	Most resources invested in populated areas.
6. Aid of he rich countries to the poor countries.	Human resources aid to developing countries.
7. Primary care facilities for the use of every human being.	Almost full coverage.
8. Weight of 2.5 kg. For 90 % of newborns.	95 %
9. Infant mortality of the disadvantaged groups less than 50 / 1000.	11 / 1000
10. Life expectancy over 60 years.	74.8
11. Literacy rate is over 70 %.	93.5 % (1986)
12. G.N.P. per capita is over $ 500	U.S.$ 8,750.

Economy	
1986 Gross Domestic Product	35 Billion U.S. Dollars
	$ 8,750 – per capita

National Expenditure on Health		
By percentages of G.N.P.	1962	5.5%
out of total expenditure	1986	7.9%
For General Hospital		43.3%
For primary Care Centers		30.0%

National Expenditure on Health and its Financing		
Percentages by financing sector	1973	1985
Govern. and Local auth.	28.2	23.2
Sick Funds	39.7	44.2
Non Profit Org.	11.4	11.9
Others	20.7	20.7

Infant Mortality (out of 1,000 births)		
	Muslims	Jews
1955	60.6	38.8
1986	18.0	44.2

Natural Increase of Population (per 1000)		
	Muslims	Jews
1955	38.3	24.5
1986	30.4	13.7

Number of Beds in Hospital by Type of Beds		
	1948	1986
Grand Total	4,626	27,420
Type of bed		
General	2,681	11,927
Tuberculosis	623	20
Mental diseases	1,197	7,670
Chronic diseases	-	7,308
Rehabilitation	125	495

Hospitals by Ownership		
	1948	1986
Total Institution	66	50
Public	35	90
Private hospitals*	31	60

*Generally of small number of beds

Beds in Hospitals (rate of 1000 persons)		
	1948	1986
Total	5.31	6.33
General Care	3.08	2.75

Average Duration of Stay in Hospital by Type of Bed		
	1960	1986
Total	18.6	12.6
General care	9.0	5.3
Tuberculosis	73.1	50.4
Mental diseases	228.8	203.5
Chronic diseases	70.1	202.2
Rehabilitation	113.9	50.5

21. Aging and architecture in Israel

International Union of Architects
U.I.A XVIth Congress – Cultures and Technologies
Montreal 1990

Abstracts

This paper deals with the problems of aging and architecture in Israel. General information on Israel and the Israeli health system is available in two other papers, ISRAEL – In view of the W.H.O. strategy – "Health for all by the year 2000" delivered in Moscow 1988 and "program and Hospital Design Guidelines in Israel" prepared for the XIIth International Public Group Seminar, Ottawa 1990. Detailed planning guidelines can also be found in my paper entitled "Health facilities in Israel" The papers mentioned here represent various facts of health architecture in Israel. When read together, they supply more complete information in a larger context than dealt with here.

This paper consists of three parts:

1. The aging population in Israel: The Israel population is aging rapidly. Out of a total population of account 4.5 million, the population aged 65+ is approximately 400,000 (8.9%) and predicted to be more than half a million by the year 2010. It is important to note that the 75+ age group, which is 40% of the 65+ age group today, is growing at a significant rate.

2. The various aspects of aging in the Israel context: The awareness of the Israel public to the old age problem and the amount of research in the various and multifaceted aspects of aging have recently increased due to the magnitude of the problem. These aspects must be understood in the Israeli context: an attitude of respect to "wisdom and old age" is rooted in traditional Judaism; different behavioral patterns within the various ethnic groups comprising Israeli society; old age in the kibbutz; and the unstable economy and burdens on the population at large. These and many other aspects, specific to the country, have all had their impact on aging and architecture in Israel.

3. The response of Israeli architecture to an aging population: The needs of the elderly called for revision in various fields of architectural design. These included: apartments specifically designed and termed "the sheltered home"; the condominium and old age home; the long-term institutions intended for semi-independent and disabled elderly; hospital planning that took into account the charge in the patients' age structure; design of public and commercial buildings appropriate for use by the elderly (elimination of architectural barriers), and many other field of architectural design that went through change and development in .... to cope with the needs of the elderly in Israel.

The aging population in Israel

The elderly population has increased considerably in the past years and will continue to grow throughout the Nineties and through the turn of the century. The number of physically infirm elderly will also increase. Demographic data, given here, define the population by age group in percent; the population aged 65+ and 75+ by age and sex in absolute numbers; and the predicted population aged 65+ until the year 2000. Changes occurred not only in the age structures of Israel society, but also in the quality of the elderly. The outcome is that the aging population is participating more actively in all aspects of life. It is the architect's task to understand these phenomena in order to be able to contribute to the design of an environment that is more adapted to the new realties.

The various aspects of aging in the Israeli context

In the framework of this paper, we can mention only a few aspects of aging specific to the country. The Israeli population is composed of a Jewish majority and non-Jewish minorities: Muslims, Christians and Druze. Each group lives in more or less confined areas and by its faith and customs, which influence the attitude toward old age. The Jewish population itself is not homogeneous. It consists of different ethnic group and origins: Israeli, Asian, African, European, American, and South American. Each ethnic group has its own behavioral pattern, which has to do among other thing, with its attitude towards old age. We must keep in mind that as a result of the "melt pot" phenomenon there are continuous changes in the social structure.

Another very important Israeli aspect concerning old age is tradition and religion. This is true for all religions practiced in Israel. Family patterns in the Jewish population, care for the elderly and the influence of the aged on Israeli society are all rooted in traditional Judaism.

One cannot overstress the importance of economic problems connected with aging populations. We shall skip this consideration here as it does not constitute a specific Israeli aspect. However, it will be of interest to mention the solution implemented in the kibbutz. In many kibbutzim, special factories have been founded to enable the elderly to work part-time and thereby to continue to give their share in productive economic support to the community and to enjoy creative employment. The few aspects described here are all connected, in one way or another, with aging and architecture in Israel. It is impossible to enumerate them all. They were mentioned merely to demonstrate some specific aspects special to the country.

The response of Israeli architecture to an aging population

An official awareness to the needs of the elderly developed only in the late Sixties. Most of the subjects mentioned here have become obligatory building regulations, especially those concerning the disabled.

The response of Israeli architecture to an aging population and design considerations concerning planning for the elderly, especially in commercial and public building, include:

1. Imparting a human scale on the building. This is always true for all ages, but it is even more so in the case of the elderly. What can be more repulsive than seeing a wise, experienced old human being entering a pompous, empty edifice.

2. Design of simple circulation routes in order to achieve the best orientation feeling and to avoid the sense of "being lost". This calls for proper signs in the most used languages, Hebrew, Arabic, and English, and use of accepted standard symbols. Use of color for the sake of orientation, written of verbal directions and other means of orienting people must be considered.

3. Elimination of architectural barrios: Non-slip floors, avoidance of steps or design of alternative routes, proper location and dimensioning of lifts, correct width of doors and passages for the free circulation of wheelchairs, counters designed to meet the limitations of the elderly, and handles and benches in corridors and waiting spaces are all of use in eliminating barriers. The architect must pay constant attention to anything that can become an architectural barrier to the elderly or handicapped.

4. Special attention must be directed to the proper location of convenience. At least one cabin of W.C., showers, etc., must be dimensioned and designed for use by the elderly.

The few suggestion mentions above are related mainly to commercial and public buildings. Other responses of Israeli architecture to an aging population are the sheltered home, condominiums for the elderly and long-term institutions. Sheltered home signifies, in Israeli terminology, an apartment designed especially for use by the elderly. In a few words, it consists of a layout allowing easy access and circulation, sufficient width of doors, special design of the kitchen and conveniences, and security measures to protect the apartment against intruders, etc. The location of the sheltered home within the neighborhood is a very important issue. Much has been done in Israel in the field of condominiums for the elderly, or if the Hebrew term is translated literally "homes for parents". Construction is carried out by the public or private initiative, mostly on a commercial basis. Condominiums are intended mainly for independent or semi-independent elderly. This kind of project consists of from tens to a few hundred apartments, a dining hall, lounge, library, reading rooms, facilities for medical treatment, etc.

The long-term institution today consists of about 16,500 beds in 157 institutions. They are intended for patients who are semi-independent (7, 130 beds), frail (2,830 beds), nursing (6,025 beds) and mentally infirm (475 beds). Some of these institutions are operated by the government, Ministry of Health, the sick fund (Kupat Holim) or other non-profit public organizations. Others arc private initiatives operated on a commercial basis. It appears to me that the subjects of long-term institutions deserve special study in an architectural workshop.

Another theme concerning the topic of this paper is geriatric hospitals, acute geriatric departments in the general hospitals, and the revisions in ward design necessitated by changes in the age structure of patients in hospitalization wards. Public awareness to the needs of the infirm and the elderly manifested itself in numerous voluntary organizations, such as the Association of Senior Citizens, the Organization of the Disabled and many others. The demands of these organizations become obligatory building regulations confirming limitations of the infirm .... the elderly. They are actually by statutory building codes.

Architectural responses to an aging population have been deployed in many fields of design. Much has been done on an experimental basis. However, if we look at the magnitude of the problem and foresee the revisions necessary in environmental design adapted to the needs of the elderly, we feel that not enough has been done.

Among the revisions that need to be considered, some of the major ones are as follows:

A) Where should sheltered homes be located within the community?

B) How are long-term institutions to be associated with medical center?

C) To what degree should the needs of the elderly be taken into account in town planning schemes and environmental design?

D) What should the priorities be in the allocation of funds in a country with economic deficits?

Answering to these questions will be made by decision-makers and influenced by various aspects of aging in Israel and by the experimental work carried out by Israeli architects. The pilot project realized in Israel, regarding the aging population, has provided sufficient information to enable us to deal with these problems of a Iarge scale.

Demographic Data (1986)	
Total Population	4,331,000
Jews	3,561,000
Non-Jews	770,000

Population by Age-Group (%)	
Total	100
0–4	11.3
5–19	30.0
20–44	34.7
45–64	15.1
65–74	5.4
75+	3.5

Population Aged 65 + by Age and Sex (absolute numbers)		
65 +	Total	380,800
65–74	Males	106,200
	Females	124,400
75 +	Males	70,400
	Females	79,800

Projected Population Aged 65+	
1990	409,800
1995	434,600
2000	462,000
2005	487,800
2010	516,600

Sheltered Housing (1987)	
No. of housing programs	6
No. of operating living units	6,020
Rat. of units (per 1,000 elderly)	16

Condominium Ownership (%)	
Public Sector	47
Voluntary Sector	43
Private Sector	10

Long-Term Care Institution 1987	
No. of institutions	157
Total No. of beds	16,460
Semi-independent	7,130
Frail	2,830
Nursing	6,025
Mentally infirm	475

Unmet Needs (1987)	
Elderly waiting for placement	1,9
Planned beds	1,8
11% of the stock beds	

22. Program and hospital design guidelines in Israel

U.I.A P.H.G
XIIth International public Health Group Seminar
Sponsored by Health and Welfare Canada
Guidelines Programming and Design in Development and Developed Countries, May 1990 – Ottawa

Abstract

Program and design guidelines of hospital planning in Israel are to be understood in the context of the country. General information on Israel and the Israel health system is available in my paper ISRAEL – in view of the W.H.O. strategy "Health for all by the year 2000", delivered in Moscow 1988. Detailed planning guidelines can also be found in my paper entitled "Health facilities in Israel".

This paper consists of two parts:
1. Historical notes on hospital planning in Israel: The historical notes distinguish the three eras of hospital design in Israel: the Ottoman era up to the end of World War I, the British Mandate era between the two world wars and the last four decades since the establishment of the State of Israel.
2. Program and hospital design guidelines in Israel: Is there an Israeli hospital concept? Numerous factors influence and shape the acceptable hospital plan in Israel. These include the heterogeneous population, religion or rather religions, the variegated customs of the different ethnic groups, medical staff coming from Europe, America and East Europe, climate, economy, security and the political situation. All these and many other factors, specific to the country, have influenced together with functional considerations the program and hospital design guidelines in Israel. The outcome of a suitable design process that takes into account the needs and constraints, specific to the country, is what can be termed the "Israeli hospital concept".

Historical Notes

One can identity three eras in Israel hospital planning: the historical era up to the First Word War, the British Mandate era between the two world wars, and the last four decades since the establishment of the State of Israel until today. Some of the health care facilities in Israel have been in existence for many centuries. These are mainly small missionary hospitals or other medical institutions controlled by non-profit organizations. They operated during the Ottoman and British epochs and some of them are still in operation today. Most of them are outdated but a few have important historical and cultural significance.

During the British Mandate period (1920–1947), the first "generation" of modern hospitals and health care facilities was founded. They were erected by the Mandatory government, the labor sick fund federation (Kupat Holim), the Hadassah Organization and private institutions. Good examples of this era are the Regional Hospital of the Valley of Israel (by Baerwalds), the Rambam Hospital (by Mendelson) and Bellinson Hospital (by Sharon). These institutions had to cope with the growing population as well as with the higher standard of living of the European immigrants. The newcomers, especially the already well-known Jewish-German physicians, brought with them up-to-date medical concepts. Hospitals built in this era had the known European wing-pattern composition.

When the state of Israel was founded, many immediate problems had to be solved by improvisation. Serious planning of health care facilities and hospitals only really commenced in the early Sixties. The hospitalization program laid down by the Ministry of Health called for the erection of hospitals with a total of approximately 5,000 beds for general hospitals, 5,000 beds for psychiatric hospitals, and 1,750 beds for rehabilitation centers and hospitals for chronic diseases. The program and planning guidelines of hospitals built during this era will be discussed later in this paper. Generally speaking, however, their functional organization and architecture were influenced on one hand by European "after the war hospital design" thinking and on the other hand by local stringent special conditions.

Program and hospital design guidelines in Israel

Planning of health services and hospitals based on a comprehensive health system and hospitalization plan, established about 30 years ago by the Ministry of Health. Since then two of three "generations" of health care facilities have been programmed, designed and built. They provide health services to the heterogeneous population of about four and a half million. Immigration and natural growth increased the population four folds in four decades, and it is still growing at a considerable rate.

In order to program and define the needs of health services, some figures, complementary to those mentioned in the Moscow paper, are necessary. The total health care expenditure is 1.5 billion U. S. dollar, about 7.5% of the gross national product and 357 dollar per capita. The percentage of the population covered by health insurance is 95.4%. The national expenditure on health by type of expenditure and service, in percent, is as follows: preventive medicine and public clinics: 32%; hospitals and research: 43.5%; dental clinic: 10.1%; and 14.4% spread over many other items. These figures demonstrate that the major part of health expenditures is allocated to hospitals, research, and other health care facilities, which amounts to about 1.2 billion dollars a year. For a tiny country like ours, with so many needs, heavy deficits and budgetary problem, this is a staggering amount. This signified the importance of an appropriate programming of hospitals and health care facilities and careful consideration of their functional design in order to save on capital investment and running costs. Numerous factors dictate capital investment and running costs. We shall deal here only with those connected with hospital design guidelines. The actual professional staff employed in health facilities is 12,000 physicians, 3,685 dentists and 27,000 nurses.

Design policy decisions can reduce or increase the number of personnel required to operate a certain facility.

The trends in general care hospitalization are to reduce the number of beds per 1,000 population, to reduce the average length of stay in hospital, and to allocate the correct number of beds to the various departments in order to maximize their use as far as occupancy is concerned.

Trends in psychiatric and geriatric hospitalization show that the rate of psychiatric beds per 1,000 population is decreasing while the geriatric rate is increasing. The increase in the rate of geriatric beds is connected, no doubt, with the phenomenon of the aging population in Israel. My paper prepared for the workshop at the Montreal congress, deals with this theme in more detail. The decrease in the rate of general hospital beds was made possible by the increase in the rate of chronic beds, the new trend of day care beds and ambulatory treatment in the outpatient departments, and mainly by more effective treatments.

Programming and design guidelines of hospitals in Israel nowadays must take into account new developments and trends. The ones mentioned here is only the tip of the iceberg. In the framework of this paper, I shall try only to make the point that as a result of specific Israeli constraints, there is an "Israeli hospital concept".

The design wise meaning of the data presented here is change in the proportion of space allocation and programming. Where did these changes occur? In the first "generation" of hospitals built during the Sixties and Seventies, the rule of thumb, in a given hospital, was that a third of the gross area should be allocated to hospitalization, a third to medical services and a third to supply and other services. In up-to-date programs, much more of the gross area in allocated to the ambulatory and day care departments.

If we look at the accepted organizational scheme of an Israeli hospital, we can distinguish five main categories of areas or services:

1. Hospitalization services.
2. Medical services.
3. Administrative services and miscellaneous.
4. Supply services.
5. Outpatient department.

Requirements for hospitalization services, or the ward block, did not change much over the years. The ward usually consists of 3 bed patient rooms with a few rooms containing 1 or 2 beds, a number of doctors' rooms, the nurses' station and utility rooms. The accepted floor area per bed was and still is about 30 sqm.

The best location of most medical services, in the Israeli context, is the ground floor. This allows their independent expansion without disturbing the functioning of the hospital as a whole. Growth and change are integral, frequent requirements for medical services. In addition, they must be designed to deal with emergency catastrophic situations. In most hospitals built during the Sixties and Seventies, we had to update and expand these services more than once, while the wards were left unchanged.

23. Chaim Sheba Medical Center – The new complex

Report 1990

The other categories of functions mentioned here are also influenced by Israeli realities. In outpatients' departments, patients prefer to wait in front of the doctors' examination room. No other waiting system works, and this reality affects the layout of the department. This department has also increased lately, because more patients receive ambulatory or day care treatment.

The trends mentioned here are true for many countries; however, one must bear in mind the specific, characteristic constraints in Israel, such as providing health services to a heterogeneous population in which anticipation of behavioral patterns is difficult to make; religious constraints, such as the holy Sabbath (the Jewish Saturday), the need for kosher kitchens, and the "laws of purity" concerning the pathology department; and the continuous concern for a state of war, which entails programming extensive casualty departments with the possibility to expand immediately and the sheltered emergency hospital, obligatory by law, for all hospitals. Added to these constraints is the unstable political and economic situation, which results in frequent changes in commission orders. All these and many other specific Israeli constraints in addition to the "nature" new developments in health services, make the picture colorful. The outcome of an architectural design process based on a given program, which takes into account the needs and constraints specific to the country, is what can be termed the "Israel hospital concept".

Many times and oft, on inauguration day of a new hospital or health care facility, it looks to me that it is a miracle that this day has arrived at all.

Chaim Sheba Medical Center, Tel Hashomer, the largest of the government central hospitals in Israel, began its operation 42 years ago in existing barracks of a former British military camp of World War II. It has now about 1,200 beds, 700 of which are located in the new medical complex (geriatric and psychiatric beds not included). It accepts patients from the greater Tel Aviv area and in special departments also from other parts of the country. Bedsides providing medical care, the hospital is also active in the training of young doctors and in the instruction of students of the Medical school of the Tel Aviv University. It does a considerable amount of clinical research work and also plays a major part in the treatment of wounded soldiers.

About 22 years ago a government decision was taken to build a new medical complex, located south of the existing one. Ground breaking took place about 15 years, but after a considerable amount of infrastructure had been carried out, building operation on site stopped due to the lack of funds.

The designer of the project, Zarhy Architects had to develop the master plan of the new medical complex on the assumption that the existing and the new campuses will run simultaneously for a long time and will have to co-exist and operate conjointly as one hospital for a certain period.

Thinking in terms of building in phases had a strong impact on design decisions. The main problems connected with this reality were; to ensure efficient operation of the hospital at any given moment, to enable relocation of medical entities right after completion of the

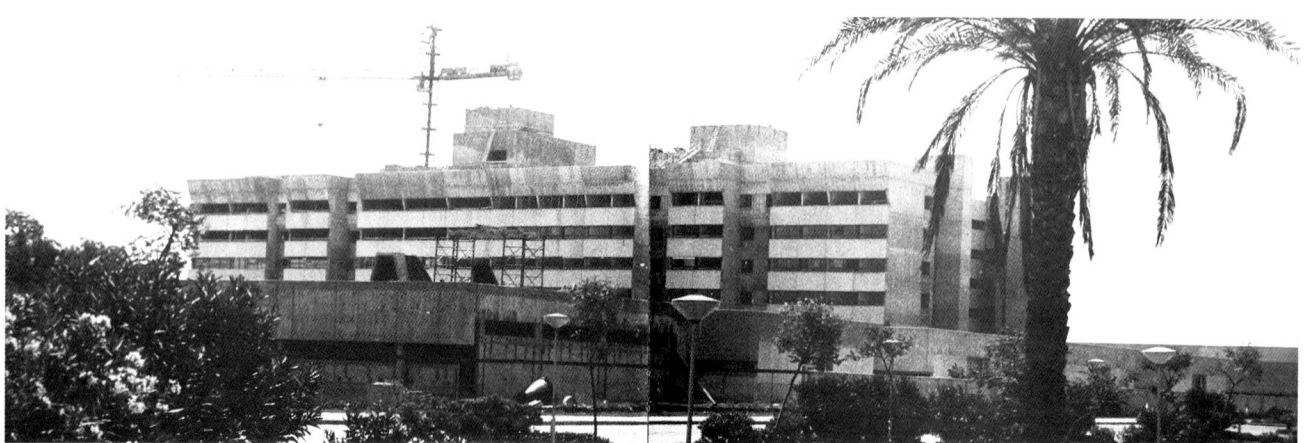

Sheba Medical Center, construction site

"wings" in the new complex designated for them and to create the proper physical and human environment in each phase of expansion.

In the first stage, the complete infrastructure of the hospital was carried out. Construction of the medical and supply services have been completed one by one and started to operate right after their completion. Hospitalization services were carried out and relocated ward by ward. The last two wards were moved from the exiting site to the new hospitalization building by the end of 1988. The general composition of the new medical complex is arranged about a main east-west axis (the spine) which is also the axis of the ward building, with secondary axes (the ribs) of the medical and maintenance services.

The wards building comprise 5 floors, 4 wards per floor, all together about 20 wards. Two circulation cores connect the various ward floors with the comprehensive medical and supply services at the ground floor. These services includes; main entrance facilities and a synagogue, casualty and admission section, operating theatres department, general intensive care unit, out-patient department, diagnostic imaging division and institutes serving both in-patients and out-patients (they comprise departments of oncology, neurology, pulmonary diseases, gastroenterology, nephrology, cardiac rehabilitation as heart institute, eye institute, maxillofacial institute and laboratory wings active in diverse disciplines of clinical and research laboratory work). The emergency hospital and all supply services are located at the lower ground floor. They include the general and medical stores, pharmacy, central sterile supply, food preparation facilities, workshops, service yard and the power plant. The total built area of the new medical complex is about 120,000 sqm. Number of in-patients, outpatient visitors, physicians, nurses, medical technicians, administrative and ancillary personnel constitute several thousand people occupied in diversified field of activity. The designers of the New Chaim Sheba Medical Center, Zarhy Architects believe that an institution so vast in scope, called upon to solve such complex problems, constitutes a human environment in itself. In the case, planning ceases to be based on the usual criteria relating to the design of building. It is more like city planning on a small scale. A medical institution such as this cannot be considered as a complete-static. Its development stems from the multiplicity of needs of the society, its serves and the changing methods and attitudes in medicine and research. Those who initiated the Chaim Sheba Medical Center and its planners tried to solve these diverse planning problems so as to produce a building which will serve society in the best possible way.

24. "Continuity in hospital design"

16th IPHS International Public Health Seminar
Florence – Italy, 30 May – 1 June, 1996
"Continuing Updating and Upgrading of Existing Health Care Facilities"

Abstract

This paper deals with the problems of continuity in hospital design and its effect on the everyday function of the medical facility. This will be illustrated by three case studies from amongst the Health Care facilities planned by Zarhy Architects. Planning a Health Care facility differs from planning other types of buildings in several areas, in addition to the basic complexity of hospital design. Its programme is determined by the country's hospitalization policy and related Health Care issues. Hospital construction often takes longer than similar sized projects and is commonly built and populated in stages. A constant feature in a hospital's life is continuous rebuilding, interior modifications and adjustments within the framework of the Master Plan, due to new medical methods and techniques. The planner provides continuous services to the hospital's management in planning of proposed interior modifications, construction of new wings and ongoing renovations, due to accelerated wear and tear of existing facilities. The problems generated by this constant need to provide architectural services to Health Care facilities have not been resolved. The architect-planner's professional conscience calls for the preservation of his creation, yet he must find solutions for current up-to-date problems. The usual client-architect work relationship does not provide answers to a situation such as described above. A proposal for solving this important issue should be formulated and should become common practice for professionals in Hospital design.

25. Keynote address

International Union of Architects
"Science and High-Tech Facilities" Work Programme
First International Meeting -Israel- May 1999

Dear Colleagues,

The UIA Council, which convened in Barcelona in January 1998, has decided on the establishment of a new Work Programme dedicated to the architecture of "Science and High-Tech Facilities".

The last quarter of the Twentieth Century has been characterized by rapid technological development in all fields. The general forecast is that, as we enter the new century, we also enter an era where hi-tech industries and services will become one of the main sources of employment worldwide.

Buildings where science and hi-tech activities can be carried out optimally are a necessity, and there is a growing demand for better and more suitable facilities. The international architectural community is aware that this forecast demands the creation of a new kind of built environment, which will naturally change life styles and behavior patterns.

The purpose of this Work Programme is to study the impact of these developments on urban pattern. With the expressed purpose of creating a "user-friendly" working environment, to promote the exchange of knowledge and practical experience in providing, designing and building Science and Hi-tech facilities.

This is the first international meeting of our Group, and it was made possible under the auspices of the UIA Israeli Chapter and the sponsorship of ISCAR Industries, which is a world renowned High-Tech firm. I want to use this opportunity to thank Mr. Stef Wertheimer, the founder of ISCAR Industries for accepting the

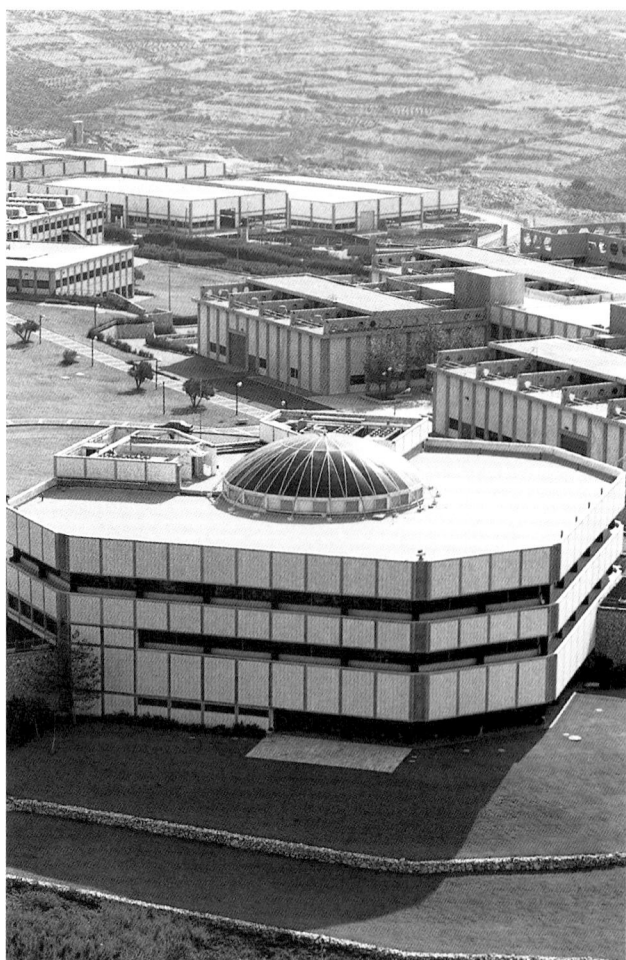

Iscar Industries, Upper Galilee

Some High-Tech Start-up companies were successful Industries which started in a small scale grew in a very short time. Other companies developed slowly, and others were liquidated. High-tech industry has a special nature. It is innovative, its scope and its goals adapt rapidly to new ideas and demands, and it attracts people of a unique kind. All this, of course, has to be taken into consideration when planning facilities which will house hi-tech research and industries.

Choosing and Developing the Site:

A high-tech campus built at the right site has a better chance of success. Proximity to a high level population and high quality of life area, enough reserve area for expansion and achievement of a "critical mass", affinity to a university or research institute, etc. contribute to the campus' success.

We are all familiar with the "Silicon Valley" and its affinity to the Stanford University and with Boston's "Route 128" and its affinity to M.I.T.

The importance of this affinity was stressed by Thomas M. Nies, President of Sincom Systems inc., who wrote: "What developers of high technology don't understand is that the university environment is the engine of technology and the driving force behind bringing technology to an area."

Besides choosing the right site for a high-tech campus, it is extremely important to develop a Master Plan and define its integration within the surrounding urban fabric, and the access routes which connect it to the main urban and national road system.

The urban character of the high-tech industrial campus is dictated by the local surroundings and by the wish to impart to the campus a unique image. It is neither a university campus nor an industrial area. The leaders of these facilities and the high-tech industry managers want the campus and its buildings to broadcast "success". In High-tech centers environmental design and landscaping enhance the quality of life and give a prestigious image to the whole campus.

sponsorship of this event and the Israeli Association of United Architects, for making this meeting possible.

Now let us turn to the substance – the theme of our meeting. High-Tech Industries deal with diverse topics: different fields of electronics, such as micro-electronics and electro-optics, software for diverse purposes, computer hardware design and manufacture, biotechnology and genetic engineering, pharmaceutics, rare chemicals, agrotechnics, research and development of office equipment, robotics, quality control, development of prosthetics and implants, bio-engineering and many other fields.

In our country, the high density population, which is a direct result of building costs and land shortage, hampers the efforts to obtain an image of spaciousness. This forces us planners to give special attention to the environmental design

Multi-purpose Buildings

A High-tech industrial campus is composed of individual industries. It is usually built in stages – one building after the other. Some of these industries will be housed in "custom made" buildings, which were planned specifically to meet the needs of the occupant. Most industries will occupy "multi-purpose" buildings, sometimes called "incubators". They are specifically designed for start-up industries. The development of a new product usually needs a relatively small working area. At this initial stage there is no certainty of the future of the enterprise. It needs immediately available housing. Such small enterprises, which are at the beginning of the road and are usually short of capital, will take advantage of the campus' services and other external auxiliary systems.

This is the reason for planning "multi-purpose buildings", which have no specific purpose, but can be adapted according to the needs of the current tenants. Planning a multi-purpose building demands a high level of sophistication. It should enable several options of division of the area to different functions, options for installation of electro mechanic supplies according to future specifc demands – planning for unknown future uses without barring any options.

The concept of a multi-purpose building was already formulated some thirty years ago and has since been performed in Israel. Many buildings have been built with this concept, and have been improved and perfected with time.

Building a High-tech Campus in Stages

The building of a high-tech industrial campus is usually carried out by stages, according to a guiding Master Plan. Each stage comprises one building or a cluster of buildings. Each stage must be executed as a whole and constitutes a whole autonomic operational unit.

The industries using the campus need joint services: restaurants, banks, post office and communication center, shops, workshops and administration services. Sometimes it is economically sound to build a joint energy plant for heating and cooling purposes.

The Envelope Building

The concept of the envelope-like building has been developed as a solution for multi-purpose uses.

The first phase is the construction of the building's shell, including the main supplies and infrastructure systems. The envelope building must be designed in such a way as to enable flexibility in the division of internal spaces. The guiding rules for planning the envelope are seemingly simple, but they are truly complex and demand extensive planning experience.

A well-designed "envelope" has to have the right dimensions of the "envelope", facilitate the division into correct "modules", and include options for electro mechanic systems, both those needed at the on start and those which will be needed in the future. The right "guesses", as close to future needs as possible, will save unnecessary expenses and will facilitate efficient functioning of the enterprise.

The second phase is the partitioning of the internal spaces and the installation of the secondary systems – according to the needs and goals specified by the users.

This phase also demands a high degree of flexibility. The dynamics of most high-tech enterprises makes a constant need for changes inevitable. Therefore, planned flexibility can be a partial answer to this difficult problem.

The finishing, furnishings and supplies, which are provided close to the actual use of the premises, should be as much mobile as possible, and adapted at all times to the needs of the users.

Another especially difficult problem is the growth of the industries and the need for additional areas. We do not always have the answer to this problem.

The Architect and High-Tech Facilities

We have to keep in mind that the driving force behind High-Tech industries are the entrepreneurs, the inventors, the men of ideas, the thinkers and the innovators. Although money is a big factor – it is not the main element.

As architects' what is our role in the process of the creation of a high-tech facility?

Some architects may think that when planning a high-tech facility they have to express modernism and emphasize futuristic architecture. It is not so. We have seen incredible failures which followed this line of thought. With all humility, we have to put architecture in the service of the subject, and not the opposite.

We have to attend to the needs to the best of our visual and conceptual abilities – and I believe that this cannot be accomplished by any other member of the building team other than the architect. We have to see the complexity of the overall picture.

The establishment of a High-tech Industries campus has an impact on the neighboring environment. There is a constant interaction between the campus and its neighboring town fabric, and the consequences of these interactions are many, but our time is too short to go into this subject. As mentioned before, we foresee that as we approach the new century we shall see many more such areas, which will provide working places for many people, and this is a direct concern to us, architects.

This is the reason why the UIA Council supported the establishment of a Work Programme. We shall strive in our group to learn and to deal with the unique problems connected with the design of High-tech facilities in the present and in the future.

I want to welcome you all to this first meeting of our group, and I wish us all fruitful deliberations and a pleasant stay.

26. Welcome address

International Union of Architects
"Science and High-Tech Facilities Work Programme"
Second International Meeting – Berlin, June 2000
"Science and High-Tech Campus in the Urban Context"

Dear Colleagues,

I have the honor and the pleasure of welcoming you all to this Second Meeting of the Work Programme.

First and foremost, I would like to thank our hosts, the BDA, Mrs. Claudia Kotte and Architect Daniel Gossler for their willingness to organize and host this meeting, and for their hospitality.

Our First Meeting took place in Israel, in the Tefen Industrial Park, in the Northern Galilee, one of the biggest in Israel in May, 1999. About thirty participants took part in the event, including WP members and Israeli architects and entrepreneurs.

The Work Group also participated in the 1999 UIA Congress which took place in Beijing by holding a Seminar and a slide presentation, which took place at the China Architectural Culture Center. We also had a display of panels at the Architectural Exhibition, depicting realizations of High-tech Facilities projects in various member countries.

Lately received a request from the UIA Secretary General, Jean Claude Riguet, that the Beijing Charter be distributed amongst all architects, and that it should not remain just a piece of paper which yellows with time (we have copies of the Charter available here – please take one and make yourselves acquainted with its contents). Just as it was with the "Carte d' Athenes" seventy years ago and with the UIA Charter which heralded the establishment of the UIA in Lausanne fifty years ago, we hope that the Beijing Charter manifests itself as a guide for future better architecture.

The theme of this Meeting is: "Science and High-Tech Campus in the Urban Context".

Hi-Tech Industries, which are "clean industries", are coming back to the cities. So much, that nowadays there are experiments that combine industrial and residential areas in the same buildings. In a way, we are closing a historical circle, and this trend will have a strong impact on the urban fabric. We deal with issues of the future, which will become more important as time goes by, and our place in these developments is crucial.

We also believe that our interdisciplinary *Abilities* give us the tools to find the optimal solutions for integrating all the innovations, and create a work environment that reflects the quality of our work. We architects *"Care about people"* – thus, within all the new scientific and technological developments, we plan for a friendlier environment for those who use them.

The first meeting in Israel was the start, and this meeting is the second step towards what I hope will become a full-fledged UIA Work Programme. The UIA Work Programmes are considered to be the backbone of the UIA, perhaps even its "raison d' etre". Most of the important work of the UIA is made in the Work Programmes, and I sincerely hope we can make our Work Programme one of the most successful ones. Of course this only depends on how dedicated we are, and how willing to spend some of our time working towards this success.

I am sure that the sessions, deliberations and learning tours of this meeting will be creative, stimulating and fruitful. Meetings, such as this one, are an integral part of what gives us architects the tools to deal with diverse planning situations by comparing and sharing experiences and diffusing knowledge.

Once again, thanks to the organizers, supporters and sponsors who have made this event possible. I wish you all fruitful deliberations and a pleasant time.

27. The search for architectural identity in Israel – Personal reflections

Genius Loci International Seminar
Under the high Patronage of the Presidency of Romania
and the International Union of Architects
Bucharest, 19–23 October 2000

Dear Colleagues,

My paper deviates slightly from the main theme of this Seminar. My words may sound subjective, but they come from my experience in the search for architectural identity, and may therefore have more than a touch of my own personal thoughts.

The search for the identity of Israeli Architecture, from the beginning to the end of the Twentieth Century, resembles the search for the identity of all plastic arts, as well as of poetry, prose, music, and all forms of expression in the endless struggle for the creation of cultural values.

Therefore, the words that I will say today are true, to all forms of art, and not only to architecture. The roads traveled in the search for identity have diverged in several directions, sometimes contradictory. At the onset of the Twentieth Century, blending into the regional culture was the preferred direction.

A land almost devoid of settlers, the deserts, the marshes infested with diseases, the middle-eastern culture with its richness of history and building styles, the wish to return to the roots, all these fed the desire to blend into the region. Several buildings of this period have survived and are witnesses to the beauty of that era. As examples of this initial period we can mention the Technion in Haifa that was built at the turn of the Century, a masterpiece of the Architect Baerwald, and other buildings he designed.

Yet, the same Baerwald, when asked to design a Hospital in the Valley of Jezreel, had to deal with the unsolved equation of the aspiration for a specific style vis a vis life styles and cultural backgrounds not compatible with the desired style.

Reality was stronger that any aspiration. Waves of immigration to the country brought people, among them artists and architects from all over the world, mainly from mid and Eastern Europe. Their imported lifestyles and their rich layers of culture produced buildings, streets and cities that are copies, somewhat blurred, of those in their old countries. During my visit to Odessa, in my capacity as UIA Vice President Region II, I had the feeling that I was walking the streets of Tel Aviv of the Thirties. Of course the truth is the other way round!

The Thirties also saw the building of the Kibbutz and the cooperative settlements, which were a direct continuation of the villages founded during the last years of the Nineteenth Century. A new and beautiful rural architecture developed at this time, especially in the Valley of Jezreel and also in other rural areas of the country. We should not neglect to mention the qualitative wave of German immigrants, which arrived more or less at the end of this era of imported style. They brought with them not only their local culture, but also the spirit of modernism and renewal that prevailed in Europe and in the Western World. Suffice to mention the "Bauhaus", its disciples and their train of thought, which built entire quarters in Tel Aviv, that are some of the best known examples of Bauhaus in the world.

At the same time, a different style of building flourished in Israel – Near Eastern architecture, as seen through western or Anglican perspective. Wonderful examples of colonial architecture are the YMCA building, the King David Hotel and the Main Post Office Building in Jerusalem, the Rockefeller Museum near the Old City of Jerusalem, Kings Street and the City Hall in Haifa, and many others. This style practically vanished after the end of the British Mandate in Israel. Chronologically, we should also mention the Second World War, which threw everything out of order. For all that, during this time some of the most beautiful buildings in Israel were built by the renowned architect Erich Mendelsohn, such as the Mount Scopus Hadassa Hospital, the Anglo-Palestine Bank and the Shoken Library House in Jerusalem; the Rambam Hospital in Haifa; the house of the first president of Israel, Chaim Weizman, in Rehovot and many others. There is no doubt that these buildings, designed by Mendelsohn had an everlasting influence on Israeli architecture.

Let us return to the post Second World War era. In its aftermath nothing could remain as it was before. The ravages of the war, the Holocaust, the struggle for national identity, the immigration waves of survivor refugees from Europe and of Arab countries created an urgent need for housing for hundreds of thousands immigrants. This could be called "the non-architecture era": – refugee camps, tin huts and housing blocks devoid of any style of identity – plain and simple shelter.

This era left deep scars, social, cultural and style wise, which have not healed to this date, and which have raised unanswered questions regarding Israeli architecture. Who are we? Should we keep the culture of the newcomer's countries of origin? Or should we renounce ancient cultures preserved in our everyday lives that are an inexhaustible source for architectural creation? All these and other questions needed immediate attention from decision makers, and had direct results in architecture and town planning.

For example, should we design residential quarters for immigrants according to their country of origin? This is no doubt the way to preserve imported style and character. Or should we try for accelerating the melting pot process, in the futile hope of creating a new society with new styles?

This is not the place to dwell on these heavy questions that are being currently asked in many countries of the world. I can only say that we, in Israel, have made all the possible mistakes – but this is a topic for a different seminar.

Let us return to our current topic – the search for identity. As previously mentioned, this era brought, inevitably, undisciplined growth of housing projects, quarters and towns.

Interestingly, after years of living in similar housing projects, these dwellings took the characteristics of their inhabitants – and I am not referring to good or bad characteristics, but in the sense that "the house takes on the appearance of its inhabitants". Two streets, built identically, keep changing. On one street the houses may take on a look of poverty, neglect and wretchedness, while on the other, houses will project prosperity and heart-warming care.

Meanwhile, a new generation of architects grew in Israel, most of them graduates of Israeli Schools of Architecture. In Europe, the post war years were characterized by massive restoration of destroyed cities and building of new ones. This is the Era of the "International Style" of architecture. This style was adopted in Israel with intolerable ease. It was too easy to imagine that we were part of the "Big World Out There", but disillusion was quick to follow, prompted by the lack of local characteristics, the absence of connection with tradition, the similarity with buildings all over the world, and above all the negative reaction of the population. After all, "vox populi vox Dei": the voice of the people is the voice of God. Too much was built in this style, which has no meaning today. When you pass by one of these buildings, you hear nothing, for they are silent.

It is evident that this is the time to reevaluate Israeli Architecture. What are the parameters of this reevaluation? The evolution of international architecture? Increased affinity with neighboring countries, or maybe a new definition of our identity?

The Israeli architectural community is extremely well informed about international events. Professional publications, visits to building sites, participation in conferences and UIA gatherings and many other activities keep us abreast with architectural news. Open borders have also facilitated the study of our neighboring countries' architecture. We are aware that nowadays the Israeli heterogeneous population follows the western patterns of life. Namely, the care of the sick is not different, medically, from what is accepted worldwide; music played here is the same music played all over the world and business in Israel is conducted in the same worldwide standards. Yet, the people who conduct these activities are uniquely different from those in other countries. Just as each country has its own unique people. We could say that the extremely diverse Israeli population has created, or is in the process of creating a "national entity" which dictates a local architectural style. What are the characteristics of this style? We do not know yet what they are, but we are keenly aware that the answer does not lie in imported clichés of post-modernism or in any other form of architecture globalization.

The search for identity in the last one hundred years, the different eras and styles that we have experienced, have not gone by without leaving their impression. Their differences and attributes notwithstanding, they constitute the layers upon which rests our rich architectural experience, and from which we can draw incessantly. When we approach a new project, we know whom we are designing for, who will dwell in these buildings and what will be their lifestyle. We do not have far to look for. We have all the tools. The way is wide open to create local architecture, fit to minister to the needs of the people and the community that we are here to create for.

28. Adapting existing hospitals for the future requirements

International Union of Architects: Public Health Programme
Architects Forum – IHF Congress
Hong Kong, May 2001

This paper attempts to identify and indicate the characteristics and the architectural solutions to the problem of adapting existing hospitals for the future requirements. It is difficult to speak in generalities due to the nature of this subject – each project has its own characteristics and information that include data on its area, its site, the existing building, and the programmatic requirements according to the medical services provided in the hospital. All these dictate architectural solutions specific to each project.

The paper refers to the subject mainly from the point of view of the Israeli prevailing situation. Most of the Israeli Hospitals are going through an extensive process of growth and internal changes, an inevitable result of the country's population growth, socio-economic changes and the trend of development of better medical services, usually connected to updating and upgrading of work methods. Israeli working methods in medical services are also affected by the country's special conditions, by the area where the hospital was built, and by the concepts of the hospital's operators.

The paper stresses the importance of keeping the Original mainframe of the Master Plan of the Medical Center, while regularly updating and adjusting it to changing requirements and developments. It depicts the guidelines for planning the changes and expansions in medical facilities.

In some cases, changes are made by the staff without consulting the architect of the Master Plan. When this process begins, there is no way to predict the rate of deterioration, both of the interior and the exterior of the building – up to a point where the Original shape is no longer recognizable. This deterioration causes undue hardship and discomfort both to the patients and the staff.

Many times the internal changes are made without knowledge or understanding of the Hospital's original Master Plan. Following the original Master Plan is a fundamental rule when planning changes and expansions.

The Master Plan of the hospital defines the main traffic routes, the location of the various buildings and wings, the connections between them, and the direction of the institution's expansion in its various building stages.

Areas being renovated look temporary and unorganized, traffic arteries are disrupted, janitorial staff are easily defeated by the confusion, danger of infection increases, medical treatment cannot be delivered properly. Architecturally speaking, the end result is a radical modification of the internal spaces.

I would like to stress the importance of the Master Plan. It forms the outline upon which the Hospital Plan is built. As time goes by, different wards and wings change their interior design or even their designation, while the main traffic axes exists, usually for the lifetime of the institution. This traffic routes system grows and branches during the years, yet it is very difficult to change the location of the main vertical and horizontal traffic axes. In other words, it is difficult to change the concept or the principles of planning after they have been set. Hence the Master Plan is of decisive importance.

The building of a Medical Center is a continuing project, that can go on for decades, During its time, it goes though social, economic and cultural changes, and is faced with scientific, technological and administrative developments, unexpected at times, Therefore the Master Plan has to be regularly updated and adapted to these developments – but the main concept, the main frame of the Master Plan is constantly valid.

These rules me hard to be implemented in the reality of the construction of Medical Centers in Israel – but the updating and adapting of the Master Plan should not be waived, under any circumstances. While planning changes and expansions, every effort has to be made to stick to the principles of the Master Plan.

Let us focus on the problems that this poses for the design of a Medical Center. The lifetime of a building is longer than the tenure of a Head of Department or the implementation of any given working method. Therefore there is no other way but to execute changes in the building when changes in the medical and supply services occur. A Medical Center is planned according to the "modus operandi" at the time of its design. When the methods change, the building must be adapted to the change.

At the time of the initial design, the architect must have in mind the fact, which changes will have to be made when the day comes. The basic design outlines the "skeleton" and the basis of the traffic routes, the passages, the supply systems etc., it must take into consideration future expansion and growth. The buildings dimensions should be plausible both during the erection stages and the foreseeable future. The departments system of the medical institution must allow for additions without spoiling the main concept of the design.

In addition to the problems of interior changes mentioned before, that take place during the lifetime of the Medical Center, we should keep in mind that hospital building in Israel is done in stages, and that during each stage the hospital has to function as one operational unit, and as an architectural whole.

From all we have said, it seems that the general list of requirements for the planning of a medical facility consist of two opposing directives. One tells us to plan each department according to its operational requirements, namely to plan for specific needs, defined by experts in the field. On the other hand, the department has to be able to function properly despite changes in working methods. It should be mentioned that we seldom find two experts who agree with each other, therefore no ward, department or service should be planned in such a way as to be suited to one individual. All departments, mainly the medical and supply departments should be planned in such a way as to be flexible enough to accommodate changes in methods and procedures.

The second directive tells us to plan schematically, so as to avoid getting "stuck" in the future, sometimes even before the end of the construction. In other words, to plan the various departments with a common denominator dictated by the general concept of the medical center building, in such a way as to enable changes and expansion of each individual department separately.

Creating a common denominator means a design based on preferred modules: design modules, functional, structural and mechanical modules; repeated use of apertures and facades, "open design" that facilitates expansion independent of other departments; and a site plan that allows for future expansions based on the design principles that were determined in the Master Plan.

Design principles do not restrict freedom of creativity. They encourage order and discipline and outline guiding lines upon which to base the design, and upon which architectural creativity can be developed and expressed.

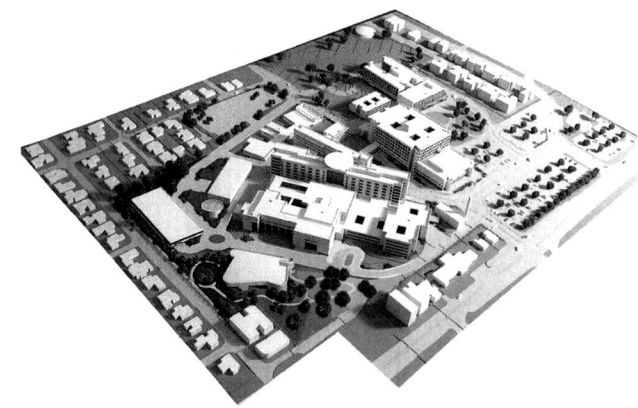

Meir Medical Center – Sapir Medical Center
Model of the master plan 2010

The main difficulty of architectural design in a health facility is that it is constantly expanding and changing. The architect has to solve the contradiction between striving for design perfection, that is basically fixed and static, and the reality of everyday operation of medical facilities that dictates frequent adjustments of the built environment. This faces the architects with difficult challenges, but we cannot change reality.

This is a challenge that every designer of health care facilities has to face and try to find the right solution for each specific problem.

Hospital Design is complex and complicated. It demands a mature attitude to problems that are both: technical and cultural. The architect plans a built environment in which an ailing patient may spend some of the most fateful times of his life. A friendly environment contributes to the well-being of the patient, or may, at least prevent unnecessary hardship.

Therefore, in addition to the challenge posed by functional problems, the architect needs to strive to create an optimal balance between the patient and the environment in which he spends his time. Today's hospitals reflect the society within which they are built. Lifestyles, social conventions, intellectual levels, the affinity to arts and aesthetics, educational and social levels, scientific and technological knowledge, and of course, health and medicine – are all reflected in hospital architectural patterns.

I would like to present to you, as a case study, a project that is in the process of being built: the Sapir Medical Center at the township of Kfar Saba in the Greater Tel Aviv Area. This is a project that I have been involved in its building for more than half a Century. Its beginnings were humble, but during the years its Master Plan has been revised and updated three times. The project presented here predicts the Sapir Medical Center in the year 2010. This project illustrates the trains of thought in the process of updating the Master Plan and adapting existing hospitals for future requirements.

29. Exchange of knowledge between developed and developing countries

International Union of Architects – Public Health Programme
XXI International Public Health Seminar
Manila, The Philippines, May 2001

This paper deals with drawing conclusions from the accumulated experience of hospital planning in Israel, from the point of view from a country that is in passage from being a developing country to being considered a developed one.

Naturally, the establishment of new medical centers in Europe and other developed countries, that have a rich tradition of providing medical services in existing small hospitals, means a transition from these historical hospitals to big medical centers. One of the newest examples is the new Georges Pompidou European Hospital (HEGP) in Paris.

On the other side, developing countries, as was Israel up until a couple of decades ago, medical centers commenced building new medical centers, at first on a small scale. Most of these medical centers have grown and branched out.

The study of the process of the growth of these centers and the results seen today enable us to draw conclusions.

· A functional scheme at the Master Plan level, which will ensure efficient use of expensive equipment and limited human resources.
· To ensure medical services in uncomplicated buildings, according to updated standards.
· Design of Medical Centers, under constant pressure of further construction and extensions.
· Consideration of environment and humanity created in everyday life of health facilities during an expansion period. (?)

30. Architecture and the information era

UIA XXI Congress – Resource Architecture
Berlin – July 26, 2001

- Most medical centers and hospitals in developing countries are built in phases because of local social, economic and political constraints that cannot be avoided.
- Another fact that has to be taken into consideration is the length of construction time.
- In order to achieve a balanced harmony, the design of the medical center has to be based on economic constraints and efficiency, and take into consideration various other factors that influence the design.
- To ensure efficient operation of the medical center at any given time, during the carrying out of extension or renovation construction.
- Reduce the amount of money needed for interest during construction. (?)
- Create the proper physical and human environment in each phase of expansion.
- Energy Conservation.
- Planning with scarce resources.

The hospital planner does not work in a vacuum. He receives feedback from many consultants. Nevertheless, a designer graced with technical leadership has to rely only on his own judgement. He has to be knowledgeable of each of the specialization areas in order to be able to balance the various requirements – which sometimes may contradict each other. This is true in every complex project, but is especially true when we plan a medical center in stages.

The last quarter of the Twentieth Century has been characterized by rapid technological development in all fields. As we enter the new century, hi-tech industries and services will become one of the main sources of employment worldwide. Buildings where science and hi-tech activities can be carried out optimally are a necessity, and there is a growing demand for better and more suitable facilities. This new kind of built environment will naturally change life styles and behavior patterns.

The most significant change that we have witnessed at the turn of the century that relates to the concept of architecture and the role of the architect is the momentous developments in the exchange of information. Accessibility, speed of transference and immediate communication has a deep influence on ways of life and creative possibilities.

The history of architecture teaches us that, at times, architects were slow to grasp the potential embodied in new technologies, for example in steel construction or reinforced concrete. Other than architects were the leaders of the progresses.

The change is not always tangible. Just as developments in building material brought new challenges, new technologies in industry and communications open new horizons in architectural thought. We have to study and understand what is happening in front of us, draw the right conclusions, and understand our place and our role as architects in the era we live in, and place ourselves at the spearhead of progress.

We are aware of the classic perception of the role of the architect and his relationship with his building team. We should define the changes in this perceived role vis a vis the developments in communications and modern industry. It is indeed true that there is some measure of architectural specialization according to the designated purpose of the building. We are not addressing the issue of one more kind of building. We are dealing with substantial alterations in the role of the architecture in this new context.

31. UIA meeting of presidents – Regions I and II

Bucharest, May 23–26, 2002

Dear Colleagues,
Last year at the Genius Loci International Seminar my paper explored the search for architectural identity in Israel, and the struggle for the creation of cultural values that would be characteristic of the local people and land.

Starting from period where the land was almost devoid of settlers, with large areas of deserts, marshes infested with diseases, the first contact with middle-eastern culture with its richness of history and building styles, the wish to return to the roots, through waves of immigration to the country that brought people from all over the world, mainly from mid and Eastern Europe, the building of the Kibbutz and the cooperative settlements during the thirties, and on through the Second World War years and their aftermath and up to the present times – Israeli Architecture has travelled a winding path.

There were many question raised regarding Israeli architecture, which remained unanswered. Who are we? Should we keep the culture of the newcomer's countries of origin? Or should we renounce ancient cultures preserved in our everyday lives that are an inexhaustible source for architectural creation in order to create architecture that is more uniform – more cosmopolitan? The Israeli dilemma exemplifies what is happening world-wide.

The last quarter of the Twentieth Century has been characterized by rapid technological development in

32. Changes in techniques, in information and in the building industry in conjunction with the role of the architect

UIA Work Programme "The Role of the Architect"
Meeting in Paris – September 28, 2001

all fields. The most significant changes that we have witnessed relating to architecture and the role of the architect are the momentous developments in the exchange of information. One cannot ignore what is happening in the world because the "world has shrunk" – there is no difficulty in experiencing the culture and the progress of countries that are half a world away from us. This proximity – although virtual in many ways – pushes for architectural globalization and blurs borders of culture, folklore and architectural style.

We are anxious witnesses to the loss of local architectural heritage, and we crave the preservation and development of national architectural identity. This is most relevant in the Countries of Region II with their rich cultural heritage, diverse national characteristics and building style. Each nation clings to its cultural heritage and yearns for continuity.

One of the challenges facing architects in the new era is how to settle the contradictions between "one world" born from the newest communication techniques and the yearn for local identity.

This challenge is an issue worthy of being discussed and looked into at a special gathering. It should also be represented in the Region II presentation in Berlin. I would like to end my paper by thanking our hosts, Alecu Beldiman, UIA Vice President Region II and Serban Sturdza, President of the Union of Rumanian Architects and the Chamber of Rumanian Architects, for their usual hospitality and warm welcome.

The purpose of this paper is to highlight the issue from different angles, mainly from the point of view of the architect as part of the planning team of hi-tech facilities, and define the role of the architect in the planning of hi-tech facilities, in conjunction with changes in techniques, in information and in the building industry, in the beginning of the Twenty First Century.

The last quarter of the Twentieth Century has been characterized by rapid technological development in all professional fields. The general forecast is that in the Twenty First Century we enter an era where hi-tech industries and services will become one of the main sources of employment worldwide.

The international architectural community is aware that this forecast demands the creation of a new kind of built environment, which will naturally change life styles and behavior patterns.

Buildings where science and hi-tech activities can be carried out optimally are a necessity, and there is a growing demand for better and more suitable facilities. It will, no doubt, change as well the role of the architect assigned to design hi-tech facilities.

High-Tech Industries deal with diverse topics: different fields of electronics, such as micro-electronics and electro-optics, software for diverse purposes, computer hardware design and manufacture, biotechnology and genetic engineering, pharmaceutics, rare chemicals, agrotechnics, research and development of office equipment, robotics, quality control, development of prosthetics and implants, bio-engineering and many many other fields.

Some High-Tech Start-up companies were successful. Industries, which started in a small scale, grew in a very short time. Other companies developed slowly, and others were liquidated. High-tech industry has a special nature. It is innovative, its scope and its goals adapt rapidly to new ideas and demands, and it attracts people of a unique kind. All this, of course, has to be taken into consideration when planning facilities, which will house hi-tech research and industries. A high-tech campus built at the right site has a better chance of success. Proximity to a high-level population and high quality of life area, enough reserve area for expansion and achievement of a "critical mass", affinity to a university or research institute, etc. contribute to the success of the campus.

We have to keep in mind that the driving forces behind High-Tech industries are the entrepreneurs, the inventors, the men of ideas, the thinkers and the innovators. Although money is a big factor – it is not the main element.

As architects, what is our role in the process of the creation of a high-tech facility?

Some architects may think that when planning a high-tech facility they have to express modernism and emphasize futuristic architecture. It is not so. We have seen incredible failures that followed this line of thought.

With all humility, we have to put architecture in the service of the subject, and not the opposite. We have to attend to the needs to the best of our visual and conceptual abilities – and I believe that this cannot be accomplished by any other member of the building team other than the architect. We are able to see the complexity of the overall picture and reach the right conclusions as far as built environment is concerned. The establishment of a High-tech Industries campus

has an impact on the neighboring environment. There is a constant interaction between the campus and its neighboring town fabric, and the consequences of these interactions are too many to list them here.

As mentioned before, we foresee that in the new century we shall see many more such areas, which will provide working places for many people, and this is a direct concern to us architects.

Besides choosing the right site for a high-tech campus, it is extremely important to develop a Master Plan and define its integration within the surrounding urban fabric, and the access routes that connect it to the main urban and national road system.

The urban character of the high-tech industrial campus is dictated by the local surroundings and by the wish to impart to the campus a unique image. It is neither a university campus nor an industrial area. The leaders of these facilities and the high-tech industry managers want the campus and its buildings to broadcast "success". In High-tech centers environmental design and landscaping enhance the quality of life and give a prestigious image to the whole campus.

A High-tech industrial campus is composed of individual industries. Some of these industries will be housed in "custom made" buildings, which were planned specifically to meet the needs of the occupant. Most industries will occupy "multi-purpose" buildings, sometimes called "incubators". They are specifically designed for start-up industries.

The development of a new product usually needs a relatively small working area. At this initial stage there is no certainty of the future of the enterprise. It needs immediately available housing. Such small enterprises, which are at the beginning of the road and are usually short of capital, will take advantage of the campus services and other external auxiliary systems. This is the reason for planning "multi-purpose buildings", which have no specific purpose, but can be adapted

33. The role of the architect

UIA Work Programme "The Role of the Architect"
Meeting in Paris-January 15, 2001

according to the needs of the current tenants. Planning a multi-purpose building demands a high level of sophistication. It should enable several options of division of the area to different functions, options for installation of electro mechanic supplies according to future specific demands – planning for unknown future uses without barring any options.

The building of a high-tech industrial campus is usually carried out in stages – one building after the other – according to a guiding Master Plan. Each stage comprises one building or a cluster of buildings. Each stage must be executed as a whole and constitutes a whole autonomic operational unit.

The industries using the campus need joint services, restaurants, banks, post office and communication center, shops, workshops and administration services. Sometimes it is economically sound to build a joint energy plant for heating and cooling purposes.

The history of architecture teaches us that, at times, architects were slow to grasp the potential embodied in new technologies, for example in steel construction or reinforced concrete. Others rather than architects were the leaders of the progresses.

New technologies in industry and communications completely alter familiar lifestyles. We have to study and understand what is happening in front of us, draw the right conclusions, and understand our place and our role as architects in the era we live in.

We are aware of the classic perception of the role of the architect and his relationship with his building team. We should define the changes in this perceived role vis a vis the developments in communications and modern industry. It is indeed true that there is some measure of architectural specialization according to the building's purpose. We are not addressing the issue of one more kind of building. We are dealing with substantial alterations in the role of the architect in this new context.

Dear Colleagues,

Through the years the Role of the Architect has been considered in the context of the wider subject of "Architecture", in a variety of commissioned charters and papers, and in numerous lectures given by illustrious architects.

Each of these were formulated through studies, long hours of work, data processing and meetings of architects worldwide.

Three of these papers are cornerstones of the UIA Philosophy formulated during the last few years, as we contemplate the end of a century – a millennium, if you like, and the beginning of a new one.

I would like to dwell upon these papers, which are definitely worth studying.

The "UIA Accord on Recommended International Standards of Professionalism in Architectural Practice" formulated the principles of professionalism, established in legislation, as well as in codes of ethics and regulations, defining professional conduct. The paper defined expertise, autonomy, commitment, accountability, requirements of the architect and policy issues.

The "International Working Group on General Policy Report", presented at the General Assembly in Beijing, defined the three UIA themes for the 21st Century – considered by most architects to be of uppermost importance: Humanity, Quality and Ability. It attempted

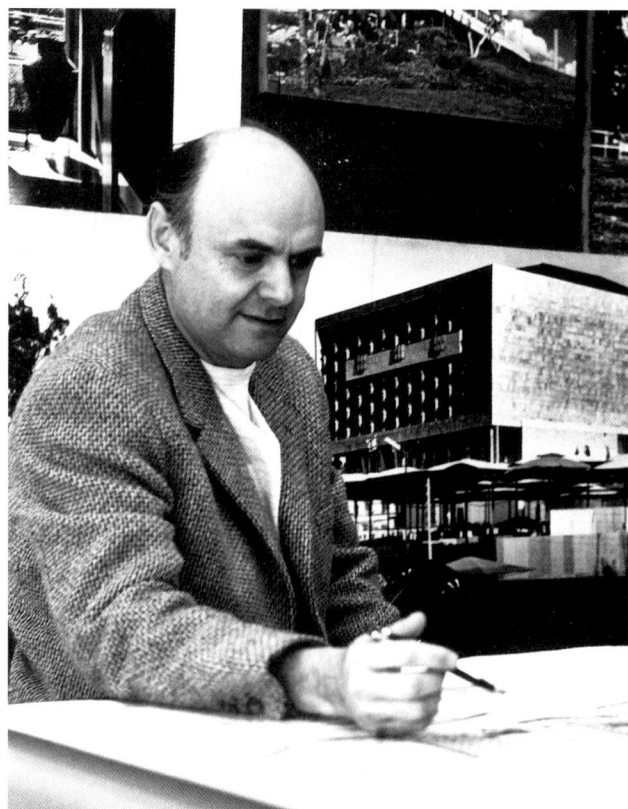

Moshe Zarhy working in his office

How controversial the issue is, can be illustrated by the paper presented by Architect Eri Goshen, member of the UIA Professional Practice Work Programme at the Seminar on 21st Century Practice which took place in Tel Aviv in September 2000. Architect Goshen offered an interesting view, and I quote from the abstract of his paper "The Architect – An endangered Species?":

"The lecture deals with the role and profession of architecture, its change over time, offering a projection for the near future. The numerous starting points (Client's needs, function, site, climate, materials, structure, style, regulations, technologies, budget, timetable, public expectations etc.,) are presented. The different layers of the architect work are detailed; as a problem solver, as an idea creator, as a three dimensional envisioned, as a team leader, as a public server and as one who creates symbols and images.

The four last revolutions of the 20th Century are listed (Computer, information, globalization and biotechnology) and their effect on architecture is explained.

The "New Architects", taking the place of the "classic one" (Client, Manager, Politician, Public) are shown as diminishing the scope, depth and impact of the architect's work".

This is, of course an interesting view, not shared by all architects. What is really the role of the architect in these changing times? Is he only a part of a building team – equal among all consultants and experts, a technician of his trade? Or should he strive to be the leader – the shaper of the initial concept and the carrier of this concept through its realization?

And if we take this one step further – can the architect take his place amongst the ones who combine new material available and conceptualize the philosophy, which will shape a sustainable built environment for the present generation, humanity through the next Century?

As I see it, this work group has a clearly defined path – to find the answers to this crucial and existential question.

"to identify and project what architects have to offer to a World Community which faces a complex, advancing and often perplexing future".

Last but not least I want to mention the "Beijing Charter", which tried to "formulate a conscious plan of action for a better and livable human habitat of the 21st Century". "In what way can an architect contribute to the future of human civilization thorough planning and design?" The Charter offered a variety of questions and partial solutions, which I will not go into.

All I have mentioned notwithstanding, until the establishment of this Work Programme, the study of the role of the architect proper has not been dealt with in depth as an independent issue, worthy of being placed in the center of the profession's concerns. This is especially true in today's ever changing New World.

34. Architecture for science and hi-tech facilities in the new millennium

UIA XXI Congress – Resource Architecture, Berlin – July 26, 2001
This paper was also presented
"Zodchestvo – 2003" Festival, Moscow October 2003

The last quarter of the Twentieth Century has been characterized by rapid technological development in all fields. The most significant changes that we have witnessed at the turn of the century relating to architecture and the role of the architect are the momentous developments in the exchange of information.

Accessibility, speed of transference and immediate communication has a deep influence on ways of life and creative possibilities.

As we enter the new century, hi-tech industries and services will become one of the main sources of employment worldwide. Buildings where science and hi-tech activities can be carried out optimally are a necessity, and there is a growing demand for better and more suitable facilities. This new kind of built environment will naturally change life styles and behavior patterns.

The history of architecture teaches us that, at times, architects were slow to grasp the potential embodied in new technologies. The leaders of the progress were other than architects.

The change is not always tangible. Just as developments in building material brought new challenges, new technologies in industry and communications open new horizons in architectural thought. We have to study and comprehend what is happening in front of us, draw the right conclusions, understand our place and our role as architects in the era we live in, and place ourselves at the spearhead of progress.

We are aware of the classic perception of the role of the architect and his relationship with his building team.

We should define the changes in this perceived role vis a vis the developments in communications and modem industry. It is indeed true that there is some measure of architectural specialization according to the designated purpose of the building, but we are not addressing the issue of one more kind of building. We are dealing with substantial alterations in the role of architecture in this new context.

What is the impact of the Information era on architecture?

There are many questions concerning this subject but no one decisive answer. Nevertheless, this is an important issue deserving of deep investigation and discussion. Let us examine some of its aspects:

One of the challenges facing architects in the new era is how to settle the contradictions between "one world" born from the newest communication techniques and the yearn for local identity.

On one hand – the swiftness of information exchange between different parts of the world, the standardization of interpersonal relationships and business management and overexposure to foreign cultures – all these push for architectural globalization and blur borders and cultural characterization between different countries.

On the other hand, we are anxious witnesses to the loss of local architectural heritage, and crave the preservation and development of national architectural identity. Each nation clings to its cultural heritage and yearns for continuity. Our challenge is to settle these two conflicting tendencies.

The modern generation is a product of decades of many areas of research that created applications in consumer goods and a revolution in the industry that produces these goods. Most of these are High-tech Industries.

Sophisticated industries deal with diverse topics: design and manufacture of computer hardware, software for diverse purposes, different fields of electronics, such as micro-electronics and electro-optics, biotechnology and genetic engineering, pharmaceutics, rare

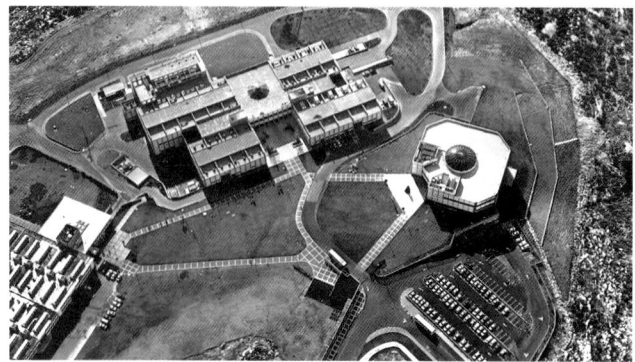

Iscar Industries, Upper Galilee

chemicals, agro-technics, robotics, bio-engineering, development of office equipment and many other fields. As mentioned before, we foresee that as we progress into the new century we shall see more and more built up areas that will provide working places for many people. These built up areas are of interest and of concern to the architectural community.

Technology-rich industry has a special nature. It is innovative, its scope and its goals adapt rapidly to new ideas and demands and it attracts people of a unique kind. We have to keep in mind that the driving force behind high-tech industries are the entrepreneurs, the inventors, the men of ideas, the thinkers and the innovators. Although money is a big factor – it is not the main element.

All this, of course, has to be taken into consideration when planning facilities to house high-tech industries and scientific research.

The location of sophisticated industries is of great importance. In many cases, such as in software development industries, we could argue that the only requirements would be comfortable and efficient office stations. This presumption is erroneous – the dynamics of the field, the teamwork, the constant interchange of personnel, the ability to grow or diminish according to present needs, the linkage of hi-tech industries to other fields, require planning a flexible facility, that includes a variety of systems.

Most high-tech industries can be planned so as to be environment friendly, therefore there is nothing to prevent its incorporation in an urban fabric. In other words, most modern industry campuses are returning to the cities and can be optimally located within urban housing schemes.

The urban character of these clusters of buildings is directed by its local surroundings and by the wish to impart to the campus a unique image. It is neither a university campus, nor is it an industrial area. The leaders of these high-technology campuses and the high-tech industry managers want the campus to broadcast "success". In high-tech centers, environmental design and landscaping enhance the quality of life and give a prestigious image to the whole campus. A high-tech campus built on the right site has a better chance of success. Proximity to an upper-level population and an area of high-quality of life, enough reserve area for expansion and achievement of a "critical mass", affinity to a university or research institute – all these factors contribute to the success of a high-tech campus.

Besides choosing the right site for a high-tech campus, it is extremely important to develop a Master Plan and define its integration within the surrounding urban neighbourhood and the access routes that connect it to the main urban and national road system. The establishment of a high-tech industrial campus has an impact on the neighboring environment. There is a constant interaction between the campus and it neighboring town fabric. The consequences of this interaction are many, but our time is too short to go into this most important subject.

Some architects may think that when planning a hi-tech facility they have to express modernism and emphasize futuristic architecture, It is not so. We have seen incredible failures that followed this line of thought. We have to put architecture in the service of the subject and not the other way round. We have to attend to the needs of the clients to the best of our visual and conceptual abilities – and I believe that this cannot be accomplished by any other member of the building team, other than the architect.

The end products of high-tech facilities are those that enable the existence of the information generation. They have become cheaper and available to all. It is hard to imagine the society, economy and culture of the Twenty-First Century generations without the constant flow of information made possible by these products.

This is a direct concern to the architectural community – we have to strive to deal with the unique problems connected with the Information Area and Architecture. The theme of the twenty first UIA Congress "Resource Architecture" was given many interpretations. In the context of our paper we can say that architecture is founded on two resources one material, the other spiritual.

The Information Area was born, and continues to develop and grow mainly on inexhaustible spiritual resources. In the course of history, radical changes in architecture happened as a result of population migration, social changes, technological discoveries, and new building materials. All these are material resources. Today, we are dealing mainly with spiritual resources and changes in lifestyle. How will they influence modern and future architecture?

Summing up our paper we can say that accessibility, speed of transference and immediate communication have a deep influence on ways of life and creative possibilities. They have and they will continue to have their impact on Architecture and Town Planning.

The ease in communications, the incredible progress in technology, the abundance of consumer products and services – all these factors necessarily change human society in all of its aspects. The present generations do not live, interact or work in the same manner as former generations – and therefore need a habitat suited to their needs. We architects are required to see the whole picture – to be able to learn from the past, see the present, look into the future and be the pioneers in creating the environment that will suit the needs of this era.

35. Hospital master planning in the country's context

International Union of Architects – Public Health Programme
XXII International Public Health Seminar
XXXIII International Hospital Federation Congress
San Francisco, USA – July/August 2003

This paper deals with the relationship between the Master Plan of a Medical Center and the people's characteristics of the country it is built in. We have dealt with the subject of the Medical Center Master Plan many times, and from several points of view. For the most part we referred to absolute data, that can be measured and defined, and with the intention of creating scientific criteria that will serve as tools in planning health care facilities.

We also have dealt with the factors that influence the Master Plan, for example healing and management methods, climate and other measurable and definable factors. The Master Plan of the hospital determines the main traffic routes, the location of the various buildings or wings, the connections between them and the direction of the institution's expansion in its various stages.

The Master Plan can be shaped in numerous ways that will fit its definition. In order to shape the pattern of the Master Plan of the Hospital, the architect has to take into account all constraints relevant to the specific project he is dealing with. These constraints include the shape of the site, its location, and its integration in the urban fabric, the client's list of requirements, administrative frameworks, economics, climate, etc. All these are quantitative constraints. They can be measured and their projection on the Master Plan can be defined.

In this paper we want to raise aspects that were not studied enough up to now, but have a lot of weight in the planning of a hospital's Master Plan. These are factors that stem from the character of those that seek medical services in a medical facility, those that provide these services and those who visit the facility. The sources of these factors are customs, beliefs, life patterns, religious practices, cultural habits and life styles. All these factors cannot always be defined or measured, and are rarely mentioned in the directives and programmes. Even we, the planners, are not entirely aware of the effect these factors have on the Master Plan and the pattern of a specific ward or wing.

It is my purpose, in this presentation, to raise the importance of these undefinable issues, that are intrinsic to the country the medical facility is located in, and to point out their effect its final pattern.

In reality, we realize, time and time again, that the process of planning the Master Plan of a health care facility is connected, interwoven and interlaced with the physical and sociological characteristics of the society which it serves, its customs and its habits. The Medial Center is a micro-cosmos which reflects the character of the people, the geographical location and the country in which it is built.

Factors of this nature, which have a strong influence on the planning, are difficult to explain and cannot be easily defined – just as a person's character cannot be scientifically defined. In this respect, the specific craftsmanship of a health care facility planner is to study, feel, sense and understand the spirit of the people he serves, their customs, their way of life, their beliefs and – taking all this into account – to plan and create the built environment in which patients, staff and visitors will feel "at home".

Israel is a land with a heterogeneous population. It is an enormous "laboratory" that enables us to study the affinity between the people's character and mentality and the pattern of the medical center. In my opinion, our role is not over and done with. By shaping the built environment we can influence, direct, refine and aspire to create improved cultural surroundings.

The case studies are presented to illustrate the projection of the country's context on the Hospital Master Plan.

36. Redesign and updating of existing hospitals

UIA International Union of Architects
24th International Public Health Work Programme Seminar
Sao Paulo – Brazil, June 2004

The paper presents several case – studies of redesign and upgrading of existing hospitals.

The life span of hospital buildings is much longer than that of medical equipment, healing and organizational methods. Therefore, in order to cope with actual problems, changes, extensions and upgrading of existing hospitals are inevitable.

The case-studies presented here are of hospitals I have designed several decades ago. Internal changes, expansion of hospital wings and upgrading the whole medical complex are ongoing ever since.

This personal experience provided me with the opportunity to study the projection of developments in medicine and management methods of redesigning existing hospitals. Out of control changes and sporadic new additions can throw into confusion the hospital complex.

The only way to guide and control hospital complex expansion is to follow the outlines upon which the hospital master plan is conceived. It is difficult to change the principles of planning after they have been set.

It is very difficult to change the location of vertical and horizontal traffic axes. The traffic system can grow and be enlarged during the years, as long as it follows the principles of the hospital master plan.

37. Location of the high-tech facility campus within the city

UIA International Union of Architects
Science and Hi-Tech Facilities Work Programme
UIA XXII World Congress – Istanbul – 2005
Cities-Grand Bazaar of Architecture / Celebrating our Cities

Dear Colleagues and guests,

Our theme "Location of the High-Tech Facility Campus within the City" is multi-faceted. Ever since the UIA Council decision – taken during the Barcelona meeting in 199 – to establish a Work Program dedicated to Architecture for "Science and High-Tech Facilities", we have held annual meetings. During each of our meetings we have presented and examined the place of High-Tech facilities from a variety of differing viewpoints. I will discuss some of these viewpoints during this lecture.

First and foremost, however, we have agreed-indisputably-that the need for buildings to be used for the purpose of High-Tech research and production is an inescapable condition of the times we live in. Constructions that are intended specifically for this purpose have been built, are being built, and will continue to be built in every country; in conjunction with the economic, urban and social development of that country. Architects and city planners must study the requirements of these buildings and sites, and contribute their knowledge and creative power to this development. In my lecture we will consider several aspects of this development and, in particular, we will reflect on the considerations in determining the Location of High-Tech Facility Campus within the City. We are all aware of the historical background of the subject before us. We all know that, urban landscape, and workers lived near their place of work. We all know, of course, of the effects and the weaknesses of the period covering the industrial revolution from an urban viewpoint. We know about air pollution, destruction and contamination of the townscape, acoustic pollution, and so on.

Even the removal of industry from within the city did not solve these problems, but created other, of impoverished neighborhoods in the vicinity of industrial areas. We now find ourselves in an era when most research and production occurs under controlled conditions. Pollution supervision is within our control. Also, city planners, the members of the community and the decision-makers are all highly aware of environmental pollution. There are no obstacles to prevent the planning of research, high-tech facilities and production sites within the city.

What exactly are the conditions needed that can ensure the success of a science-based, High Tech campus? The main problem is that of human resources. Science-based and High-Tech facilities are operated by and attract 'unique' people. These are primarily people with 'special' thought processes, creative skills, high levels of devotion and determination to their ideas, and a deep knowledge of science and technology in their specialized field of expertise. For us, the architects and city planners, this means proximity to urban population centers and to a general public requiring culture, education, knowledge and art. Often, this also requires proximity to universities or places where basic research is conducted, since there are those among the researchers who divide their time between basic and applied research. It is true that there are also examples of high-tech campuses in natural environments, perhaps with the intention of stimulating the imagination of the inventors who populate these sites. However, here we are dealing with the reciprocal relationship between the city and the research site, and the application of that research in production.

It is also possible to see this problem from the other side – and there are many examples where we have witnessed the selection of a site in an area which has deteriorated, with the express intention of restoring the area and elevating it to an urban level. Observing examples, we note how this happens in practice. Many people choose to live next to or near the campus, thus increasing property value, and result in the construction of buildings to be used for education, culture and commerce.

Let us now return to the main theme of this discussion – reciprocal relations connecting the location of the campus with the city. One should bear in mind that the campus is built in stages. The site is composed of building clusters, where each building or cluster has its own purpose, and is involved only with its own particular field. Mostly, it is an enclosed unit, with its own lines of information and communication, and entrance to the building (or cluster) is limited and controlled. However, all of the buildings require common services in the fields of energy, employee services, site management and administration, and so forth. For efficient operation of the entire campus a "critical mass" of buildings is needed, and for the operations which take place in them. As we have said, normally development of the campus is conducted in stages, which means for us – the planners – the preparation of a Master Plan at the earliest possible opportunity.

We must be able to anticipate and plan the creation of an infrastructure that will operate faultlessly during each and every stage, right through to the completion of the entire project. One notes, therefore, the conflict between the different requirements and conditions that lead up to the choice of a particular location – and the campus where research and production of science-rich products are undertaken. On the one hand, the endeavors to ensure future developments – which are expressed in the need for relatively large areas of ground – but on the other hand, areas such as this are difficult to find in centrally located urban districts.

Due to this conflict of interests we must sometimes compromise with the situation as it is, or find an alternative solution. One possible solution is to open up areas on the outskirts of the city, and at the same time, develop effective means of public transportation in the necessary directions. Thus we see the reciprocal relations and the inter-dependency between the structure of the city and the location of the research and production campus within the city; bearing in mind that the high-tech campus is a place of work for thousands among the city's population. Its location shapes the built environment, as well as the character of the urban area adjacent to it. It appears to us that in the future the necessity for such sites will increase, and will become an important component of city planning and renovation.

Architects and city planners are directly involved with decision making and urban design, and therefore they have an obligation to study the architectural and planning matters connected with the development and location of the High-Tech Facility Campus within the City, and to take an active part in their design.

We, the architects, have a particular problem regarding the subject under discussion – that is the matter of "local identity".

Since science and technology are subjects that all of the nations in the world share in common, one could presume that buildings in which science-related research and production are conducted would be identical in all those countries. That is, however, not the case. According to our beliefs and our professional integrity – and based on the experience we have accumulated in our work – we find that the lifestyles, habits and character of the people in each country also affect the design and the structure of the buildings. Therefore it is the objective of the planners to incorporate these differences, so to speak, and to design an identity that will meld with the urban environment – thus weaving the character of the campus into the fabric of the city.

Hereunder a short report on the activities of the Science and Hi-Tech Facilities Work Programme, as well as a number of case studies and lessons that we have learned during our Seminars, which represent some of the principals that we have looked at during this lecture. The Work Programme members met for the first time in Israel in 1999: this was the founding meeting, intended to delineate the purposes of the Work Programme and the subjects to be studied by the group. The general topic was: "Architecture for Science and High-Tech Facilities – A Comprehensive Outlook".

A study tour was conducted at the 'Atidim' campus, a High-Tech Industrial Park affiliated with the Tel Aviv University and the municipality of Tel Aviv. The campus area totals 90,000 m² – which includes a built floor area of about 100,000 m² – where approximately 5,000 people are employed. The Park, which was erected at the time in a run-down urban neighborhood, favorably altered the aspect of that area.

We conducted a tour of the Tefen Industrial Park in the Upper Galilee. This 'industrial city' comprises a Technological Park of high-tech industry, located at the summit of a hillside and surrounded by nature on all sides. Particular attention was paid to incorporating the industrial site into the natural landscape.

We toured the Technological Garden in Jerusalem, which is situated in a central location within the city. This is an outstanding example of how a research and production site can be built inside a city, and yet still blend seamlessly into the urban environment.

A tour was arranged to the High-Tech Industrial Park situated next to the world-renowned research facility, the Weizmann Institute of Science in Rehovot. This is a good example of how to integrate a research institute and a high-tech industrial park.

During that same year the Work Programme group participated in the UIA World Congress in Beijing, China, where we held our Seminar and displayed an exhibition of High-Tech research and production Facilities.

In 2002 we held our Meeting and Seminar in Berlin, and the theme of that seminar was "Science and High-Tech Campus in the Urban Context Today". The seminar was held at the Berlin-Adlershof campus, which is a Science and Applied Research and Production Facility in the city of Berlin – located on a site that was in the past an east-German airfield. This is a unique example of a large space that became available within the confines of a city – resulting from political events – enabling the location and integration of an industrial campus in the heart of the city.

Our meeting in 2001 was held in Moscow, and the theme for that event was „Thechnopolis -The City of Science". In Russia, during the Second World War, a number of „science towns" were created. We visited one such town – Chevhoglovka – which at the time was a closed city and is now dilapidated. This example illustrates the difficulty of situating a technological city in an isolated area, far from a high-density population. When visiting research and high-tech sites located within Moscow, we observed ongoing growth and development.

In 2002 we actively participated in the twenty-first UIA World Congress of Architecture held in Berlin. The Seminar and Exhibition emphasized the increasing relevance and importance of the Architectural issue of planning for Science and Hi-Tech Facilities in our era.

The 2003 Annual Seminar and Members' Meeting was held in the United States, in Phoenix, Arizona: the theme of that meeting was „The Principles of Architecture for Science and High-tech Facilities". We also had the opportunity during that event to visit several High-Tech campuses in the city. Tours were made of state-of-the-art high-tech industrial sites in Phoenix, which demonstrated how pollution-controlled industry can be located in an urban area. Our Seminar was held in the Arizona State University and the winter session at the Frank Lloyd Wright Foundation at Taliesin West, Arizona.

The theme of the 2004 annual session that took place in Macau, China, was „Science and Hi-tech Facilities contribution for regional environment". This seminar also included visits to Science and High-Tech enterprises in mainland China.

38. Science and hi-tech facilities work programme

UIA International Union of Architects
Presented 2005 in Paris, UIA Office

Hereunder some of the lessons we have learned during the Seminars and Meetings of the "Architecture for Science and Hi-Tech Facilities Work Programme".

The Work Programme met for the first time in Israel in 1999: this was the founding meeting, intended to delineate the purposes of the Work Programme and the subjects to be studied by the group. The general topic was: "Architecture for Science and High-tech Facilities – A Comprehensive Outlook".

Study Tours were organized to visit the campus of the Tel Aviv University – the Atidim High-Tech campus where a presentation and explanation were provided; the campus of the Tefen Industrial Park in the Upper Galilee (presentation and explanation); the Technological Garden in Jerusalem (presentation and explanation); the Weizmann Science Park, Weizmann Research Institute in Rehovot (presentation and explanation)

During that same year the Work Programme group participated in the UIA World Congress in Beijing, China, where we held our Seminar and displayed an exhibition of High-Tech research and production Facilities.

The theme of the Berlin-Adlershof / Germany meeting in 2000 was: "Science and High-Tech Campus in the Urban Context Today", where we made a presentation and provided background information.

Our meeting in 2001 was held in Moscow / Russia, and the theme for that event was "Technopolis …. The City of Science". We arranged a presentation and an overview.

In 2002 we actively participated in the twenty-first UIA World Congress of Architecture held in Berlin / Germany. The Seminar and Exhibition emphasized the increasing relevance and importance of the Architectural issue of planning for Science and Hi-Tech Facilities in our Era.

The 2003 Annual Seminar and Members' Meeting was held in Arizona USA – the theme of that meeting was "The Principles of Architecture for Science and High-Tech Facilities". We also had the opportunity during that event to visit several High-Tech campuses in the area.

The theme of the 2004 annual session that took place in Macau, China, was "Science and Hi-Tech Facilities contribution for regional environment". This seminar also included visits to local Science and High-Tech enterprises nearby.

39. The hospital in the city – The Israeli experience

UIA PHG Seminar – Istanbul – July 2005

When deliberating the location of the Hospital in the City, we must take into account that any specific hospital – and its location within any specific city – is a case unto itself; it has its own history, and will be noteworthy in its own right. Nevertheless, there are common rules of consideration that all hospitals share.

My presentation will discuss the rules of consideration that have evolved in Israel during the course of the twentieth century regarding the Location of the Hospital in the City.

Firstly it should be noted that at the beginning of the previous century there were only a handful of hospitals in Israel. Some of these had existed for hundreds of years, and had sufficed to serve the sparse population that lived in the region during that time. Most of the hospitals existing in Israel today were constructed throughout the twentieth century, and nearly all of them were built in cities that had also come into existence during that time. Therefore, considerations relating to the location of the city hospitals were free from historical and other limitations, and hospitals could, for the most part, be located in accordance with practical considerations. Thus, this is an excellent theme for discussion by planners of city hospitals – a sort-of practical laboratory where we may examine the subject over a historical timespan.

Experience teaches us, that every medical campus must have three points at which it connects with the infrastructure of the city roads: One to serve as the Main Entrance; the second as a Service Entrance, and the third for the exit of funerals – if this is to be an existing function within the hospital. The Emergency Entrance branches off from the Main Entrance. These three Entrances connect the infrastructure of transportation within the medical campus with the city transportation network. These Simple guidelines dictate the projected location of the city hospital, which must be next to a main thoroughfare in order to enable accessibility by car, proximity to public transportation, and as near as possible either to the city center, or centrally located for the sector of the population that most requires hospital services. Examples included in this paper will demonstrate how these guidelines were implemented in a number of hospitals located in the largest Israeli cities. Most of the larger hospitals have Outpatients Departments that, in addition to examination and follow-up, also serve as outpatients' clinics for the local community. The practical significance is that there is a constant traffic of patients from the community and from the hospital – with all that this entails: movement of vehicles, movement of people, welfare services and the creation of an image of support that the hospital projects among the local populace. To this one must add the preventative medical activities that increase the reciprocal relations between the city population and the hospital, expressed in training, in hygienic supervision of school activities, and among, the youth.

I want to point out that all of the hospitals in Israel are constructed in stages. This is both because of the budgetary limitations, and because of the inevitable connection between the size of the population – which continually increases – and between the size of the hospital and the services that it must provide. The practical interpretation of this fact – which is incontrovertible and unchanging – is that the hospital must be designed on the basis of a Master Plan, allowing for an ever-growing campus. Obviously it is difficult to target areas within the city centers that are large enough to accommodate a Medical Center. In most of the medical campuses in Israel we are currently facing a situation of insufficient grounds, resulting in the building of high-rise hospitals or, sometimes, the demolition of existing structures in order to allow reconstruction, and maximum utilization of every inch of land.

We are witness to an ongoing dialog between the municipality and its residents, and the city hospital.

Let us present examples of this dialog in various cities in Israel, with the objective of learning from current conditions and educating ourselves in accordance with the reality of the situation as it is today. Let us nevertheless recall, that the hospital is often the largest employer in the city, and for many it is perceived as the place in which some of the most important and significant events of their lives take place. All of these have direct implications on architectural planning, and on the atmosphere that architects are supposed to provide to the medical campus by means of building design.

Meir Medical Center is located in the City of Kfar Saba, in the Sharon Valley area.

The Master Plan is designed to allow implementation in stages according to management priorities and financial resources.

The main pedestrian internal axis is the Hospital Street, which connects all major buildings and facilities, providing the shortest way of getting around the Campus.

The Ring Road will provide full vehicle access to all Campus buildings on the perimeter, keeping the center of the Campus for pedestrians only. The Ring Road will provide access to emergency vehicles and to parking areas adjacent to the different buildings.

The network of transportation on the perimeter of the campus connects with the municipal network of transportation at two points.

The Main Entrance – A – leading in from the north from the inter-urban route, and from the east, from the urban network.

Service Entrance – B – coming from the north and the west.

Rebecca Sieff Regional Hospital – Upper Galilee

The Master Plan enables a large General Hospital to be built in stages, so that all medical and technical services can be expanded with minimum interference to the running of the Hospital.

The building is situated on a mountain ridge on the outskirts of Safed. Despite the steep slopes, the site was ideal in terms of location, climate and view. The crucial architectural problem was to relate the scale of this very large building with the more intimate one of the town. To achieve this, the building was conceived as a superstructure containing the wards, atop a base of inter-connected pavilions on different levels, which blend into the site. Medical and technical service areas are unobtrusively located in the lower part of the building.

The transcription network and the connection to urban networks. Because of the topographical conditions, entrance to the site is possibly only from the north. The entrance road separates into one road leading to the main entrance (A) a road to the Emergency Department (B), and a road leading to the service entrance (C).

Sheba Medical Center

The Sheba Medical Center is the central hospital for Israel. It is located in the Greater Tel-Aviv area. The Medical Center includes a number of hospitals: A General Hospital, a Pediatric Hospital, a Gynecology & Obstetrics Hospital, a Psychiatric Hospital, a Rehabilitation Hospital, a Geriatric Hospital, and a number of other buildings serving a variety of purposes in the field of medicine.

We will concentrate on the General Hospital. The general layout of the Hospital is composed of a main east-west axis (the spine) which is the axis of the ward-block, with secondary axes (the ribs) which are the axes of the medical and maintenance service wings.

There are three entrances to the Hospital: the Main Entrance A, Patient & Casualty Entrance to the Admission Section B and a Service Entrance C.

Access to all entrances to the General Hospital is from the ring road, which surrounds the Women's, Pediatrics and the General Hospital. The perimeter road of the Medical Center is connected with the urban network of transportation at two points.

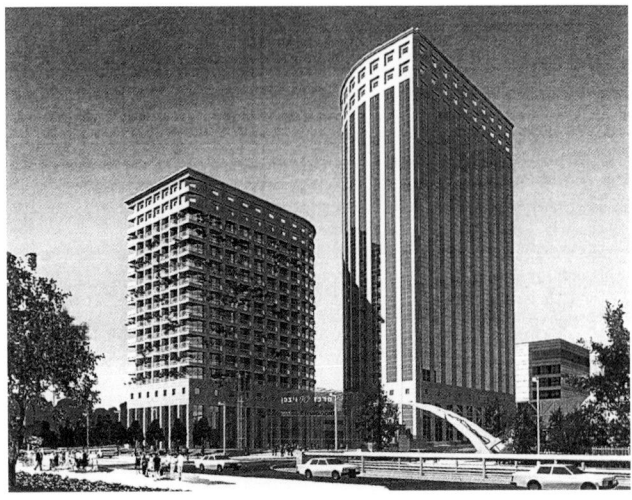

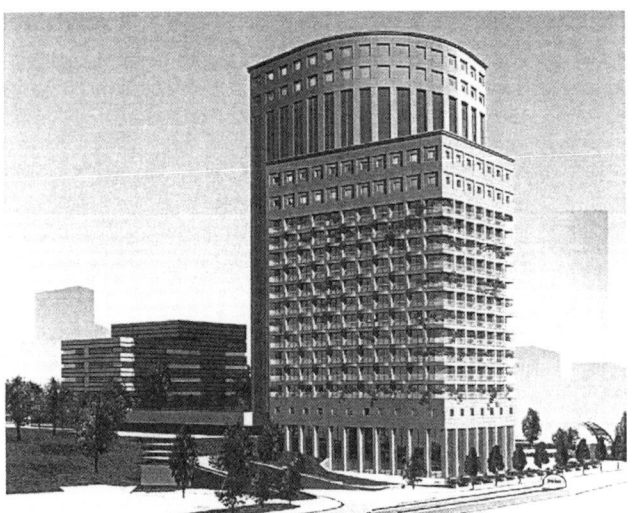

The Weizman Multi Use Center, Tel Aviv

Weizmann Multi-Use Complex

At the Souraski Medical Center, Tel Aviv

The Weizmann Complex, adjacent to the Tel Aviv Municipal Medical Center, includes a Geriatric Hospital, doctors' clinic, hotel, commercial areas and underground parking for the entire Medical Center. The Main Entrance (A) is from the west. Weizmann Boulevard and the Service Entrance (B) is from the east. In order to meet the list of requirements, high-rise buildings were the only possibility due to site limitations.

The Berlin-Adlershof Campus

In 2002 we held our meeting and seminar in Berlin, and the theme of that seminar was: "Hi-tech Campus in the urban context today."

The Berlin-Adlershof campus, which is a Science and Applied Research and Production Facility in the city of Berlin – located on a site that was in the past an East-German airfield. This is a unique example of a large space that became available within the confines of a city.

40. Architecture for science and high-tech facilities

UIA International Union of Architects
A New UIA Work Programme
Presented in 2005 in Paris in the UIA office

The UIA Council, which convened in Barcelona in January 1998, has decided on the establishment of a new Work Programme dedicated to the architecture of "Science and High-Tech Facilities". The last quarter of the Twentieth Century has been characterized by rapid technological development in all professional fields. As we enter the new century, we also enter an era where hi-tech industries and services will become one of the main sources of employment worldwide. The international architectural community is aware that this forecast demands the creation of a new kind of built environment, which will naturally change life styles and behavior patterns. Buildings where science and hi-tech activities can be carried out optimally are a necessity, and there is a growing demand for better and more suitable facilities. The purpose of this WP is to study of the impact of these developments on urban pattern and, with the expressed purpose of creating a "user-friendly" working environment, promote the exchange of knowledge and practical experience in providing, designing and building Science and Hi-tech facilities. The "Science and High-Tech Facilities" Work Programme works in the framework of the statutes and by-laws of the International Union of Architects. The first meeting of the Work Programme took place in Israel and included tours of facilities for high-tech industries and dialogues with entrepreneurs and architects. Twenty countries have already nominated their representatives to the "Science and High-Tech Facilities Work Programme". If you are interested, please contact Moshe Zarhy, the Work Programme Director – Israel, by telephone number 972-3-5223111 or fax 972-3-5223588

41. Architecture for science and high-tech facilities work programme

UIA International Union of Architects
Annual International Seminar and Members' Meeting
October 2006 – Budapest, Hungary
Introductory Remarks

Dear Colleagues,
Firstly, in my own name and on behalf of all of the participants in this event, I would like to thank our member and friend Gabor Becker, the Association of the Hungarian Architects, and the Budapest University of Technology and Economics for organizing and coordinating the Seminar here in Budapest this year.
Our Work Programme group has held nine study seminars since its inception seven years ago. The themes of these meetings were:

Israel, 1999: "Architecture for Science and High-Tech Facilities – A Comprehensive Outlook"
China, 1999: Participation in the UIA Congress
Germany, 2000: "Science and the High-Tech Campus in the Urban Context Today"
Russia, 2001: "Thechnopolis – the Town of Science"
Germany, 2002: Participation in the UIA Congress and holding a Seminar on the theme: "Architectural issue of planning for Science and High-Tech facilities in our Era"
USA, 2003: "The Principles of Architecture for Science and High-Tech Facilities"
China, 2004: "Science and High-Tech Facilities' Contribution for Regional Environment"
Turkey, 2005: "Location of the High-Tech Facility Campus within the City"

We can learn much from the discussions held during our Work Programme meetings, the study tours that we have participated in, and from the papers that were presented by members of our Group during our Seminars.

One of the main lessons that we have learned is the importance of the correct location of the high-tech industry campus within the city, and the interrelationship of the campus and the city. The proper location of the campus contributes much to the prosperity of the campus, and to its success. Furthermore, the neighborhoods of the city in which the high-tech industries are situated will flourish, and will bring prosperity to the built environment.

The high-tech campus is a place of employment for thousands of city dwellers. Its location affects the built surroundings, and influences the character of the urban areas adjacent to it. We believe that in the future the need for sites such as this will increase, and will become an important component of planning and urban renewal. We need to be aware of the fact that we are discussing a historical process that alters urban patterns. As a consequence of the development of scientific and technological products, the "era of communications" completely changes our way of life and behavior. This must also have a direct influence on architecture and town planning. Architects and town planners are directly involved in decision-making and urban design; they must therefore be familiar with matters of architecture and planning that are connected with the development and the location of high-tech installations and facilities within the city, and must take an active part in planning them.

An assertion that is sometimes heard against the integration of high-tech industries in cities is connected with the dangers of environmental pollution. Nowadays we know that it is possible to exert control over matters of pollution in most high-tech industries.

This brings us to the theme of our Meeting this year in Budapest, which is:

"The High-Tech Campus in the City – The Eco-Technological Dilemma"

Our intention is to learn about this subject, as well as any restrictions that are applicable. We should note that the theme under discussion is of utmost relevance and importance, primarily with regard to the implications for architecture of the buildings and installations that will function as high-tech industries. I would like to wish us all fruitful and interesting presentations and discussions.

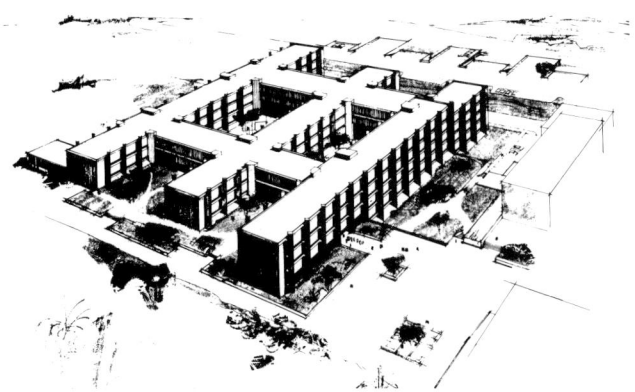

**Hebrew University of Jerusalem, The Institute of Life Sciences
View from north-east**

42. Designing for sustainable healthcare facilities – Israeli experience

UIA International Union of Architects
UIA Public Health Group
Symposium – August 2006, Pretoria, South Africa

Let us imagine an optimal situation where there are no constraints; where we have an appropriate and suitable location a practical client who knows what he wants, and we have the necessary programme and the list of requirements to establish a hospital in a developing country. How would we design, arrange and organize the layout of the hospital? What are the priorities and the references that would guide us? Even in such an ideal situation – which, of course, we know doesn't actually exist! – the central problem would be the 'so far unknown'.

Unknown developments in medicine during the coming decades, as well as in education and economics, unknown technological innovations and developments in the foreseeable future; requirements that hospitals will have in the coming era; all of these are matters for educated conjecture.

From this we can conclude that anyone wishing to plan a sustainable healthcare facility needs to take into account the 'unknown' factors, as well as everything that might be connected with that. It has already been said many times during meetings of our Work Programme group, that planning for growth, planning for ongoing change; preparation of Master Plans at as early a stage as possible; must all be prepared taking into account options for future electro-mechanical systems, modular design, flexibility of design, and an attempt to anticipate the foreseeable future. There must be differentiation between the fixed components of the plan and the variable components. Remember that during the planning you must be able to ensure an appearance of completion during all stages of development. The main categories of functions to be considered when planning a general hospital are:

1) Hospitalization services
2) Medical services,
3) Administrative and miscellaneous services
4) Supply services
5) Outpatient's department.

If we learn from the lessons of the past we will see that hospitalization services have not changed for decades. Physical dimensions of the human body have not changed, and thus the beds and hospital wards are also not expected to change during the coming years.

However, medical services have undergone considerable transformation and are constantly changing, striving to improve. This also applies to supply services which are frequently being industrialized and upgraded, as well as to administration and social services that have also advanced steadily over the years.

We have learned even more from lessons of the past – especially from developing nations – about how hospitals are created piecemeal and built in stages, according to the resources available, although the objective is that at any given time, the hospital will function as one operative unit.

We have learned that horizontal and vertical pedestrian paths of traffic cannot be changed, while the various departments – that are dependent on that flow of traffic – change constantly, and many of them will also grow and expand in the future. There is also the latent difficulty in designing the Master Plan in such a way as it must enable expansion of every functional division independently of all of the other functional divisions. This is by no means similar to expanding an office building in which the expansion is of the entire functional area. Thus, also medical services need to be divided into subdivisions that have the capability of increasing independently of each other. In addition to all

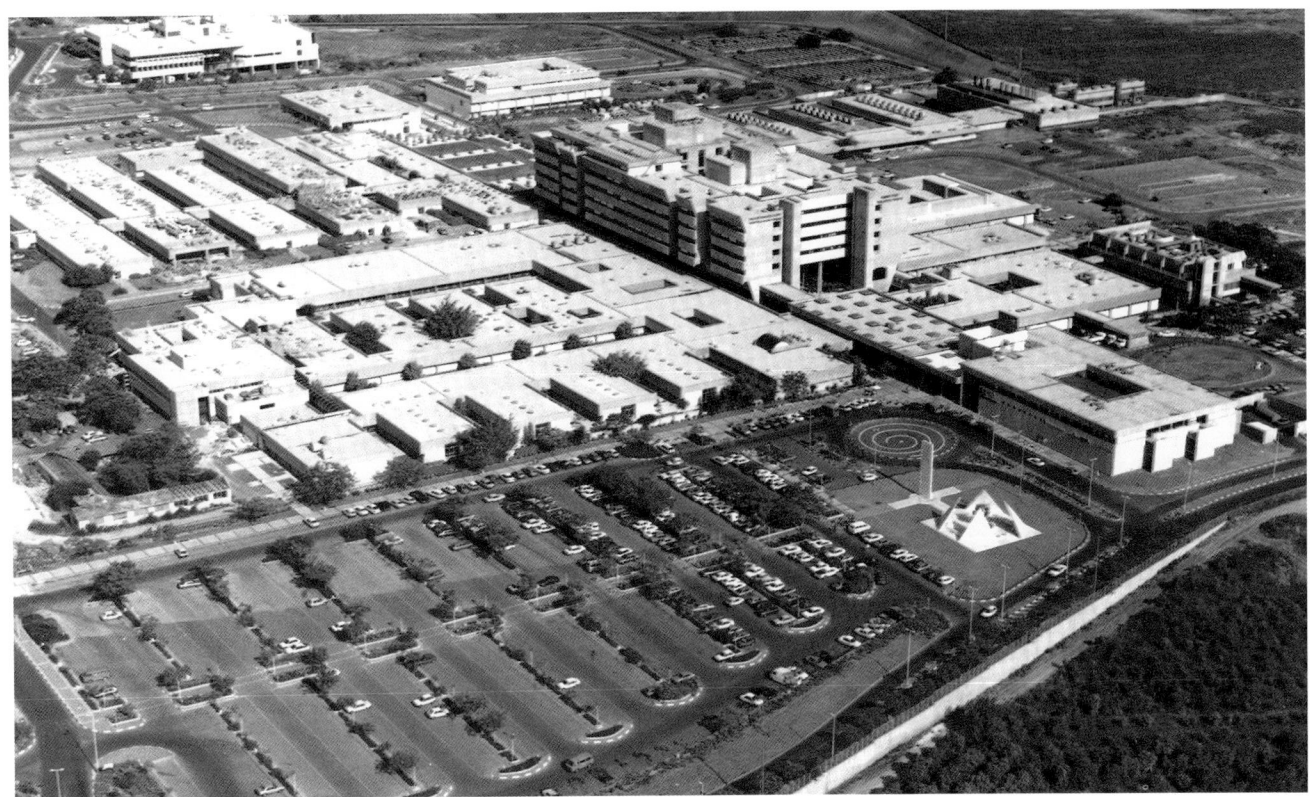

Sheba Medical Center
View of the General Hospital

of the above-mentioned, we must relate to the subject of the nature and lifestyle habits of the specific population for whom the hospital is designed. The character of the population has direct effect and implication on the design that will be proposed to the hospital. Medicine is common to all populations of the world, but the education of those dealing with medicine, habits and way of life for those requiring medical assistance, religious beliefs, waiting habits, food services and so on which are characterized by many of the populations in different countries, have a considerable influence on the Master Plan of the hospital. I would even say that they have a decisive impact on the Master Plan.

What should also be mentioned is that when planning a hospital in a developing country the Master Plan should be designed in such a way that the largest possible number of medical staffers will have maximal access to the medical equipment: This will result in the lowest possible expenditure for medical equipment. This rule has implications and must be taken into account when designing the reciprocal relations and the location of the departments, thus helping to minimize costs.

In conclusion let me say that I apologize for describing a complex and complicated problem – which requires much experience and knowledge – in an abbreviated way, much in the style of 'rules of thumb'. I am, of course, taking into account the circumstances, the location and the time available, and I also acknowledge that all of the participants in this discussion are experienced, and will therefore relate to what I have said as headings of subjects for discussion.

8

Appendix

Projects Chronology

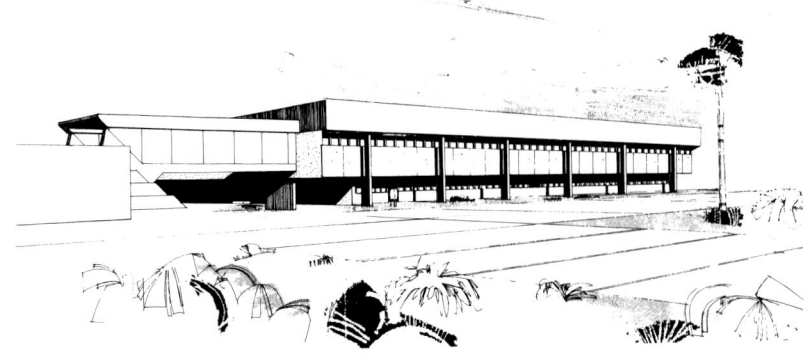

Hospitals and Health Care Facilities				
Start	Open	Project	Location	Remark
1967	2010	**Sheba Medical Center, Tel Hashomer** - The General Hospital - Women Hospital - Rehabilitation Hospital - Psychiatric Hospital - Medical Training and Teaching Institute - Oral and Maxillofacial Institute - Administation and Management Building - Public Health Research Institute - E.N.T. and Audiology Institute	S.M.C. Ramat Gan, Tel Aviv	150,000 sqm
1952	2010	**Meir Medical Center** - Meir Medical Center-Master plan - School for Nurses - The Synagogue	Sharon Area, Kfar Saba	80,000 sqm
1962	1973	**Ziv Hospital** - The General Hospital - The Nurses Training School	Safed, Upper Galilee	30,000 sqm
		- The Synagogue		decorated by artwork "Zeigermacher"
1972	1975	**Tel Aviv University** - School of Dental Medicine	Tel Aviv	6,000 sqm
1965	1969	**Government Hospital**	Dimona	Project was stopped in 1969
1980	1983	**Home for mentally retarded**	Ramat-Hasharon, Greater Tel Aviv Area	395 sqm
1980	1960	**Private Clinics**	Tel Aviv	
1981	1984	**Home for autistic children and adults**	Tel Aviv	2,500 sqm
1981	1973	**Tel Giborim Hospital**	Tel Giborim	not realized

Residential – Private Homes

Start	Open	Project	Location	Remark
	1953	**Moshe Zarhy Residence**	Ramat HaSharon	
	1970	**Mr. + Mrs. Ne'eman**	Tel Aviv	
	1975	**Mr. + Mrs. Naor**	Jerusalem	
	1979	**Shoken House**	Herzlia	
	1980	**Stef Wertheimer Residence**	Naharia	
	1981	**Advocate + Mrs. Porat**	Tel Aviv	
	1981	**Mr. + Mrs. Lahover**	Carmei Yosef	
	1994	**Semi detatched single-family houses**	Ramat HaSharon	3,600 sqm
	2011	**Arlozorov 150**	Tel Aviv	1,500 sqm

Residential – Housing Estates

Start	Open	Project	Location	Remark
1956	1959	**1.000 Dwelling Units**	Maoz Aviv	
	1973	**350 Dwelling Units**	Carmiel, Upper Galilee	
	1975	**300 Dwelling Units**	Mitzpe Ramon, Negev	
	1977	**500 Dwelling Units**	Acre	
	1979	**300 Dwelling Units**	Naharia	
1976	1980	**300 Dwelling Units**	Beit Hakerem, Jerusalem	
	1980	**500 Dwelling Units**	Tsur Shalom, Haifa	
	1985	**400 Dwelling Units**	Ein Sarah, Western Galilee	
	1985	**300 Dwelling Units**	Givat Savyon, near Tel Aviv	
	1987	**300 Dwelling Units**	Nazareth	
1984	1994	**Six Residential Blocks, 350 units**	Ramat-Aviv, Tel Aviv	6,400 sqm

Mixed Uses

Start	Open	Project	Location	Remark
1967	1969	**ATIDIM** Industrial Park f. Science-Based Industries	Tel Aviv	100,000 sqm
	2007	**Weizman Center** The Weizman Multi Use Center	Tel Aviv	140,000 sqm

8. Appendix

Public and Education

Start	Open	Project	Location	Remark
1973	1977	**Hebrew University of Jerusalem** - Life Sciences Complex Microbiological Teaching and Research Laboratories	Jerusalem	25,000 sqm
		Technion – The Israel Institute of Technology	Haifa	
1970	1973	- Solid State Physics Research Building		4,000 sqm
1978	1985	- Faculty of Nuclear Engineering, Research Building		6,000 sqm
1979	1980	- Technion Sport Center / Swimmingpool		4,000 sqm
1984	1989	- Microelectronics Building		3,000 sqm
1961	1971	**Convention / Congress Facilities**	Jerusalem, Binyanei HaUma	National auditorium
	1994	**Weizman Institute of Science** Physics Library	Rehovot	1,500 sqm
1980	1980	**Zionist Archive**	Jerusalem	6,000 sqm
1981	1982	**Janco Dada Museum**	Ein Hod, Haifa	1,600 sqm
1993	1998	**Synagoge and Jewish Memorial**	Moscow / Russia	
1980	1985	**Ha'Hatzer Synagoge and Yeshiva**	Jerusalem	
1979	1985	**Hilton Hotel**	Jerusalem	
1980	1990	**Public Plaza**	Jerusalem	

Hi-Tech and Science-Based Industries

Start	Open	Project	Location	Remark
1985	2000	**Iscar Industries** - Hi-Tech Research and Prod. Plant - Research + Hard Metals Prod. Plant - Jet Aircraft Engine Blades Prod. Plant	Teffen, Upper Galilee Teffen, Upper Galilee Naharia	9,000 sqm 15,000 sqm 10,000 sqm
		Weizmann Institute of Science	Rehovot	Industrial Park
1967	1969	- Industrial Park Rehovot		85,000 sqm
1967	1969	- Animal Breeding Plant Rehovot		5,000 sqm
	1969	- The Sub-Micron Building		
		Pecker Industries		
1965	1971	- Production Plant	Kfar Shaba	10,000 sqm
1975	1981	- Packing Production Plant	Kiriat Malakhi	6,000 sqm
		RAFAEL – Israel Armaments Devel. Authority		
1979	1981	- Development Control Plan	Upper Galilee	90,000 sqm
		Lesham Industrial Complex		
1961	1963	- Research + Semi-Conductor Pro.Fac.	Upper Galilee	20,000 sqm
		National Semiconductor (Israel)		
1965	1967	- Research and Production Plant	Migdal Ha'emek	10,000 sqm

		Nuclear Research Center	Tel Aviv Area	
1966	1969	- Development Control Plan of new Research Center		
		Hot Laboratories		
1985	1989	- Research Building	Tel Aviv Area	Tel Aviv Area
		Hanita Metal Works		
1981	1983	- Koor Industries	Shlomi, Upper Galilee	10,000 sqm
		Israel Military Industries		
1967	1969	- Production Facility	Tel Aviv Area	20,000 sqm
		Teva Pharmaceuticals Copaxon		
1992	2005	- Copaxon OSD plant	Kfar Saba	25,000 sqm

List of Papers

Year	Title	Place	Presented to / Published in
1970	The High Tech laboratory – Design architectural considerations	Jerusalem / Israel	I.D.F. authority
1970	The High Tech laboratory – An Israeli experience	Jerusalem / Israel	I.D.F. authority
1970	Change of scale in building in Israel	Tel Aviv / Israel	Ministry of Housing
1970	Science industries	Jerusalem / Israel	Tel Aviv Municipality and Tel Aviv University
1972	Comments on Israel architecture and housing	Jerusalem / Israel	TAC (Technological advisory commitee)
1974	Professional education in View of expected social and economic developments	Jerusalem / Israel	TAC (Technological advisory commitee)
1974	Residential development in Israel	Jerusalem / Israel	
1974	Competition for the design of a residential development – Summary	Tel Aviv / Israel	Engineers and architects newspaper
1975	Modul beton Israel housing schemes	Jerusalem / Israel	Ministry of Housing
1974	Community design responsibility	Paris / France	TAC (Technological advisory commitee)
1975	Proposal for the 1975 / 78 triennal activities of the U.I.A. – Planning with scare resources	Paris / France	UIA
1977	On modernisation of hospitals in urban areas – Meir Hospital case	Tokio / Japan	World Hospitals volume XVII
1981	Aspects of the modernisation and existing health and hospital-care facilities in Israel	Warsaw / Poland	
1981	Living environment based on a comprehensive pre-cast concrete building system	Warsaw / Poland	

8. Appendix

1981	Planning, building and organization of medical research facilities – Three developments in Israel	Worl Hospitals volume XVII	
1981	The precast concrete industry and the environment	Jerusalem/Israel	
1983	The balanced hospital concept	Lausanne/Switzerland	
1985	Future hospital design	Budapest/Hungary	
1984	10th international public health seminar	Tel Aviv/Israel	
1988	Israel – In view of the W.H.O. strategy "Health for all by the year 2000"	Moscow/Russia	
1990	Aging and architecture in Israel	Montreal/Canada	
1990	Guidelines programming and design in development and developed countries	Ottawa/Canada	
1990	Chaim Sheba Medical Center – The new complex	Tel Aviv/Israel	University and municipality of Tel Aviv
1991	On disarity in health and hospital care facilities	Washington/USA	
1996	Continuity in hospital design	Florence/Italy	
1997	Program and hospital design guidelines in Israel	Tel Aviv/Israel	
1999	"Science and High-Tech facilities" – Work programme	Tefen Upper Galilee/Israel	
2000	Science and High-Tech campus in the urban context	Berlin/Germany	
2000	The search for Architectural Identity in Israel – Personel reflections	Bucharest/Romania	
2001	Adapting existing hospitals for the future requirements	Hong Kong/China	
2001	Exchange of knowledge between developed and developing countries	Manila/The Phillipines	
2001	Architecture and the information era	Berlin/Germany	
2002	UIA Meeting of presidents – Region I and II	Bucharest/Romania	
2001	Changes in techniques, in information and in the building industrie in conjunction with the role of the architect	Paris/France	
2001	The role of the architect	Paris/France	
2002	Architecture and the information era	Berlin/Germany	
2003	Hospital master planning in the countries context	San Francisco/USA	
2003	Architecture for science and Hi-Tech facilities in the new millennium	Moscow/Russia	
2004	Redesign and updating of existing hospitals	Sao Paulo/Brazil	

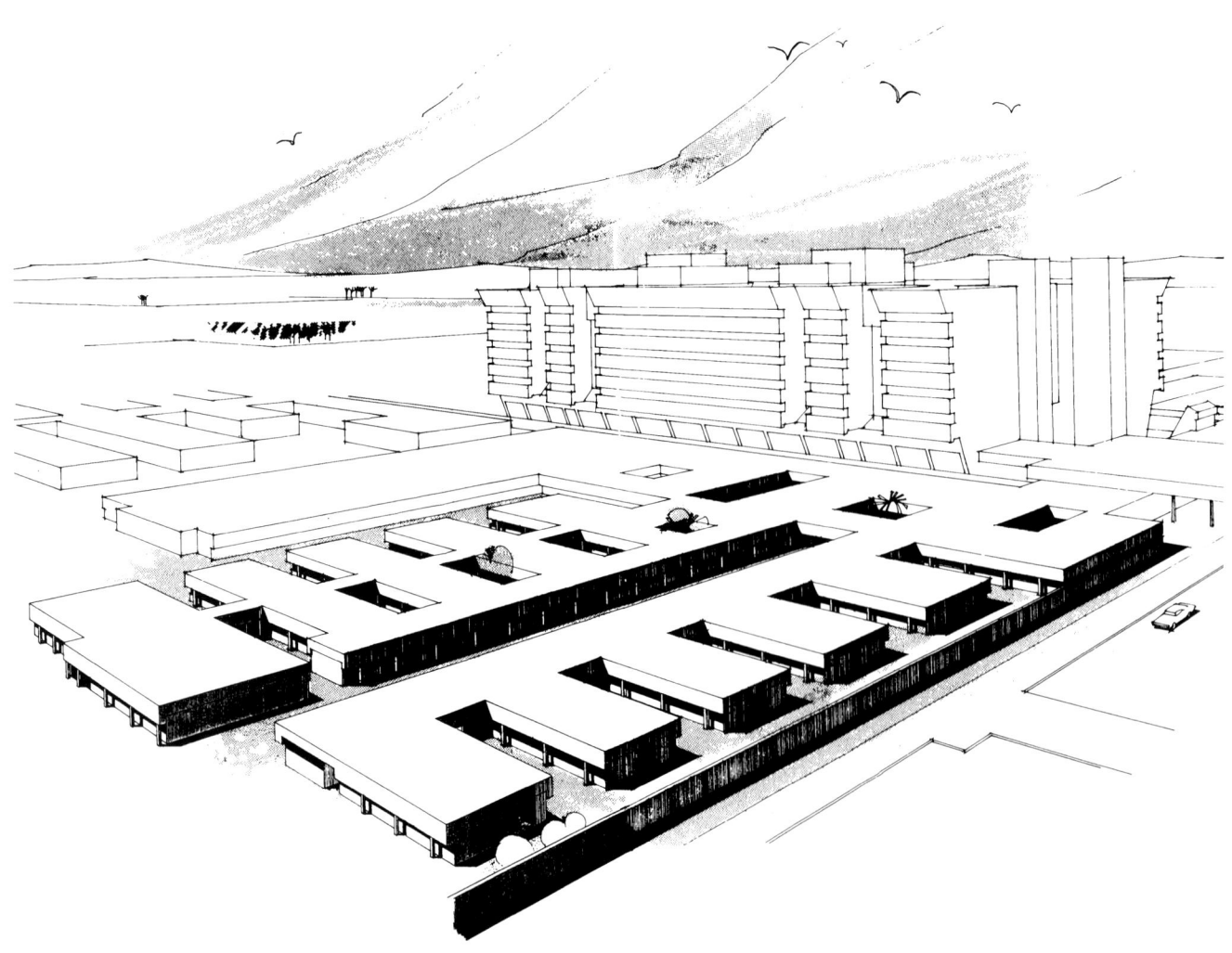

8. Appendix

Chronological Table

1899
David Zarhy, father of Moshe Zarhy, was born in Vitecs, Russia.

1899
Zeev Rechter was born in Ukraine. He became a famous Israeli architect, later Moshe Zarhy's father-in-law and partner.

1904
Moshe Zarhy's Mother, Rebecca Flexer was born in Kamenez-Podolsk / Ukraine (later Poland).

1919
David Zarhy immigrated to Palestine. He settled in Jaffa / Tel Aviv. His profession was Mechanical Engineer. In Israel he worked as a driver of an excavator on different building sites.

1921
Moshe's first wife, Aviva Rechter, was born on 21st January in Tel Aviv. Her later profession was child and family therapist.

1923
Moshe Zarhy was born in Jerusalem, Palestine on 24th November as first child of David and Rebecca Zarhy.

1930
Vera Ronnen, Moshe's second wife, was born on 27th June 1930 in Cluj / Transylvania. With her parents and brother she was deported to KZ Bergen-Belsen in 1943, liberated in 1944 by R. Kastner (see the Kastner Train), transported to the Swiss border where the RED CROSS took over and received them in Basel / Switzerland.

Her profession: Artist, working in vitreous enamel on steel, on site-specific installations in architecture. Studies: Ecole des Arts et Métiers, and at the Beaux Arts in Geneva, Switzerland. Practical work: Professor at the Bezalel Academy of Art in Jerusalem (1950–1977, 1984–1993), Vitreous Enamel in Architecture.

1932
Moshe's brother Zvi Zarhy was born in Tel Aviv. He later studied at the M.I.T. (Massachusetts Institute of Technology) in Boston / USA. His profession was Naval Architect. He lived for several years in Sweden, where he built ships. He lives in Haifa. Death of Moshe's mother Rebecca in a car accident. The taxi, she and her family travelled in on the way to Tel Aviv, got in collision with a train. His father, Moshe and the baby Zvi survived. The brothers were well brought-up by their grandmother, Haia Flexer, the mother of Rebecca.

1939
Matriculation of Moshe, High School-Palestine, Jerusalem.

1939–1945
Study of Architecture at Technion, The Israel Institute of Technology, Viazman 87, Kesalsaba Haifa, Palestine.

1940–1943
Moshe served in the British Army in the Haifa Region, which enabled him to continue his studies at the Technion.

1941
Moshe's father died in a car accident, near the place where the brothers lost her mother nine years earlier.

1944
First Marriage of Moshe Zarhy, to Aviva Rechter.

1945–1949
Moshe worked as an architect in the office of Zeev Rechter in Tel Aviv, Rabin Square. First Hospital Projects for Moshe: school for nurses in Kfar Saba. Planning of a Tuberculosis-hospital in Kfar Saba, later transformed into a General Hospital (Meir hospital).

1948
Birth of Yael in Tel Aviv, first daughter of Moshe and Aviva. Later she studied comparative literature in New York / USA. At Tel Aviv University she teaches comparative literature, especially British theatre in the 1960.

1949–1950
Post Graduate Studies of Moshe in Town planning at Ecole D'Urbanisme, Sorbonne, Paris / France; adoption by and friendship with the internationally known artist Chana Orloff.

1951–1959
Moshe becomes partner in the office of Zeev Rechter. They operate under "Rechter-Zarhy-Rechter" in Tel Aviv, Rabin Square. Partners: Zeev Rechter, Moshe Zarhy, Yaakov Rechter (son of Zeev).
First Hospital Projects for Moshe: school for nurses in Kfar Saba. Planning of a Tuberculosis-hospital in Kfar Saba, later transformed into a General Hospital (Meir hospital).

1951
Moshe's second child, David, is born. Later he attended High school in Tel Aviv and studied architecture at the Technion, the Israel Institute of Technology in Haifa, like his father. From 1974 to 1979 David worked in the IDF as an Architect and joined the office of Zarhy Architects as partner in 1979.

1953
Moshe Zarhy built his own residence in Ramat Hasharon. He lived there for over 60 years untill 2013.

1954
Rivi, the third child of Aviva and Moshe, is born. She is a scientist.

1956–1959
Building of 1.000 dwelling units in Maoz Aviv.
1959 Ruthi is born, the last of 4 children of the Moshe and Aviva. Later she studied in London AA School of Architects and is now working in the field of Industrial Buildings in Tel Aviv.

1960
Zeev Rechter died. The partners Moshe Zarhy and Yaakov Rechter continued the office work together with Michael Peri, an engineer, who was married to the younger daughter of Zeev Rechter, Tuti. They operated under "Rechter-Zarhy-Peri".

1961
Start of work for the Lesham Industrial Complex in Upper Galilee. Building of the Convention Center in Jerusalem (finished in 1971). 1962 The Hospital Project in Kfar Saba, the Meir Hospital started. Zarhy Architects have continued to work on these projects up to the recent. In the same year, work on the Ziv Hospital in Safed, Upper Galilee, began(finished in 1973).

1967
Start of the project Sheba Medical Center, Tel Hashomer in Tel Aviv. Ongoing through Projects for the Israel Military Industry were started.

1970
Beginning of planning of the Solid State Physics Research Building at Technion in Haifa. Start of paper presentations in different countries. This lasted till

2006. Start of projects for the Weizman Institute of Science in Rehovot: the industrial park and the Animals Breeding Plant.

1972
Start of the project "School of Dental Medicine" at the Tel Aviv University (finished 1975).

1973
Moshe Zarhy founded Zarhy Architects Ltd. In Tel Aviv, 150 Arlozorov (4 floors, later extended to six floors). The reason for the separation from Rechter and Peri: 80 people in the existing office. The partners decided to split, but remained on friendly terms. One of the first projects on the industrial site of ATIDIM was started: the Hospital's Main Laboratories for the Tel Aviv region (finished in 1980).

1976
Beginning of the planning and building of 4.000 Dwelling units in 11 different places (till1994).

1979
Moshe's son David and his daughter-in-law, Anat Patrycha-Zarhy, became partners in Zarhy Architects Ltd. Anat, born in Warsaw, Poland, had studied together with David Zarhy at the Technion in Haifa and later at the Ecole Nationale des Beaux-Arts in Paris. Anat and David have 2 children: Daughter May is a dancer and Choreographer. She lives in Frankfurt/Germany and works in Europe. Son Daniel is an architect. He worked in several European offices (Herzog de Meuron, Basel/Switzerland and Rem Koolhaas/Netherlands). He works as a freelance architect and also in association with Zarhy Architects, continuing the family tradition in the fourth generation. Start of work for the RAFAEL-Israel Armaments Development Authorities in Upper Galilee.

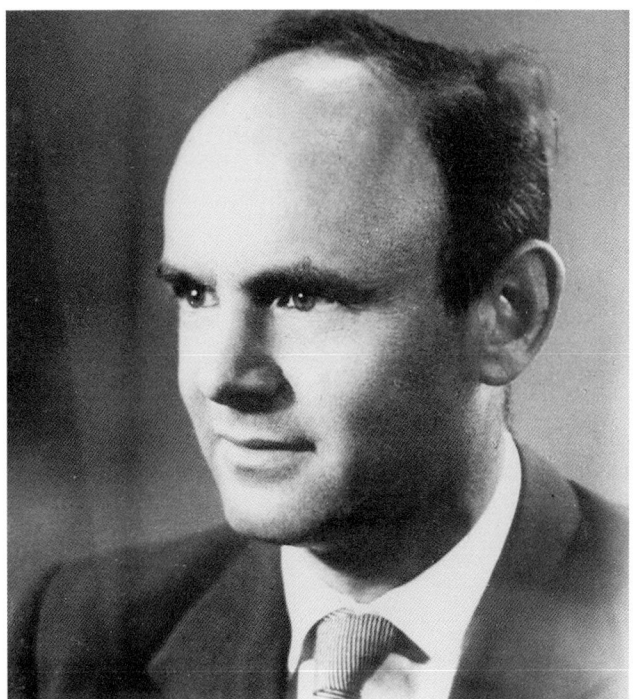

Portrait Moshe Zarhy

1980
Building of the Stef Wertheimer residence in Naharia; building of a Home for Mentally Retarded People in Ramat Hasharon (finished in 1983) and Zionist Archives in Jerusalem (finished 1987).

1981
Start of planning of a home for autistic children and adults in Tel Aviv (finished in 1984) and Janco Dada Museum in Ein Hod (finished 1982).

1985
Start of several Hi-Tech Industrial projects in Tefen for ISCAR Industries.

1992
Planning and building for Teva Pharmaceutical Copaxon in Kfar Saba (till 2005).

1993

Aviva Zarhy, Moshe's wife died. Start of planning of the Synagogue and Jewish Memorial in Moscow / Russia.

1993–1999

Moshe Zarhy was elected as Vice President of UIA Region 2.

1994

2nd Marriage of Moshe Zarhy in Tel Aviv to Vera Ronnen Zarhy. Start of building of the Synagogue and Jewish Memorial in Moscow / Russia (finished 1998).

1996

Moshe Zarhy decorated with the Silver badge of Catalonian Architects. Receives a Letter of evaluation of the Architects of Russia and honored in the same year with the Insignia of the Higher Council of Spanish Architects.

1998

Becomes an honorary member of the Moscow Branch of the International Academy of Architecture. Receives a Letter of evaluation of the Academy of the Architects of Russia.

2000

Receives a Letter of evaluation from the Israeli Architects Association. Elected Vice President of the UIA Region 2, The Industrial-Parc project.

2004

Receives the Honorary Fellowship of the American Institute of Architects. Becomes an Honorable Member of the "KAZGOR" Design Academy of the Republic of Kazakhstan.

2009

Becomes a Senior Member of Israeli Top Executive Business Leadership of 2009.

2012

Moshe Zarhy was honored with an Award, given at the 1st International Conference on Medicine and Architecture in the 21st Century at his old University of Technion / Tel Aviv.

2013

Moshe and Vera move from the house in Ramat Hasharon to their new home at Arlozorov 150.

8. Appendix

Index of Adresses

Index of Persons

Bibliography

Books and publications

Cohen, Nahoum .... Bauhaus in Tel Aviv (2003)
Dursthoff, Wiebke .... Kibbutz und Bauhaus. Arieh Sharon und die Moderne in Palästina
Gatermann, Hans Evert (Editor) .... UIA – Programming, Guidelines and Masterplanning
           for Hospitals (2003)
Hoffmann, Jérémie .... Three Animals (Docomomo No. 40, 2009)
Pawlik, Peter R. .... Von Bergedorf nach Germania – Hermann Distel (1875–1945) –
           Ein Architektenleben in bewegter Zeit (2009)
Pawlik, Peter R. .... Von Saarow nach Alexandria – Ernst Kopp (1890–1962) –
           Die Umwege eines großen Krankenhaus-Baumeisters (2013)
Sharon, Arieh .... Kibbutz+Bauhaus, an architect's way in a new land (1972)
Unknown .... Health Services in Israel (World Hospitals Vol. 1, 1964)

Brochures

Zarhy Architects .... Government Hospital Dimona
Zarhy Architects .... Memorial Synagogue at the Memorial
Zarhy Architects .... Tel Giborim Hospital – Competition Projects
Zarhy Architects .... The Institute of Life Sciences. The Hebrew University of Jerusalem
Zarhy, Moshe .... Health Facilities in Israel
Zarhy Architects .... Chaim Sheba Medical Centre, Tel Hashomer
Zarhy Architects .... Meir Medical Center, Master Plan 2010
Zarhy Architects .... Safed Government Hospital
Zarhy Architects .... Modul Beton Israel Building System

Websites

www.rechter-arch.com
www.zarhy.com

The Deutsche Bibliothek lists this publication in the
Deutsche Nationalbibliografie; detailed bibliographic
data is available on the internet at *http://dnb.d-nb.de*

ISBN 978-3-86922-340-7

© 2014 by DOM publishers, Berlin
www.dom-publishers.com

Translation
Harald Pawlik

Proofreading
Peter R. Pawlik

Design
Masako Tomokiyo

Picture Credits
Courtesy Moshe Zarhy and Peter R. Pawlik

Printing
Tiger Printing (Hong Kong) Co., Ltd
www.tigerprinting.hk

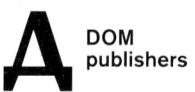
DOM
publishers